Methods for Serum-Free Culture of Cells of the Endocrine System

Cell Culture Methods for Molecular and Cell Biology

David W. Barnes, David A. Sirbasku, and Gordon H. Sato, *Editors*

Volume 1: Methods for Preparation of Media, Supplements, and Substrata for Serum-Free Animal Cell Culture

Volume 2: Methods for Serum-Free Culture of Cells of the Endocrine System

Volume 3: Methods for Serum-Free Culture of Epithelial and Fibroblastic Cells

Volume 4: Methods for Serum-Free Culture of Neuronal and Lymphoid Cells

Methods for Serum-Free Culture of Cells of the Endocrine System

Editors

David W. Barnes

Department of Biological Sciences
University of Pittsburgh
Pittsburgh, Pennsylvania

David A. Sirbasku

Department of Biochemistry
and Molecular Biology
University of Texas Medical School
Houston, Texas

Gordon H. Sato

W. Alton Jones Cell Science Center
Lake Placid, New York

Alan R. Liss, Inc., New York

Address all Inquiries to the Publisher
Alan R. Liss, Inc., 150 Fifth Avenue, New York, NY 10011

Copyright © 1984 Alan R. Liss, Inc.
Printed in the United States of America.

Library of Congress Cataloging in Publication Data

Main entry under title:

Methods for serum-free culture of cells of the endocrine system.
   (Cell culture methods for molecular and cell biology; v. 2)
   Includes index.
   1. Cell culture.   2. Culture media (Biology)
3. Endocrine glands.   I. Barnes, David W. (David William),
1949-   .   II. Sirbasku, David A. (David Andrew),
1941-   .   III. Sato, Gordon.   IV. Title: Serum-free
culture of cells of the endocrine system.   V. Series.
QH585.M464 1984   591.1'42'0724   84-7202
ISBN 0-8451-3801-4

Contents

Contributors vii

Contents of Volumes 1, 3, and 4 ix

Preface xv

1   Growth of GH₃, a Rat Pituitary Cell Line, in Serum-Free,
    Hormone-Supplemented Medium
    Izumi Hayashi 1

2   Growth of Adrenocortical Cell Cultures in Serum-Free Medium
    Michael H. Simonian and Mark L. White 15

3   Primary Culture of Testicular Somatic Cells
    J.P. Mather and D.M. Phillips 29

4   Isolation and Growth of Adult Human Prostatic Epithelium in
    Serum-Free, Defined Medium
    Mukta M. Webber, Donna M. Chaproniere-Rickenberg, and
    Robert E. Donohue 47

5   Growth of Functional Primary and Established Rat Ovary
    Cell Cultures in Serum-Free Medium
    Joseph Orly 63

6   Growth of Rat Mammary Tumor Cells in Serum-Free,
    Hormone-Supplemented Medium
    Tamiko Kano-Sueoka 89

7   Growth of Normal Mammary Epithelium on Collagen in
     Serum-Free Medium
     William R. Kidwell, Mozeena Bano, and David S. Salomon 105

8   Isolation and Serum-Free Cultivation of Mammary Epithelial
     Cells Within a Collagen Gel Matrix
     Walter Imagawa, Yasuhiro Tomooka, Jason Yang, Raphael Guzman,
     James Richards, and Satyabrata Nandi 127

9   Serum-Free Culture of the Isolated Whole Mammary Organ
     of the Mouse: A Model for the Study of Differentiation
     and Carcinogenesis
     Mihir R. Banerjee and Michael Antoniou 143

10   Growth of Human Mammary Epithelial Cells in
     Monolayer Culture
     Martha Stampfer 171

11   Definition of Hormones and Growth Factors Required for
     Optimal Proliferation and Expression of Phenotypic
     Responses in Human Breast Cancer Cells
     Marc E. Lippman 183

12   Serum-Free Cell Culture of MCF7 Human Mammary Carcinoma
     David W. Barnes 201

13   General Methods for Isolation of Acetic Acid- and Heat-Stable
     Polypeptide Growth Factors for Mammary and Pituitary
     Tumor Cells
     Tatsuhiko Ikeda, David Danielpour, Peter R. Galle, and
     David A. Sirbasku 217

     Index 243

Contributors

Michael Antoniou, Tumor Biology Laboratory, School of Biological Sciences, University of Nebraska at Lincoln, Lincoln, NE 68588 **[143]**

Mihir R. Banerjee, Tumor Biology Laboratory, School of Biological Sciences, University of Nebraska at Lincoln, Lincoln, NE 68588 **[143]**

Mozeena Bano, Laboratory of Pathophysiology, National Cancer Institute, National Institutes of Health, Bethesda, MD 20205 **[105]**

David W. Barnes, Department of Biological Sciences, University of Pittsburgh, Pittsburgh, PA 15260 **[xv,201]**

Donna M. Chaproniere-Rickenberg, Division of Urology, Department of Surgery, School of Medicine, University of Colorado Health Sciences Center, Denver, CO 80262 **[47]**

David Danielpour, Department of Biochemistry and Molecular Biology, University of Texas Medical School, Houston, TX 77225 **[217]**

Robert E. Donohue, Division of Urology, Department of Surgery, School of Medicine, University of Colorado Health Sciences Center, Denver, CO 80262 **[47]**

Peter R. Galle, Department of Biochemistry and Molecular Biology, University of Texas Medical School, Houston, TX 77225 **[217]**

Raphael Guzman, Cancer Research Laboratory, University of California at Berkeley, Berkeley, CA 94720 **[127]**

Izumi Hayashi, Division of Cytogenetics and Cytology, City of Hope National Medical Center, Duarte, CA 91010 **[1]**

Tatsuhiko Ikeda, Faculty of Nutrition, Kobe-Gakuin University, Kobe 673, Japan **[217]**

Walter Imagawa, Cancer Research Laboratory, University of California at Berkeley, Berkeley, CA 94720 **[127]**

Tamiko Kano-Sueoka, Department of Molecular, Cellular, and Developmental Biology, University of Colorado, Boulder, CO 80309 **[89]**

William R. Kidwell, Laboratory of Pathophysiology, National Cancer Institute, National Institutes of Health, Bethesda, MD 20205 **[105]**

Marc E. Lippman, Medical Breast Cancer Section, National Cancer Institute, National Institutes of Health, Bethesda, MD 20205 **[183]**

Jennie P. Mather, Center for Biomedical Research, The Population Council, New York, NY 10021 [29]

Satyabrata Nandi, Cancer Research Laboratory and Department of Zoology, University of California at Berkeley, Berkeley, CA 94720 [127]

Joseph Orly, Department of Biological Chemistry, Institute of Life Sciences, The Hebrew University of Jerusalem, 91904 Jerusalem, Israel [63]

David M. Phillips, Center for Biomedical Research, The Population Council, New York, NY 10021 [29]

James Richards, Cancer Research Laboratory, University of California at Berkeley, Berkeley, CA 94720 [127]

David S. Salomon, Laboratory of Tumor Immunology and Biology, National Cancer Institute, National Institutes of Health, Bethesda, MD 20205 [105]

Gordon H. Sato, W. Alton Jones Cell Science Center, Lake Placid, NY 12946 [xv]

Michael H. Simonian, Department of Physiology and Biophysics, University of Iowa, Iowa City, IA 52242 [15]

David A. Sirbasku, Department of Biochemistry and Molecular Biology, University of Texas Medical School, Houston, TX 77225 [xv,217]

Martha Stampfer, Division of Biology and Medicine, Lawrence Berkeley Laboratory, Berkeley, CA 94720 [171]

Yasuhiro Tomooka, National Institute of Environmental Health Sciences, Research Triangle Park, NC 27709 [127]

Mukta M. Webber, Division of Urology, Department of Surgery, School of Medicine, University of Colorado Health Sciences Center, Denver, CO 80262 [47]

Mark L. White, Department of Physiology and Biophysics, University of Iowa, Iowa City, IA 52242 [15]

Jason Yang, Cancer Research Laboratory, University of California at Berkeley, Berkeley, CA 94720 [127]

Contents of Volumes 1, 3, and 4

Volume 1: Methods for Preparation of Media, Supplements, and Substrata for Serum-Free Animal Cell Culture

METHODS FOR PREPARATION OF BASAL NUTRIENT MEDIA

1   Formulation of Basal Nutrient Media
    Richard G. Ham

2   Preparation and Use of Serum-Free Culture Media
    Charity Waymouth

3   Preparations and Uses of Lipoproteins to Culture Normal Diploid and
    Tumor Cells Under Serum-Free Conditions
    Denis Gospodarowicz

METHODS FOR PREPARATION OF MITOGENIC PEPTIDES

4   Preparation of Human Platelet-Derived Growth Factor
    Elaine W. Raines and Russell Ross

5   Purification of Multiplication-Stimulating Activity
    Lawrence A. Greenstein, S. Peter Nissley, Alan C. Moses,
    Patricia A. Short, Yvonne W.-H. Yang, Lilly Lee, and
    Matthew M. Rechler

6   Preparation of Guinea Pig Prostate Epidermal Growth Factor
    Jeffrey S. Rubin and Ralph A. Bradshaw

7   Purification of Human Epidermal Growth Factor From Urine
    C. Richard Savage, Jr. and Robert A. Harper

8   Isolation of Growth Factors From Human Milk
     Yuen W. Shing and Michael Klagsbrun

9   Purification of Type β Transforming Growth Factors From Non-
     neoplastic Tissues
     Anita B. Roberts, Charles A. Frolik, Mario A. Anzano,
     Richard K. Assoian, and Michael B. Sporn

10   Preparation of Endothelial Cell Growth Factor
     Thomas Maciag and Robert Weinstein

         METHODS FOR PREPARATION OF SUBSTRATA

11   Use of Basic Polymers as Synthetic Substrata for Cell Culture
     Wallace L. McKeehan

12   Preparation of Cellular Fibronectin
     Kenneth M. Yamada and Steven K. Akiyama

13   Isolation of Laminin
     Steven R. Ledbetter, Hynda K. Kleinman, John R. Hassell,
     and George R. Martin

14   Isolation of Chondronectin
     Hugh H. Varner, A. Tyl Hewitt, and George R. Martin

15   Human Serum Spreading Factor (SF): Assay, Preparation, and Use in
     Serum-Free Cell Culture
     Janet Silnutzer and David W. Barnes

16   Purification of Epibolin From Human Plasma
     K.S. Stenn

17   Preparation of Extracellular Matrices Produced by Cultured Bovine
     Corneal Endothelial Cells and PF-HR-9 Endodermal Cells: Their
     Use in Cell Culture
     Denis Gospodarowicz

18   Analysis of Basement Membrane Synthesis and Turnover in Mouse
     Embryonal and Human A431 Epidermoid Carcinoma Cells in
     Serum-Free Medium
     David S. Salomon, Lance A. Liotta, Mounanandham Panneerselvam,
     Victor P. Terranova, Atul Sahai, and Paula Fehnel

19   Cell Attachment and Spreading on Extracellular Matrix-Coated Beads
     Shing Mai and Albert E. Chung

Volume 3: Methods for Serum-Free Culture of Epithelial and Fibroblastic Cells

SERUM-FREE CULTURE OF EPITHELIAL CELLS

1   Growth of Primary and Established Kidney Cell Cultures in Serum-Free Media
     Mary Taub

2   Hormonally Defined, Serum-Free Medium for a Proximal Tubular Kidney Epithelial Cell Line, LLC-PK$_1$
     Milton H. Saier, Jr.

3   Serum-Free Organ Culture of Embryonic Mouse Metanephros
     Ellis D. Avner, William E. Sweeney, Jr., and Demetrius Ellis

4   Primary Culture of Hepatocytes
     H.L. Leffert, K.S. Koch, and H. Skelly

5   Selective Growth of Human Small Cell Lung Cancer Cell Lines and Clinical Specimens in Serum-Free Medium
     Desmond N. Carney, Martin Brower, Virginia Bertness, and Herbert K. Oie

6   Primary Tissue Cultures of Human Colon Carcinomas in Serum-Free Medium: An In Vitro System for Tumor Analysis and Therapy Experiments
     Jürgen van der Bosch

7   Growth and Differentiation of Human Bronchogenic Epidermoid Carcinoma Cells in Serum-Free Media
     Kaoru Miyazaki, Hideo Masui, and Gordon H. Sato

8   Serum-Free Cell Culture of A431 Human Epidermoid Carcinoma
     David W. Barnes

9   Growth and Differentiation of Embryonal Carcinoma Cells in Defined and Serum-Free Media
     Angie Rizzino

10   α_2-Macroglobulin, a Contaminant of Commercially Prepared Pedersen Fetuin: Isolation, Characterization, and Biological Activity
     David S. Salomon, Kathryn B. Smith, Ilona Losonczy, Mozeena Bano, William R. Kidwell, Giulio Alessandri, and Pietro M. Gullino

SERUM-FREE CULTURE OF FIBROBLASTIC CELLS

11   On Deciding Which Factors Regulate Cell Growth
      Arthur B. Pardee, Paul V. Cherington, and Estela E. Medrano

12   Purification of Pituitary and Brain Fibroblast Growth Factors and Their
      Use in Cell Culture
      Denis Gospodarowicz

13   Preparation of Bovine Pituitary Fibroblast Growth Factor
      Sandra K. Lemmon and Ralph A. Bradshaw

14   Preparation of Pituitary Acidic FGF
      Angelo A. Gambarini, Mari C.S. Armelin, and Hugo A. Armelin

15   Growth of SV40 BALB/c-3T3 Cells in Serum-Free Culture Medium
      G.A. Rockwell

16   Use of Hormone-Toxin Conjugates and Serum-Free Media for the
      Isolation and Study of Cell Variants in Hormone Responses
      Nobuyoshi Shimizu

17   Growth of Human Fibroblast Cultures in Serum-Free Medium
      Richard G. Ham

18   Serum-Free Cell Culture for Growth of NIH 3T3 and 10T1/2 Mouse
      Embryo Fibroblast Cell Lines, SV40 Virus Propagation and Selection of
      SV40-Transformed Cells
      Lin-Chang Chiang, Janet Silnutzer, James M. Pipas, and David W. Barnes

      Volume 4: Methods for Serum-Free Culture of Neuronal and
                 Lymphoid Cells

SERUM-FREE CULTURE OF NEURONAL CELLS

1   Culture Methods for Growth of Neuronal Cell Lines in Defined Media
      Jane E. Bottenstein

2   Preparation of a Chemically Defined Medium for Purified Astrocytes
      Richard S. Morrison and Jean de Vellis

3   Growth and Differentiation of Pheochromocytoma Cells in
     Chemically Defined Medium
     R. Goodman

4   Differentiated Mouse Fetal Hypothalamic Cells in Serum-Free
     Medium
     A. Faivre-Bauman, J. Puymirat, C. Loudes, and A. Tixier-Vidal

5   Regulation of Pigmentation and Proliferation in Cultured
     Melanocytes
     John M. Pawelek

6   Neuron-Glia Interaction in Mammalian Brain: Preparation and
     Quantitative Bioassay of a Neurotrophic Factor (NTF) From
     Primary Astrocytes
     Wilfried Seifert and Hans Werner Müller

7   Preparation and Assay of Nerve Growth Factor
     Thomas L. Darling and Eric M. Shooter

SERUM-FREE CULTURE OF LYMPHOID CELLS

8   Production and Purification of Interleukin-2 for the Initiation and
     Maintenance of T-Cell Lines
     Diane Mochizuki and James D. Watson

9   Methods for Production and Purification of Human T-Cell Growth
     Factor
     M.G. Sarngadharan, R.C. Ting, and R.C. Gallo

10   Preparation of Thymosins
     Teresa L.K. Low and Allan L. Goldstein

11   Culture of Lymphocytes and Hemopoietic Cells in Serum-Free
     Medium
     N.N. Iscove

12   Growth of Lymphoid Cells in Serum-Free Medium
     Frederick J. Darfler and Paul A. Insel

13   Serum-Free Cultivation of Plasmacytomas and Hybridomas
     Hiroki Murakami

14   Culture of Human Lymphocytes in Serum-Free Medium
     John Mendelsohn, Alendry Caviles, Jr., and Janice Castagnola

15   Studies of Growth and Differentiation of Human Myelomonocytic
      Leukemia Cell Lines in Serum-Free Medium
      Theodore R. Breitman, Beverly R. Keene, and Hiromichi Hemmi

16   Serum-Free Growth of SP2/0-AG-14 Hybridomas
      Kathelyn Sue Steimer

Preface

The growth in vitro of a variety of endocrine-responsive cells can be achieved using serum-containing culture medium. However, results of studies using these conventional culture systems often have been less than satisfactory. If in vitro experiments in the areas of biochemical and molecular endocrinology are to be meaningful, the culture medium must be as defined as is possible in order to eliminate substances that might interfere with hormone responses, as well as to eliminate endogenous hormones that would mask or otherwise prevent the identification of expected cellular responses. Further, nontarget cells must be eliminated from the cultures to prevent measurement of secondary or unrelated effects.

The serum-free approaches to endocrine cell cultures described here are workable solutions to these problems, and do provide for identification of cellular responses that are not identifiable in serum-containing culture medium. For example, the growth-promoting effects of estrogens described in this volume are observed in serum-free, defined media, while these same responses may not be easily demonstrable in serum-containing medium. The effect described in this volume of ACTH on normal adrenal cell steroid biosynthesis is another area of biochemical endocrinology that is more easily characterized under serum-free conditions. Methods are detailed for the establishment of fibroblast-free cultures of normal human prostate cells through serum-free techniques that will be valuable to many researchers interested in function and growth regulation of this major site of endocrine-related cancer in man. Although defined media for many cell types have important components in common (i.e., transferrin, insulin, and many nutrients), it is possible to design restrictive serum-free media that make possible the growth of only selected cell types from primary cultures. Other methods described further demonstrate the importance of the substratum and matrix composition in chemically defined media for endocrine target cells and the use of serum-free assay conditions to identify new growth factors for human and rat normal and malignant mammary cells.

Also detailed are the preparation and use of chemically defined media specifically developed for the culture of fibroblast-free monolayers of normal functional endocrine target cells from breast, ovary, testes, and adrenals and serum-free organ culture of mammary tissue. The methods for establishing these cultures from tissues are presented, and when applied along with the general approaches to formulation of serum-free, defined media described in Volume 1 of this series, suggest ways to approach the culture of other endocrine target cells not described in these volumes.

The methods given here are intended for those wishing immediate directions for application of a previously formulated medium for a given cell type and for those investigators with the need for developing new types of defined media, or having the need for modification to suit a new cell type. We hope that, in addition to the immediate usefulness of the methods presented, that they will also provide a working base for new applications.

David W. Barnes
David A. Sirbasku
Gordon H. Sato

Methods for Serum-Free Culture of Cells of the Endocrine System, pages 1–13

1
Growth of GH₃, a Rat Pituitary Cell Line, in Serum-Free, Hormone-Supplemented Medium

Izumi Hayashi

GH₃ is a functional rat pituitary cell line [Yasumura et al., 1966] originally developed from a transplantable pituitary tumor MtT/W5 [Takemoto et al., 1962] carried in female Wistar/Furth rats. A cloned cell line, GH₃ secretes both prolactin and growth hormone into culture medium [Tashjian et al., 1968, 1970]. Using serum obtained from thyroidectomized cows, Samuels et al. [1973] demonstrated the dependence of GH₃ cells on thyroid hormone for growth. The other growth-promoting factors for GH₃ that were supplied by the hypothyroid cow serum were eventually identified, and now GH₃ cells can be maintained in a completely defined culture medium supplemented with hormones and purified growth factors. There are a number of approaches one can take to derive the complete elucidation of growth requirements for a given cell line [Bottenstein et al., 1979; Barnes and Sato, 1980]. This chapter describes the process that was taken to identify the growth factors for GH₃, as one such example.

DERIVATION OF THE SERUM-FREE MEDIUM
Studies in Thyroid Hormone-Depleted Medium

The effect of 3,3,5-triiodothyronine (T₃), the biologically active form of thyroid hormone, on the growth of GH₃ cells can be clearly demonstrated by using either hypothyroid serum obtained from propyl thiouracil-treated rats, or serum extracted with activated charcoal (Fig. 1). Initially, the basal medium

Division of Cytogenetics and Cytology, City of Hope National Medical Center, Duarte, California 91010

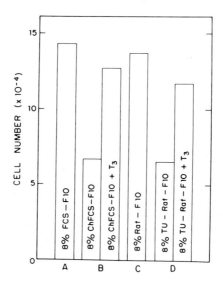

Fig. 1. Effect of T_3 on the growth of GH_3 cells in thyroid hormone-depleted media. Medium F10 supplemented with 8% FCS (A), 8% ChFCS (B) with or without T_3 (1×10^{-9} M), 8% rat serum obtained from a normal Wistar-Furth rat (C), 8% hypothyroid rat serum (TU) obtained from a propyl thiouracil-treated rat (D). The inoculum was 3.5×10^4 cells per 35-mm plate. The cells were counted on day 4.

used to demonstrate the effect of T_3 consisted of Dulbecco's modified Eagle's medium (DME) or Ham's F-10 medium (F10) supplemented with charcoal-extracted fetal calf serum (ChFCS) or calf serum (ChCS). When T_3 is added at 1×10^{-9} M to ChFCS, growth equivalent to that in rich medium (DME supplemented with 12.5% horse serum [HS] and 2.5% FCS) is obtained (Fig. 2). However, unexpectedly, the effect is not observed when T_3 is added to ChCS, indicating the requirement of GH_3 cells for substance(s) other than T_3. Since FCS seemed to serve as a better indicator serum, this serum was chosen over calf serum for the medium in which to further investigate the growth requirements for GH_3 cells. Since charcoal extraction is an empirical method used for the removal of steroids, thyroid hormones, and other aromatic compounds, ChFCS was subjected to a repeated treatment with activated charcoal (2ChFCS) to minimize the background. The effect of T_3 at varying concentrations was examined in medium supplemented with either 8% FCS, ChFCS, or 2ChFCS. The result is shown in Figure 3. The optimal dose for T_3 is 1×10^{-9} M in all serum supplements. Although the basal cell number is lower for cultures supplemented with 2ChFCS than with ChFCS, the addition of T_3 at higher concentrations did not enhance the growth of cells

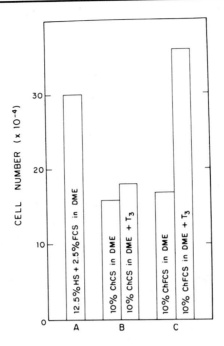

Fig. 2. Effect of T$_3$ on the growth of GH$_3$ cells in charcoal-extracted sera. DME supplemented with 12.5% horse serum and 2.5% FCS (A), 10% charcoal-treated calf serum with or without T$_3$ (B), 10% charcoal treated FCS, with or without T$_3$ (C). The inoculum was 1×10^5 cells per 60-mm plate. T$_3$ was used at a final concentration of 1×10^{-9} M.

in medium supplemented with 8% 2ChFCS to the level equivalent in 8% ChFCS with 1×10^{-9} M T$_3$. This finding confirmed the earlier indication (Fig. 2) that there is an additional substance (or substances) required by GH$_3$ cells for growth that is removed by the second charcoal extraction of serum. Survey of some 15 hormones led to the result shown in Figure 4. Growth is recovered to the rich medium level only by supplementing the depleted medium with T$_3$ and thyrotropin-releasing hormone (TRH). This finding strongly suggested that the role of serum in cell culture medium is to provide hormones [Sato, 1975] and that the cells could grow in an infinitely serum-depleted medium if the lacking serum components were replaced with hormones.

Discovery of Additional Hormone Requirements

The feasibility of this idea was examined. Since the simplest method of depletion is dilution, the concentration of ChFCS was reduced to 0.2% and

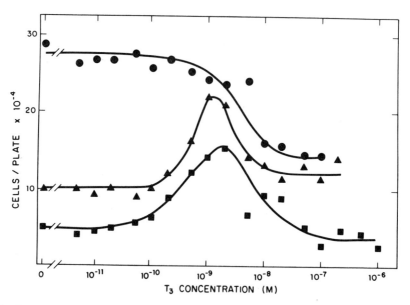

Fig. 3. Effect of T_3 at various concentrations on the growth of GH_3 cells in F10 supplemented with FCS, ChFCS, or 2ChFCS. The cells were suspended in F10 medium supplemented with 8% 2ChFCS after trypsinization and inoculated into each experimental condition. The inoculum was 1×10^5 cells per 60-mm plate. The cells were counted on day 4. ●, 8% FCS; ▲, 8% ChFCS; ■, 8% 2ChFCS.

the effects of additional hormones on growth were examined. Also, the medium F10 was changed to F12, a nutritionally richer medium in the same series, to assure an adequate nutrient supply. Some 30 hormones were tested for their growth-stimulating effect, individually and in various combinations in the presence of T_3 and TRH. The greatest stimulation was observed when insulin and transferrin were added with T_3 and TRH (Fig. 5). The remaining 0.2% serum was finally eliminated when the cells were grown in F12 supplemented with T_3, TRH, transferrin, parathyroid hormone (PTH), and a partially purified somatomedin preparation [Hayashi and Sato, 1976].

Refinement of the Serum-Free, Hormone-Supplemented Medium

It was found that the partially purified somatomedin preparation (kind gift of Dr. Knut Uthne, Ab Kabi, Sweden) could be replaced by insulin and the three isoelectric focusing fractions of blood meal. Blood meal (Bandini, Los Angeles, CA, a commercial fertilizer) is prepared by drying cow blood in a furnace at a temperature above 100°C, hence making it a very desirable source of heat-stable peptides. Such peptides were extracted from blood meal

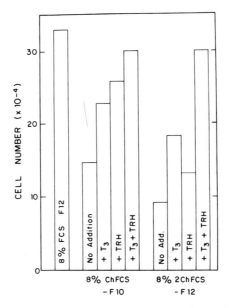

Fig. 4. Effect of T$_3$ and TRH on the growth of GH$_3$ cell. The effect of T$_3$ and TRH was tested alone and in combination in F10 medium supplemented with either 8% ChFCS or 8% 2ChFCS. The conditions are shown in the figure. The inoculum was 1 × 10^5 cells per plate. The cells were counted on day 4.

with 1 M acetic acid and purified by carboxymethyl cellulose (CMC) column chromatography and isoelectric focusing (IEF). The growth-stimulating activity of IEF fractions on GH$_3$ cells were examined in the presence of T$_3$, TRH, transferrin, PTH, and insulin. Three active peaks were present, corresponding to pI 8.5, 9.5, and 10.0 (Fig. 6). When all of the three fractions were combined, together with the other hormones, the growth equivalent to that in serum-supplemented medium was achieved (Fig. 7). Since the pI values suggested the active fractions of IEF to be similar to fibroblast growth factor (FGF) and somatomedin C, the effect of these factors was tested under the same conditions. FGF and somatomedin C (the pure preparations were generous gifts of Dr. Denis Gospodarowicz, University of California at San Francisco and Dr. Judsen Van Wyk, University of North Carolina, Chapel Hill, respectively) in combination could replace the effect of three IEF fractions.

Figure 8 shows the growth of GH$_3$ cells in the completely defined medium supplemented by T$_3$, 10^{-11} M; TRH, 1 ng/ml; transferrin, 5 μg/ml; PTH, 0.5 ng/ml; insulin, 5 μg/ml; FGF, 1 ng/ml; and somatomedin C, 1 ng/ml. The growth rate in the defined medium is identical to that in the serum-

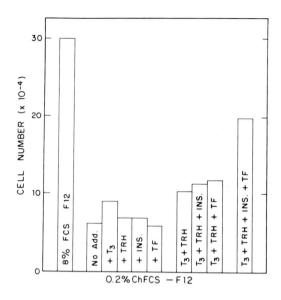

Fig. 5. Effect of T_3, TRH, insulin (INS), and transferrin (TF) on the growth of GH_3 cells. Growth-stimulating effects of the hormones either alone or in combination were tested in F12 medium supplemented with 0.2% ChFCS. The conditions are shown in the figure. The cells were suspended in F12 medium containing 0.2% ChFCS after trypsinization, and inoculated at 1×10^5 cells per 60-mm plate. The final concentrations of hormones used are as follows: T_3, 1×10^{-9} M; TRH, 1×10^{-9} M; insulin, 0.5 μg/ml; and transferrin, 5 μg/ml. The cells were counted on day 4.

supplemented medium. When the cells in the defined condition were subcultured on day 7 into fresh serum-free, hormone-supplemented medium, they continued to grow at the same rate, indicating the complete replacement of serum components for GH_3 cells [Hayashi et al., 1978]. Approximately 30 other hormones and factors such as steroids, pituitary and hypothalamic hormones, peptides of the gastrointestinal tract, catecholamines, and prostaglandins were examined individually and in various combinations for growth-stimulating effect on GH_3 cells. No such effect was observed by any of these substances. Macromolecular substances such as bovine serum albumin, fetuin, fibronectin, and polyvinylpyrrolidone, which are known to improve culture conditions in serum-free medium, also failed to show any additional effect.

METHODS
Cell Culture

GH_3 cells were maintained in DME supplemented with 12.5% HS and 2.5% FCS, in which they grew with a doubling time of 40-48 h, and were

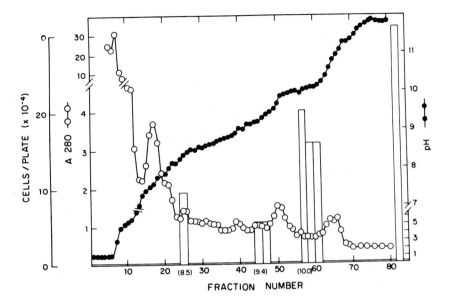

Fig. 6. Isoelectric focusing patterns of blood meal and the growth-stimulating activities of the IEF fractions on GH₃ cells. Blood meal (Bandini) was first washed with water to eliminate salts, and then extracted with 1 N acetic acid for 2 h. The extract was lyophilized to eliminate acetic acid and then redissolved in water at pH 6.8. This was then applied to a carboxymethyl cellulose column equilibrated with 0.05 M sodium phosphate buffer at pH 6.8. The column was washed once with the buffer and then eluted with 0.2 M ammonium formate at pH 8.0. The eluate was lyophilized, stored in the freezer, and used as a substitute for somatomedin preparation. The eluate was purified further by isoelectric focusing (pH range 7.0–10.0). Growth-stimulating activity of the fractions was examined in the presence of T_3, TRH transferrin, PTH, and insulin. The concentration of each hormone is indicated in Figure 7. The inoculum was 0.5×10^5 cells per 35-mm plate. The cells were counted on day 5. The IEF fractions are shown here. O-O, Absorption at OD 280; ●-●, pH gradient. The bar graphs represent the number of cells on day 5. Only the three fractions at pI 8.5, 9.5, and 10.0 showed growth-stimulating activity on the GH₃ cells. The bar at the extreme right shows the effect of CMC ammonium formate eluate, the starting material for IEF, at 10 μg/ml.

subcultured every 4–5 days from subconfluent plates. All sera were heat-inactivated at 55°C for 30 min prior to use. For experiments, Ham's nutrient mixture F10 or F12 was used. In all cases, medium contained 15 mM N-2-hydroxyethylpiperazine-N'-2-ethane sulfonic acid (HEPES), 192 units/ml penicillin, 200 μg/ml streptomycin, and 25 μg/ml ampicillin. The cells were grown on Falcon tissue culture dishes in a humidified atmosphere of 95% air and 5% CO_2.

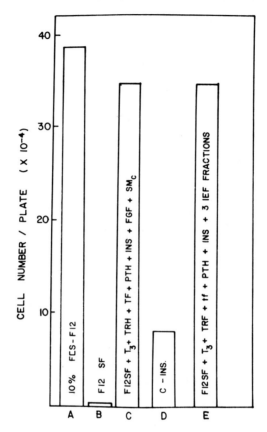

Fig. 7. Growth of GH$_3$ cells in hormone-supplemented serum-free medium. F12 medium supplemented with 10% FCS (A); without addition (B); with T$_3$ (3 × 10^{-11} M), TRH (1 ng/ml), transferrin (5 μg/ml), PTH (0.5 ng/ml, insulin (5 μg/ml), FGF (1 ng/ml), and somatomedin C (1 ng/ml) (C); with C minus insulin (D); with C minus FGF and somatomedin C, which were replaced by three IEF fractions of blood meal (1 μg/ml each of pI 8.5, 9.5, 10.0 materials) (E). The inoculum was 1 × 10^5 cells per 60-mm plate. The cells were counted on day 4.

For growth experiments in serum-free medium, exponentially growing stock cells were trypsinized (1 mg/ml in phosphate-buffered saline [PBS], trypsin 1:250, Difco Laboratories, Detroit), followed by a treatment with soybean trypsin inhibitor (1 mg/ml in phosphate-buffered saline, Sigma, St. Louis). Single cells thus obtained were collected by centrifugation, resuspended in serum-free medium, and inoculated into hormone-containing experimental plates at either 0.5 × 10^5 (35 mm) or 1 × 10^5 (60 mm) cells per dish. On appropriate days, the cells were trypsinized, collected in serum-

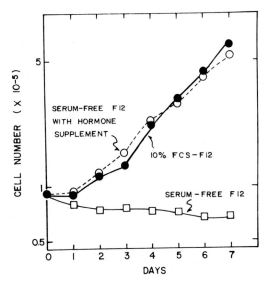

Fig. 8. Growth curve of GH₃ cells in defined medium and in medium supplemented with serum. The hormones and their concentrations are indicated in Figure 7. The inoculum was 0.9 × 10⁵ cells per 35-mm plate. On day 4, the cells were fed with fresh F12 medium with the appropriate supplementation.

containing phosphate-buffered saline, and immediately counted by Coulter Counter.

Hormones

Insulin was dissolved at 1-2 mg/ml in 0.05 N HCl in water, and diluted further with PBS to make a 500-μg/ml working stock solution. The stock solutions were stored at 4°C, as freezing is not recommended. The insulin solution thus stored at 4°C remains active for over 6 months. T_3 was initially dissolved into 0.05 N NaOH at a concentration of $(1-10) \times 10^{-3}$ M. The working stock solution of 3×10^{-9} M was made by diluting the concentrate with PBS. All T_3 solutions were stored frozen. Other hormones and factors were dissolved in PBS and stored frozen. In every case, the working stock solutions were 100-fold concentrates of the final concentrations of hormones and factors in the experimental medium. These stocks were stored in small aliquots to avoid repeated freezing and thawing, and were kept at -20°C no longer than 3 months.

Medium

The choice of medium is of importance for growing cells in serum-free condition supplemented with defined components. Serum provides many trace elements such as vitamins and minerals that had not been discovered in the past studies of the nutritional requirements of cells using dialyzed serum [Eagle, 1955]. These elements, though required in minute quantities, are nevertheless essential for cell growth [McKeehan et al., 1976; Ham and McKeehan, 1978]. When severely deprived or depleted for an extended period, cell growth slows down, leading eventually to cell death. Thus, DME is a nutritionally rich medium when supplemented with high concentrations of serum, but it becomes inadequate for supporting cell growth when serum concentration is lowered. On the other hand, F10 or F12, which were originally developed for the purpose of growing cells in serum-free medium [Ham, 1963, 1965], continue to support the growth of cells in low or no serum supplementation. How various media can affect the growth of cells in serum-free, hormone-supplemented conditions is illustrated in Figure 9. The results are in agreement with many other serum-free systems for which F12 is the sole or a partial choice of synthetic medium.

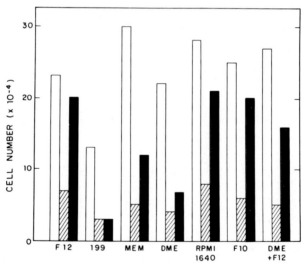

Fig. 9. Growth of GH$_3$ cells in a variety of serum-free media supplemented with T$_3$, TRH, transferrin, PTH, and somatomedin preparation. The cells were trypsinized, treated with trypsin inhibitor, suspended in phosphate-buffered saline, and then inoculated under each experimental condition at 1×10^5 cells per 60-mm plate. Three sets of bars are shown for each medium tested. The open and closed bars are for serum-free medium supplemented with 8% ChFCS and the hormones (T$_3$ + TRH + transferrin + PTH + somatomedin preparation), respectively. The hatched bars in the middle show the cell number in serum-free medium without any addition. The hormones were used at the final concentrations of 3×10^{-11} M T$_3$, 1×10^{-9} M TRH, 5 μg/ml transferrin, 0.5 ng/ml PTH, and 50 mU/ml somatomedin preparation. The cells were counted on day 4.

Serum Depletion

Although the primary purpose of this chapter is to describe an approach and a method for growing GH$_3$ cells in a defined culture medium, serum-free culture need not be the only means to that end. The study of a particular hormone or a factor may be conducted by using a specifically depleted serum as a medium supplement. For this reason although widely used, methods for obtaining hypothyroid serum and charcoal extraction of serum are worth mentioning here again. Hypothyroid serum may be obtained from rats or rabbits treated with 0.05% propyl thiouracil in their drinking water for 6 weeks. The animals are bled at the end of 6 weeks and the serum is obtained by clotting and centrifugation. The procedure for charcoal extraction is as follows: A stock charcoal solution is made by adding 10 g Norit A (Sigma) and 1 g of Dextran T-40 (Pharmacia Fine Chemicals) to 100 ml of PBS. One part of this stock charcoal solution is mixed to nine parts of serum, and extraction is carried out for 30 min at 55°C in a water bath with a shaker. The treated serum is centrifuged at 7,000 rpm (Sorvall centrifuge) for 10 min at 4°C to remove the charcoal. The residual charcoal is eliminated by paper and membrane filtration. This method was shown to remove more than 90% of the steroids and about 30% of thyroid hormones effectively from serum, but it extracts less than 2% of the total serum protein [Armelin and Sato, 1973].

DISCUSSION

At the time the hormonal requirements for GH$_3$ were investigated, studies on cellular growth control were still generally based on the a priori assumption that serum provided a few macromolecular components that are irreplaceable and essential for the growth of cells in culture. The successful replacement of serum with a group of defined components for many cell lines eventually have shown that this is not the case. Many of the hormones and factors that replaced serum are small molecules normally associated with the macromolecular components of serum. Thus, the past attempts to purify growth-stimulating macromolecular components resulted in the loss of activity, or at best, variability in results [Brooks, 1975]. Much of this incoherence may be avoided by using appropriately depleted medium and/or by lowering the serum concentration in a stepwise manner and finding, one by one, the substances that restore the optimal cell growth. Now that the hormonal requirements for many cell types have been established, it is possible to attempt the replacement of serum for cells for which the complete elucidation of the growth factors is unknown, by directly transferring the cells to serum-free medium and examining the effects of various combinations of hormones and factors. However, the methodical stepwise depletion of serum and the replacement of the eliminated serum components by known hormones and defined factors have certain advantages, because the process of depletion itself may provide clues as to the nature of the growth-promoting substances. This knowledge becomes especially critical if the activity under question is caused by a factor whose existence has not yet been revealed. One of the reasons why these factors have not been discovered is probably that they do not have storage organs and/or that the lack of them does not result in severe endocrine disorder. Many of the growth factors discovered in the last decade attest to such reality. Although the physiological significance and specificity for many of the factors discovered by means of in vitro systems await further study, cell culture in hormone-supplemented, serum-free conditions provides an ideal system for the discovery and establishment of the essential nature of these factors. For the pituitary GH_3 cells, as mentioned above, the requirements for somatomedin C and FGF have been derived from the results obtained with the IEF fractions. In the past 5 years, the biochemistry of growth factors has seen much progress. Some of the factors previously difficult to obtain may now be obtained through commercial sources. One such factor is platelet-derived growth factor (PDGF). PDGF has a similar stimulatory effect as FGF on the DNA synthesis of many cell lines. Although FGF and somatomedin C can replace the effects of IEF fractions, considering the heat-resistant nature of the IEF material, PDGF (which, unlike FGF, is known for its heat-stable property) may well be just as effective, if not more.

The optimal doses for most of the hormones and factors are within the physiological range of concentration. The apparently high dose of insulin (1–5 μg/ml) is necessary owing to the presence in the medium of cysteine, one of the classic reducing agents for insulin. The concentration of insulin added at 1 μg/ml to F12 will be reduced to less than 100 ng/ml by radioimmunoassay detection test within 1 h. It is of interest that the optimal concentration for T^3 shifts from 1×10^{-9} in serum-supplemented medium (Fig. 3) to 3×10^{-11} M in serum-free medium. These figures are in agreement with the total concentration of T^3 ($\sim 10^{-9}$ M) and that of biologically active unbound T_3 ($\sim 10^{-11}$ M) in the blood [Samuels et al., 1973].

Although hormonally defined medium for GH_3 cells has been thus developed, this system proved to be difficult for studying the actions of hormones and factors for the regulation of growth. One of the reasons for such difficulty is the long G1 period for GH_3 cells. However, the defined culture system for GH_3 cells has other potential uses, especially in studying the regulation of the production of growth hormone and prolactin, and in identifying other pituitary factors yet to be discovered that are possibly produced by these cells. The hormone-supplemented serum-free system may also be used as a basis for the selective growth of pituitary cells in primary cultures.

REFERENCES

Armelin HA, Sato GH (1973): Cell culture as model systems for the study of growth control. In Ts'o P, DiPaolo J (eds): "World Symposium on Model Studies in Chemical Carcinogenesis, Part B." New York: Marcel Dekker, pp 97-104.

Barnes D, Sato GH (1980): Serum-free cell culture: A unifying approach. Cell 22:649-655.

Bottenstein J, Hayashi I, Hutchings S, Masui H, Mather J, McClure DB, Ohasa S, Rizzino A, Sato G, Serrero G, Wolfe R, Wu R (1979): The growth of cells in serum-free hormone-supplemented media. In Jacoby WB, Pastan IH (eds): "Methods in Enzymology," Vol 58: "Cell Culture." New York: Academic, pp 94-109.

Brooks RF (1975): Growth regulation in vitro and the role of serum. In Allison AC (ed): "Structure and Function of Plasma Proteins." New York: Plenum, pp 1-112.

Eagle H (1955): Nutrition needs of mammalian cells in tissue culture. Science 122:501-504.

Ham RG (1963): An improved nutrient solution for diploid Chinese hamster and human cell lines. Exp Cells Res 29:515-526.

Ham RG (1965): Clonal growth of mammalian cells in a chemically defined synthetic medium. Proc Natl Acad Sci 53:288-293.

Ham RG, McKeehan W (1978): Development of improved media and culture conditions for normal diploid cells. In Vitro 14:11-22.

Hayashi I, Sato GH (1976): Replacement of serum by hormones permits growth of cells in a defined medium. Nature 259:132-134.

Hayashi I, Sato GH, Larner J (1978): Hormonal growth control of cells in culture. In Vitro 14:23-30.

McKeehan W, Hamilton WG, Ham RG (1976): Selenium is an essential trace nutrient for the growth of WI-38 diploid human fibroblasts. Proc Natl Acad Sci 73:2023-2027.

Samuels HH, Tsai JS, Clinton R (1973): Thyroid hormone action: A cell culture system responsive to physiological concentrations of thyroid hormones. Science 181:1253-1256.

Sato GH (1975): The role of serum in cell culture. In Litwack G (ed): "Biochemical Actions of Hormones." New York: Academic, pp 391-396.

Takemoto H, Yokoro K, Furth J, Cohen AJ (1962): Adrenotropic activity of mammo-somato-tropic tumors in rats and mice. I. Biological aspects. Cancer Res 22:917-924.

Tashjian AH Jr, Yasumura Y, Levine L, Sato GH, Parker ML (1968): Establishment of four functional clonal strains of animal cells in culture. Endocrinology 82:342-352.

Tashjian AH Jr, Bancroft FC, Levine L (1970): Production of both prolactin and growth hormone by clonal strains of rat pituitary tumor cells. J Cell Biol 47:61-70.

Yasumura Y, Tashjian AH Jr, Sato G (1966): Establishment of four functional clonal strains of animal cells in culture. Science 154:1186-1189.

Methods for Serum-Free Culture of Cells of the Endocrine System,
pages 15–27

2
Growth of Adrenocortical Cell Cultures in Serum-Free Medium

Michael H. Simonian and Mark L. White

A normal cell culture system from the zona fasciculata-reticularis of the bovine adrenal cortex has been established and used for studies on the regulation of differentiated function (steroidogenesis) and cellular growth [Gospodarowicz et al., 1977; Gill et al., 1979]. In serum-supplemented medium, bovine adrenocortical cells have a finite life span of 60 population doublings in culture and maintain an inducible steroidogenic pathway that is stimulated by adrenocorticotropin (ACTH) [Hornsby and Gill, 1978; Simonian et al., 1979]. To gain full advantage of this normal endocrine cell culture system in studies of cellular physiology, more-defined culture conditions that reflect those in vivo are required.

A serum-free, defined culture medium has been developed for bovine adrenocortical cells in culture that supports not only sustained cellular proliferation but also the full differentiated function of steroidogenesis [Simonian et al., 1982]. Maximum cell proliferation in the absence of serum required a fibronectin-coated substratum and a medium composed of a 1:1 mixture of Ham's F-12 medium and Dulbecco's modified Eagle's medium (DMEM) supplemented with fibroblast growth factor (FGF), insulin, thrombin, low-density lipoprotein (LDL), transferrin, fatty acid-free bovine serum albumin (FAF-BSA), ascorbic acid, α-tocopherol, and selenium. This report describes the preparation and use of this defined medium for normal bovine adrenocortical cells in culture.

Department of Physiology and Biophysics, The University of Iowa, Iowa City, Iowa 52242

MATERIALS AND METHODS
Preparation and Storage of Medium Components

Basal medium. Powdered Ham's F-12 medium and DMEM (4.5 g/liter glucose) obtained from Grand Island Biological Co. (Grand Island, NY) were prepared separately. Initially, triple-glass-distilled water was used to dissolve the media; however, the solutions described here used water that was pretreated with activated charcoal, ion exchange, and reverse osmosis before final purification by a four-cartridge Nanopure system (Barnstead Co., Boston, MA). Both media were made to 1.2 g/liter sodium bicarbonate and 15 mM HEPES [Barnes and Sato, 1980] before sterilization through a 0.2-μm filter cartridge. The DMEM was stored at 4°C and the Ham's F-12 at -20°C.

Fibronectin. Fibronectin was purified from freshly collected bovine plasma by a modification of the procedure of Ruoslahti et al. [1978]. Pooled plasma from two adult animals was prepared from blood that contained 11 mM sodium citrate and 0.1% EDTA. The fibronectin was purified according to the above procedure except that the plasma was not first passed over an underivatized Sepharose (Pharmacia Inc., Piscataway, NJ) column, and the gelatin was coupled to Sepharose CL 6B packing. The cross-linked packing is more resistant to the urea in the elution buffer, and therefore the column can be reused. The fibronectin has been stored in a 1 M urea–10 mM phosphate (pH 7.4) solution at 4°C for nearly 1 year. The fibronectin can be further purified by gel filtration [Simonian et al., 1982], but for routine growth of bovine adrenocortical cells this is not necessary. The fibronectin was sterilized by filtration with a 0.2-μm membrane (Gelman, Ann Arbor, MI). Human fibronectin from outdated plasma has also been purified by this procedure and was as effective as the bovine fibronectin for growth of these cells. The fibronectin, as are all other protein components, was stored in sterile polypropylene tubes.

FGF. Bovine brain FGF was purified in collaboration with Dr. Denis Gospodarowicz (University of California, San Francisco) according to the published procedure [Gospodarowicz et al., 1978]. The FGF-2 peak fraction collected from the Sephadex G75 column can be used for routine growth of the adrenocortical cells in the serum-free medium. A stock solution of FGF (5 μg/ml) was prepared from lyophilized protein in Dulbecco's phosphate-buffered saline (PBS) [Dulbecco and Vogt, 1954] containing 5 mg/ml FAF-BSA and was stored at -20°C for several months.

LDL. Although LDL is at a lower concentration in adult bovine blood than in human blood [Puppione, 1978], possible species differences in the apoproteins prompted purification of bovine LDL. Pooled plasma from at least two animals was prepared as described for fibronectin. The LDL was fractionated by differential ultracentrifugation [Miller et al., 1977]; NaBr was used to adjust the density. The density of the plasma was adjusted to 1.030 g/ml and centrifuged in a Beckman 60Ti rotor at 50,000 rpm for 24 h. The supernatant, which contains very low density lipoprotein and chylomicrons, was discarded and the infranatant density was adjusted to 1.070 g/ml and recentrifuged. The supernatant from this density centrifugation contained the LDL. The LDL was further purified by successive centrifugations in a Beckman SW41 rotor at 38,000 rpm for 24 h to remove remaining contaminants and yield a washed LDL fraction of density 1.019-1.063 g/ml. Bovine blood contains a high-density lipoprotein (HDL) species with a lower density range of approximately 1.063 g/ml [Puppione, 1978]. To minimize contamination of LDL with this HDL species, the final wash centrifugation of LDL into the supernatant had an overlay solution of density 1.060 g/ml. All purified LDL preparations were assayed for protein concentration [Lowry et al., 1951] and cholesterol concentration [Rudel and Morris, 1973]. The average cholesterol:protein ratio for the LDL was 1.70 ± 0.05 (n = 15). Although this ratio was relatively constant among preparations, the absolute concentrations of protein and cholesterol would vary among the preparations. In addition, each purified LDL preparation was analyzed for relative purity from other lipoproteins by agarose gel electrophoresis stained for lipid by sudan black [Noble, 1968]. This analysis was kindly performed by the Lipid Research Center at the University of Iowa (Iowa City, IA). Analysis by sodium dodecyl sulfate-polyacrylamide gel (3-20%) electrophoresis [Laemmli, 1970] of select LDL preparations verified the apoprotein purity for bovine LDL [Forte et al., 1981]. The LDL in 50 mM phosphate-buffered saline with 0.3 mM EDTA (pH 7.2) was sterilized by filtration through a $0.2\text{-}\mu m$ membrane and stored at 4°C for 1 month. After this length of time, a noticeable precipitate occurred.

Insulin. Bovine insulin was commercially obtained (Sigma Chemical Co., St. Louis, Catalog No. I5500), and a 1 mg/ml solution in 0.01 M HC1 was stored at 4°C for a period of 3 months.

Thrombin. Bovine thrombin was commercially obtained (Sigma) and stocks of 10 U/ml in Dulbecco's PBS were aliquoted and stored at −20°C for several months. Two thrombin preparations that differ in specific activity, 2,000 NIH U/mg protein (Catalog No. T7531) and 600 NIH U/mg protein (Catalog No. T6634) have been used, and the dose-response characteristics based on U/ml added to the medium were identical.

Transferrin. The transferrin used in the defined medium was the only nonbovine protein component. Human transferrin was purchased (Sigma, Catalog No. T4515), stock solutions were prepared at 10 mg/ml in PBS, and aliquots were stored at −20°C for several months.

FAF-BSA. This preparation of BSA (fatty acids $<0.005\%$) was obtained commercially (Sigma Catalog No. A7511), and a 45-mg/ml solution in PBS was prepared and sterilized with a 0.2-μm membrane filter. This solution was aliquoted and stored at $-20°C$.

Selenium. Selenium in the form of sodium selenite (Na_2SeO_3, Difco Laboratories, Detroit) was prepared as a stock solution at 5×10^{-6} M in water and stored at $4°C$. A fresh stock was made every 3 months.

α-Tocopherol. The d-isomer of α-tocopherol was obtained commercially (Supelco, Bellefonte, PA) and a stock solution of 10 mM in acetone was prepared. This stock was stored at $4°C$ and renewed every 3 months.

Ascorbic acid. Ascorbic acid was purchased (Sigma, Catalog No. A7506) and a 10 mM solution in water was prepared fresh from the powder for each medium change.

Antibiotics. Penicillin G (Sigma, Catalog No. Pen K) and gentamycin sulfate (Sigma, Catalog No. 3632) were purchased, and a stock solution containing both antibiotics at 10 and 5 mg/ml, respectively, in PBS was prepared and stored at $-20°C$ for several months.

Use of Medium Components

Fibronectin coating of culture dishes. The fibronectin was diluted in Ham's F-12 medium to a concentration on 10 μg/ml and dispensed into tissue culture dishes (Falcon, Oxnard, CA) at a concentration of 2 μg/cm^2 of surface area. The dishes were incubated at $37°C$ for 30 min and then washed twice with sterile, warm PBS. The dishes were used immediately for culturing of the cells.

Nonprotein components. The required volumes of Ham's F-12 medium and DMEM were mixed in a 1:1 ratio into either a sterile glass or plastic vessel just prior to use. The following components were added to the medium mixture from the above stock solutions so that the final concentration per culture (shown in parentheses) was a 100-fold dilution of the stock: penicillin (100 μg/ml), gentamycin sulfate (50 μg/ml), Na_2SeO_3 (5×10^{-8} M), and ascorbic acid (10^{-4} M). The α-tocopherol was added as a 10,000-fold dilution, so that the final medium concentration was 10^{-6} M. This mixture was aliquoted to 90% of the final volume into fibronectin-coated culture dishes.

Protein components. All protein components except the LDL were premixed in a sterile polypropylene tube that contained a volume of Ham's F-12 medium and DMEM (1:1) that was dispensed to the cultures as 9% of the final volume in the dish. The stock of insulin was diluted fresh 100-fold into 0.01 M HCl, and this was then added to the protein mixture so that the final concentration per culture was 10 ng/ml, or a 1,000-fold dilution of the fresh stock. The other protein components were added to the protein solution so that the final concentration in the culture (shown in parentheses) was a 100-fold dilution of the stock preparation: FGF (50 ng/ml + 50 μg/ml FAF-BSA), FAF-BSA (450 μg/ml), thrombin (100 mU/ml), and transferrin (100 μg/ml). This protocol of mixing the proteins minimizes the acid-labile effect of the insulin solution on FGF [Gospodarowicz et al., 1978] and permits the use of polypropylene tubes and pipette tips for dispensing the proteins, a procedure that decreases the problem of protein loss by adsorption.

The LDL was added directly to the culture as 1% of the final volume in the dish at a concentration of 10 μg/ml of protein. When the LDL was combined with the other protein components and then aliquoted into the cultures, the final cell number was 30% lower than when the LDL is added alone directly to the medium in the culture dish (unpublished observation). This may be due to inactivation of one of the other protein mitogens by the EDTA in the LDL buffer when all the protein components are premixed. The LDL must be added 24 h after plating of cells, when they are firmly attached to the dish. When LDL at this concentration was added prior to this, cell attachment was inhibited [Simonian et al., 1982].

Cell Culture Methods

The preparation and storage of primary bovine adrenocortical cells from the zona fasciculata-reticularis has been previously described [Gospodarowicz et al., 1977; Hornsby and Gill, 1977]. A frozen vial of primary cells was thawed, diluted, and plated into four 6-cm culture dishes that contained Ham's F-12 medium with 10% newborn bovine serum (Irvine Scientific, Irvine, CA) and 50 ng/ml FGF. The cell cultures were maintained in this medium for 4 days with a complete change of medium after 2 days, which eliminates the unattached cells and tissue debris from the frozen cell suspension. After 4 days, the cells were removed in the absence of serum according to the subculture method described below and were aliquoted into fibronectin-coated culture dishes (1×10^3 to 1.5×10^3 cells per cm^2) that contained the defined medium. The defined medium was replenished every 2 days. The cultures were maintained in a humidified incubator at 37°C containing 85% N_2, 10% air (2% oxygen), and 5% CO_2. This lowered oxygen concentration as compared to conventional conditions of 19% oxygen helps preserve the 11β-hydroxylase activity of the steroid pathway in these cells [Hornsby, 1980] without affecting the rate of cell proliferation in the defined medium (unpublished observation).

To subculture adrenocortical cells grown in the defined medium, the medium was removed, and the cells were washed twice with PBS and then treated at room temperature with 500 μg/ml trypsin in PBS that contained 0.1% glucose. When the cells began to detach, they were suspended in 4 ml of 1 mg/ml soybean trypsin inhibitor and 1 mg/ml FAF-BSA in Ham's F-12 and then aliquoted into culture dishes that contained the defined medium. The trypsin solution used for subculture did not contain EDTA, because with EDTA present the cells no longer contained intracellular granules as observed in primary cultures (unpublished observations). The trypsin and trypsin inhibitor were stored in frozen aliquots prepared as follows. Bovine pancreatic trypsin was obtained commercially (Sigma, type III, Catalog No. T8253) and a tenfold concentrated trypsin solution in PBS-glucose was filtered through a 0.2-μm membrane. This sterile solution was diluted to the final working concentration with sterile PBS-glucose, and 1 ml aliquots were stored at $-20°$C. Soybean trypsin inhibitor was purchased (Sigma, type II-S, Catalog No. T9128) and a tenfold concentrated solution was prepared in FAF-BSA in Ham's F-12, sterilized with a 0.2-μm filter, and diluted tenfold with sterile FAF-BSA in Ham's F-12. The trypsin inhibitor was stored in 4-ml aliquots at $-20°$C for several months. Both the trypsin and trypsin inhibitor solutions were thawed and used only once.

Cell number was quantitated by removing the cells from dishes by incubation with PBS containing 0.05% trypsin and 0.025% EDTA (obtained lyophilyzed from Grand Island Biological Co.) for 1–2 min at 37°C. Cells were diluted and immediately counted in a Model Z_B Coulter Counter (Coulter Electronics, Inc., Hialeah, FL).

RESULTS WITH THE DEFINED MEDIUM
Growth in the Defined Medium

The dose-response characteristics of the protein factors in defined medium were determined by varying the concentration of each factor in the presence of a constant concentration of the other factors. The results are shown in Table I. The FAF-BSA concentration was the total of that added from the FGF and the FAF-BSA stock solutions. If the FAF-BSA was not present, the half-maximal and maximal concentrations of FGF were ten times higher than that shown [Simonian et al., 1982]. The FAF-BSA stabilized the FGF and possibly other factors in the defined medium and also had a slight growth effect. All protein components of the defined medium increased the cell number by at least 20% over that in absence of the protein, which was the original criterion used for screening of the factors [Simonian et al., 1982]. Bovine HDL had a slight growth effect on these cells; however, this was less than half that observed with LDL.

**TABLE I. Concentration Effects of Protein
Factors on Cell Proliferation in the
Defined Medium**

Protein factor[a]	Maximal concentration	Stimulation over control[b]
Fibronectin	$2\ \mu g/cm^2$	18.6
FGF	50 ng/ml	2.2
Insulin	10 ng/ml	2.5
Thrombin	100 mU/ml	1.2
LDL	$10\ \mu g/ml$	1.7
Transferrin	$100\ \mu g/ml$	1.2
FAF-BSA	$500\ \mu g/ml$	1.3

[a]Secondary cultures of bovine adrenocortical cells were
subcultured at 15,000 cells per 3.4-cm dish that
contained a 1:1 mixture of Ham's F-12 and DME
media, 100 μM ascorbic acid, 1 μM α-tocopherol, and
50 nM Na_2SeO_3. The concentration of one protein
factor was varied in the presence of a constant
contraction of the other factors. Except when varied, the
concentration of the protein factors was $2\ \mu g/cm^2$
fibronectin, 50 ng/ml FGF, 10 ng/ml insulin, 100 mU/
ml thrombin, 10 μg/ml LDL, 10 μg/ml transferrin, and
50 μg/ml FAF-BSA. The LDL was added starting on
day 1 after plating of the cells. The medium was
replenished every 2 days.
[b]Cell numbers were determined from triplicate plates on
day 6 for each concentration of an addition. For each
protein factor, except FAF-BSA, the control plates
lacked the factor being studied. The FAF-BSA control
plates contained 50 μg/ml FAF-BSA.
Reprinted with permission from the Endocrine Society
[Simonian et al., 1982].

Maximum proliferation of adrenocortical cells in the defined medium required a substratum of fibronectin, which is the most potent mitogen for serum-free growth. Although these cells would proliferate in the absence of any single protein factor, maximum proliferation required all these components. In the absence of the polypeptide factors added to the defined medium, the cells would survive but they did not grow on fibronectin-coated dishes containing medium with only ascorbic acid, α-tocopherol, and Na_2SeO_3 (Table II).

The growth effects of maximal concentrations of the antioxidants ascorbic acid, α-tocopherol, and Na_2SeO_3 are shown in Table III. In the absence of any antioxidants, or with only α-tocopherol or Na_2SeO_3 present, the cells did

TABLE II. Effect of Protein Growth Factors in the Defined Medium on Cell Proliferation

Additions	Number of cells[b]	
to medium[a]	Day 1	Day 6
Ascorbic acid	30,677 ± 164	32,300 ± 1,189
+ α-tocopherol		
+Na$_2$SeO$_3$		
Complete mix	33,373 ± 660	489,333 ± 2,667

[a]Second-passage cells were added to fibronectin-coated dishes containing medium and 100 μM ascorbic acid, 1 μM α-tocopherol, and 50 nM Na$_2$SeO$_3$ without and with 50 ng/ml FGF, 10 ng/ml insulin, 100 mU/ml thrombin, 100 μg/ml transferrin, and 500 μg/ml FAF-BSA; 10 μg/ml LDL was added to the complete mix on day 1 after plating of the cells. The medium was replenished on all cultures every 2 days.
[b]Number of cells was determined for cultures on day 1 and day 6 after starting the cultures. Mean ± SEM for triplicate dishes are shown [Simonian et al., 1982].
Reprinted with permission from the Endocrine Society [Simonian et al., 1982].

TABLE III. Effect of Antioxidants on Cell Proliferation in the Defined Medium

Additions to medium[a]	Final number of cells[b]
None	9,013 ± 1,097
α-Tocopherol	9,433 ± 542
Na$_2$SeO$_3$	7,348 ± 810
α-Tocopherol + Na$_2$SeO$_3$	55,467 ± 481
Ascorbic acid	161,080 ± 10,832
Ascorbic acid + α-tocopherol	181,387 ± 9,416
Ascorbic acid + Na$_2$SeO$_3$	186,320 ± 5,127
Ascorbic acid + Na$_2$SeO$_3$ + α-tocopherol	185,333 ± 9,340

[a]Second-passage cells were subcultured into fibronectin-coated (2 μg/cm$_2$) dishes (3.5 cm) containing a 1:1 mixture of Ham's F-12 and DME media and 50 ng/ml FGF, 10 ng/ml insulin, 100 mU/ml thrombin, 100 μg/ml transferrin, 500 μg/ml FAF-BSA without and with 100 μM ascorbic acid, 1 μM α-tocopherol, and/or 50 nM Na$_2$SeO$_3$; 10 μg/ml LDL was added to all cultures on day 1 after subculturing of the cells. Medium was replenished every 2 days.
[b]The starting cell density was 15,000 cells per 3.5-cm dish and the final cell number was determined on day 6 after starting the cultures. Mean ± SEM for triplicate dishes are shown.

not survive after 6 days in the defined medium. Cultures containing both Na_2SeO_3 (50 nM) and α-tocopherol (1 μM) survived and nearly doubled once in this time. However, in the presence of only ascorbic acid (100 μM) the cells doubled 3.4 times in the defined medium. The addition of ascorbic acid plus α-tocopherol and/or Na_2SeO_3 in the defined medium supported maximal cell proliferation (3.6 population doublings).

As shown in Figure 1, the growth rate of bovine adrenocortical cells in the defined medium was equivalent to that in medium containing serum and FGF, which has been previously demonstrated to be optimal for proliferation of these cells in culture [Gospodarowicz et al., 1977]. The addition of 10 nM adrenocorticotropin to the defined medium on day 2 inhibited cell proliferation over the next 4 days with an average generation time (52.4 h) that was twice that for cultures in the defined medium without ACTH (24.6 h). The complete inhibition of cell proliferation by ACTH indicates that the defined medium supports proliferation of only the adrenocortical cells. ACTH has been shown to inhibit cell proliferation in serum-supplemented medium of bovine, rat, mouse, and human adrenocortical cells [Hornsby and Gill, 1977; Ramachandran and Suyama, 1975; Masui and Garren, 1971; Simonian and Gill, 1981].

Bovine adrenocortical cells have been subcultured for 10 passages (35 generations) in the defined medium without any serum intervention. The same final cell density (3 $\times$ 10^4 to 4 $\times$ 10^4 cells per cm^2) was observed for each passage. Therefore, the defined medium for bovine adrenocortical cells supports proliferation at the same rate as in serum-supplemented medium and long-term culturing.

Function in Defined Medium

Adrenal-specific steroid production was also supported by the defined medium. The maximal steroid production with ACTH in the defined medium required 10 μg/ml LDL, with a half-maximal concentration of 1.1 μg/ml [Simonian et al., 1982]. Previous studies have shown that, for maximal stimulated steroidogenesis by bovine adrenocortical cells in culture, the cholesterol substrate was provided for exogenously by LDL [Simonian et al., 1979; Kovanen et al., 1979]. Bovine adrenocortical cells have high-affinity LDL receptors but not similar HDL receptors [Kovanen et al., 1979], which has been confirmed in the defined medium for these cells from comparison of effects of LDL and HDL on growth and function [Simonian et al., 1982]. ACTH stimulated steroid production in the defined medium with a maximum concentration of 10 nM and a half-maximal concentration of 0.5 nM, which is the same effective concentration range observed in serum-containing medium [Hornsby and Gill, 1978].

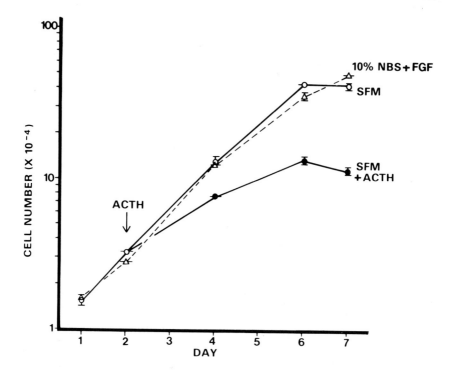

Fig. 1. Effect of ACTH on cell proliferation in the defined medium. Primary cultures of bovine adrenocortical cells were plated into 3.5-cm dishes containing a 1:1 mixture of Ham's F-12 and DME medium supplemented either with 10% newborn bovine serum (NBS) plus 50 ng/ml FGF (△--△) or the serum-free medium (SFM) consisting of fibronectin-coated (2 μg/cm^2) dishes with 50 ng/ml FGF, 10 ng/ml insulin, 100 mU/ml thrombin, 10μg/ml LDL, 100 μg/ml transferrin, 500 μg/ml FAF-BSA, 100 μM ascorbic acid, 1 μM α-tocopherol, and 50 nM Na$_2$SeO$_3$ (○—○ and ●—●). The LDL was added to the defined medium starting on day 1. All media were replenished every 2 days. Starting on day 2, 10 nM ACTH was added with each medium change to a set of the defined medium cultures (●—●). Cell numbers were determined at the times indicated. The mean ± SEM for triplicate plates is shown. Reprinted with permission of the Endocrine Society [Simonian et al., 1982].

The effect of the defined medium on maintaining adrenal-specific ste-roidogenesis was determined by reverse-phase high-performance liquid chro-matography analysis of the Δ^4,3-ketosteroid products [O'Hare et al., 1976]. Control second passage cells grown to confluence in the defined medium synthesized progesterone, 20α-dihydroprogesterone, 17α-hydroxyprogester-one, 11-deoxycortisol, and cortisol (Fig. 2). When ACTH was added for 24

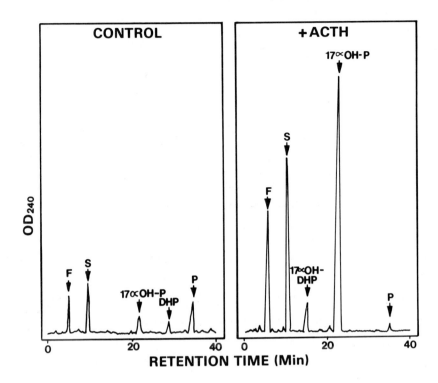

Fig. 2. High-pressure liquid chromatogram of steroids secreted by cultures of bovine adreno-cortical cells grown in the defined medium. Confluent cell cultures grown in the defined medium as described in Figure 1 were incubated with or without 1 μM ACTH. After 24 h, media from triplicate cultures were pooled and extracted with dichloromethane. Steroids were separated by high-pressure liquid chromatography with a concave exponential gradient of acetonitrile-water. The retention times of the steroid standards are indicated by the arrows: F, cortisol; S, deoxy-cortisol; 17αOH-P, 17α-hydroxyprogesterone; DHP, 20α-dihydroprogesterone; 17αOH-DHP, 17α-hydroxy-20α-dihydroprogesterone; P, progesterone. Attenuation was 0.02 absorption units full scale. Reprinted with permission of the Endocrine Society [Simonian et al., 1982].

h, there was marked stimulation of 17α-hydroxyprogesterone, 17α-hydroxy-20α-dihydroprogesterone, 11-deoxycortisol, and cortisol. Thus the defined culture medium supports the hormone-stimulated differentiated function of bovine adrenocortical cells.

ACKNOWLEDGMENTS

The authors thank Dr. Gordon Sato for advice on development of the serum-free medium, Dr. Denis Gospodarowicz for the gift of highly purified

FGF, and Dr. Gordon Gill for his support of this work. In addition we are grateful to Patty Hardy for typing the manuscript. This research was supported by Research Grant IN-122B from the American Cancer Society and a Wellcome Research Travel Grant from the Burroughs Wellcome fund.

REFERENCES

Barnes D, Sato G (1980): Serum-free growth of cells in culture. Anal Biochem 102:255-270.

Dulbecco R, Vogt M (1954): Plaque formation and isolation of pure lines with poliomyelitis viruses. J Exp Med 99:167-182.

Forte TM, Bell-Quint JA, Cheng F (1981): Lipoproteins of fetal and newborn calves and adult steer: A study of developmental changes. Lipids 16:240-245.

Gill GN, Hornsby PJ, Simonian MH (1979): Regulation of growth and differentiated function of bovine adrenocortical cells. In Sato GH, Ross R (eds): "Cold Spring Harbor Conferences on Cell Proliferation," Vol 6: "Hormones and Cell Culture." Cold Spring Harbor, NY: Cold Spring Harbor Laboratory, pp 701-715.

Gospodarowicz D, Ill CR, Hornsby PJ, Gill GN (1977): Control of bovine adrenal cortical cell proliferation by fibroblast growth factors. Lack of effect of epidermal growth factor. Endocrinology 100:1080-1089.

Gospodarowicz D, Bialecki H, Greenburg G (1978): Purification of the fibroblast growth factor activity from bovine brain. J Biol Chem 253:3736-3743.

Hornsby PJ (1980): Regulation of cytochrome P-450-supported 111β-hydroxylation of deoxycortisol by steroids, oxygen, and antioxidants in adrenocortical cell cultures. J Biol Chem 255:4020-4027.

Hornsby PJ, Gill GN (1977): Hormonal control of adrenocortical cell profliferation. J Clin Invest 60:342-352.

Hornsby PJ, Gill GN (1978): Characterization of adult bovine adrenocortical cells throughout their life span in tissue culture. Endocrinology 102:926-936.

Kovanen PT, Faust JR, Brown MS, Goldstein JL (1979): Low density lipoprotein receptors in bovine adrenal cortex. I. Receptor-mediated uptake of low density lipoprotein and utilization of its cholesterol for steroid synthesis in cultured adrenocortical cells. Endocrinology 104:599-609.

Laemmli UK (1970): Cleavage of structural proteins during assembly of the head of bacteriophage T4. Nature 227:680-685.

Lowry OH, Rosebrough NJ, Farr AL, Randall RJ (1951): Protein measurement with the Folin phenol reagent. J Biol Chem 193:265-275.

Masui H, Garren LD (1971): Inhibition of replication in functional mouse adrenal tumor cells by adrenocorticotropin mediated by adenosine 3':5'-cyclic monophosphate. Proc Natl Acad Sci USA 68:3206-3210.

Miller NE, Weinstein DB, Carew TE, Koschinsky T, Steinberg D (1977): Interaction between high density and low density lipoproteins during uptake and degradation by cultured human fibroblasts. J Clin Invest 60:78-88.

Noble RP (1968): Electrophoretic separation of plasma lipoproteins in agarose gel. J Lipid Res 9:693-700.

O'Hare MJ, Nice EC, Magee-Brown R, Bullman H (1976): High-pressure liquid chromatography of steroids secreted by human adrenal and testis cells in monolayer culture. J Chromatogr 125:357-367.

Puppione DL (1978): Implications of unique features of blood lipid transport in the lactating cow. J Dairy Sci 61:651–659.

Ramachandran J, Suyama AI (1975): Inhibition of replication of normal adrenocortical cells in culture by adrenocorticotropin. Proc Natl Acad Sci USA 73:113–117.

Rudel LL, Morris MD (1973): Determination of cholesterol using o-phthalaldehyde. J Lipid Res 14:364–366.

Ruoslahti E, Vuento M, Engvall E (1978): Interaction of fibronectin with collagen in radioimmunoassay. Biochim Biophys Acta 534:210–218.

Simonian MH, Gill GN (1981): Regulation of the fetal human adrenal cortex: Effects of adrenocorticotropin on growth and function of monolayer cultures of fetal and definitive zone cells. Endocrinology 108:1769–1779.

Simonian MH, Hornsby PJ, Ill CR, O'Hare MJ, Gill GN (1979): Characterization of cultured bovine adrenocortical cells and derived clonal lines: Regulation of steroidogenesis and culture life span. Endocrinology 105:99–108.

Simonian MH, White ML, Gill GN (1982): Growth and function of cultured bovine adrenocortical cells in a serum-free defined medium. Endocrinology 111:919–927.

Methods for Serum-Free Culture of Cells of the Endocrine System,
pages 29–45
© 1984 Alan R. Liss, Inc., 150 Fifth Avenue, New York, NY 10011

3
Primary Culture of Testicular Somatic Cells

J.P. Mather and D.M. Phillips

Primary cell cultures have played a major role in the application of tissue culture to studies of cell and organ physiology. With the establishment of clonal cell lines that maintained functional properties of the cell type of origin many laboratories chose to investigate the properties of these cell lines rather than work with primary cultures. However, primary cell cultures can still contribute significantly to our understanding of animal physiology. The development of hormone-supplemented serum-free media for a number of cell lines led to the realization that primary cultures of these cell types could often be grown in the same, or similar, hormone-supplemented medium as that devised for an established cell line derived from the same cell type [Mather and Sato, 1979]. The use of hormone-supplemented medium can be devised to partially or completely select for the cell type of interest [Bottenstein et al., 1980; Taub and Sato, 1979; Ambesi-Impiombato et al., 1980]. This has eliminated fibroblast overgrowth, one of the major problems in previous work with serum-supplemented medium [Purvi and Turner, 1978; Barnes et al., 1981]. In addition, work on several different organs has shown that serum is capable of suppressing the expression of many differentiated functions of cells in primary culture [Orly et al., 1980]. This work has extended the usefulness of primary cultures and allowed the isolation of new nontransformed cell lines. We will discuss the preparation of testicular somatic cell types for primary culture in serum-free medium. Two methods of cell isolation are discussed in detail.

The Population Council, New York, New York 10021

GENERAL CONSIDERATIONS FOR PRIMARY CULTURE

The decision to use primary cell culture as a model system for the study of a specific problem will depend on several considerations. Cells in primary culture, at least initially, express many of the functions and properties of the same cell in vivo. This situation may then be considered to reflect the operation of that cell in the animal. Several aspects of the in vivo environment, however, change immediately when a cell is placed in vitro. These may become major considerations in designing the culture system to be used. While tissue culture incubators are designed to provide an atmosphere with pH, pO_2, pCO_2, temperature, and humidity similar to those found in the blood, these parameters may be radically different in the microenvironment of the cell in vivo. Thus, steroidogenesis has been shown to be maintained better in primary adrenal cell cultures when the cells are placed in a low-oxygen atmosphere with anti-oxidants included in the medium [Hornsby, 1980; Crivello et al., 1982]. Likewise, Leydig cell cultures from the pig [Mather et al., 1983] and mouse [Murphy and Moger, 1982] maintain function better in such an environment. Testicular cells are frequently cultured at 32°C (the temperature of the human testis) rather than 37°C, which is generally used for most cell types.

The three-dimensional configuration of cells in monolayer culture is quite different from that of most cells in vivo. Culture on collagen gels [Elsdale and Bard, 1972] or on floating collagen rafts [Emerman et al., 1977] has been shown to improve the function of many cell types. It is to be expected that those cellular functions that depend on the maintenance of a cuboidal or spherical shape or three-dimensional cellular structures may be lost in monolayer culture.

Cell-cell and tissue interactions are also lost when a single cell type is placed in culture. While known trophic hormones and growth factors can be provided in culture, the full complexity of paracrine control in the testis has only begun to be understood. It may thus be difficult to provide all the factors required for the complete maintenance of cell function or to maintain them in adequate concentrations. In addition most cells are associated with extracellular matrix material in vivo. The importance of this matrix in controlling or maintaining cell function is a major area of research [Reid, 1982; Gospodarowicz and Ill, 1980].

Finally, the effect of a hormone on cell function may depend not only on its concentration but on the timing of pulsatile variation in hormone and nutrient levels. These variations are extremely difficult to reproduce in tissue culture.

The above considerations should not be taken as a discouragement to using primary culture. The major advantage of cell culture is that it simplifies and allows control of the cellular environment. The use of progressively more complex defined cell culture systems will help define the parameters required for the expression of specific cell functions and provide valuable information impossible to obtain in vivo.

SELECTION OF MODEL SYSTEM

The selection of species and age of the animals used to place cells in primary culture, as well as the type of isolation procedure used, should reflect the problem to be studied. The cost and availability of animals and housing is often a consideration. In vivo studies on the animal in question facilitate comparison of results obtained in vivo and in vitro. The availability of inbred strains of animal and/or mutations that affect the function of the cell type to be studied may be of importance. The stability of chromosomes in cultured cells may vary widely from one species to another and may be of considerable importance if one of the goals of the work is to establish normal cell lines from primary cultures. The anatomy of the testis varies widely from one species to another [Setchell, 1978] and will affect the purity and yield of a cell preparation, as well as the procedure used for cell separation. The interstitial tissue of the rat and mouse is separated from the seminiferous tubules by lymphatic spaces. It can thus be isolated by nonenzymatic mechanical separation, although more damage is sustained by rat than mouse Leydig cells when this procedure is used [Aldred and Cooke, 1980]. Tubular segments can also be mechanically dissected out by hand [Parvinen and Vanha-Perttula, 1972]. In contrast, porcine testicular tissue has densely packed interstitial tissue and tubular elements arranged in lobes connected to the central mediastinum. Isolation of both interstitial tissue and tubular tissue from this species requires more extensive enzymatic digestion. However, rat and mouse testis contain only a very small number of Leydig cells (3-4%) [Mori and Christensen, 1980], whereas the immature porcine testis is composed of 50% Leydig cells and the testis itself is much larger than that of the mouse. Thus the disadvantages of the requirement for enzyme digestion may be offset by high cell yields and purity if large numbers of cells are required.

The age of the animal from which the cells are obtained is also important. In the testis the Sertoli cells undergo division in the immature animal but reach a nondividing state at puberty, when the germinal cells begin rapid proliferation and differentiation. Thus, in an adult animal, a large proportion of the testicular mass is germ cells. The morphology, pattern of protein secretion, and hormone response of Sertoli cells in vivo and in vitro changes from birth to maturity [Rich et al., 1983; Solari and Fritz, 1978]. A higher yield of Sertoli cells can be obtained from an immature animal, with little germ cell contamination. However, these cells function as immature Sertoli cells and are thus not the optimal model system for studying the function of the mature Sertoli cell in an adult animal.

Finally cells of the same type but from different species can behave very differently under the same culture conditions. Thus a comparison of the maintenance of gonadotropin responsiveness in mouse, rat, and pig Leydig cells over the first week in culture shows that porcine Leydig cells maintain response over weeks, rather than days, in culture [Mather et al., 1981, 1982a].

PREPARATION OF THE CELLS FOR CULTURE

Since most tissues, including the testis, are composed of several cell types and adjacent connective tissue, some type of dispersion and cell selection is required to obtain a primary culture that is predominately of a single cell type. As discussed above, the type of tissue and the age and species of animal from which it is obtained will play a role in determining the method of cell isolation. Various types of mechanical and/or enzymatic dispersion techniques are the usual first step. This can be followed by purification of a single cell type by size or density. Percoll [Hunter et al., 1982] and metrizimide [Dufau et al., 1978] gradients have been used to further purify Leydig cells from interstitial tissue. Immunologic selection may be employed 1) to label a subpopulation of cells with fluorescence-tagged antibody followed by fluorescence cell sorting [Auerbach et al., 1982]; 2) to specifically kill an undesired cell type; or 3) to coat tissue culture dishes with an antibody to a specific cell surface component that will cause the desired cell population to rapidly adhere to the dish [Wysocki and Sato, 1978]. Finally, as discussed above, the hormone supplements added to the medium can be selected so as to optimize the survival and growth of the desired cell type, while being insufficient for the survival of other types of cells in the cultures. Various combinations of the above techniques can be used.

A method of identifying the desired cell type in culture is required to monitor purity of the original cell suspension plated and to follow changes in the cell population with time in culture. Ideally this identification method should be rapid, inexpensive, and specific for the cells to be cultured. Histochemical staining for 3-β-ol-dehydroxysteroid dehydrogenase activity is frequently used to assess the purity of Leydig cell preparations [Bilinska, 1979].

Phenylesterase staining has also been used as a Leydig cell marker [Hunter et al., 1982]. Purity of Sertoli cell preparations has been shown on the basis of morphologic criteria at the electron microscope level [Solari and Fritz, 1978]. This is obviously not a technique that can be routinely used to monitor each cell preparation. Secreted products known to be produced by a specific cell type may be assayed in the culture medium. Thus transferrin and androgen-binding protein (ABP) are secreted by Sertoli cells and testosterone by Leydig cells. These measurements may tell which cells are present (or not present) but are usually not quantitative, as they may vary as a function of cell density, the presence of other cell types, and/or time in culture. Where no specific methods for quantitatively detecting the desired cell type exist, one can assay for the presence of possible contaminating cell types. Thus, while there are presently no specific markers for peritubular myoid cells, the myoid-enriched preparations may be monitored for Leydig or Sertoli cell contaminants. This procedure at best only yields information on what is not included in the cell preparation, not on what cells are there. In addition to Sertoli, Leydig, myoid, and germ cells, the testis contains vascular, lymphatic, and connective tissue. Cells from these tissues contribute to the possible cell types in testicular cultures and should not be ignored in interpretation of data or in assessing cross-cell contamination of cultures.

Generally speaking, the goal is to obtain the desired cell type in high yield, with minimum contamination by other cell types and minimal damage to the cells. In practice, most procedures will require some compromise in one or two of these areas. The protocol chosen should reflect the requirements of the experiments to be performed. Thus, if long-term culture is desired, minimal cell damage is of prime importance. If characterization of a specific cell's function (e.g., protein secretion) is desired, maximal cell purity is required. If the response to be measured is specific to only one cell type and requires large amounts of tissue, cell purity may be sacrificed for large yield. In no case should it be forgotten that the isolation procedure can alter cell function and that very few primary cell cultures contain only one cell type.

The two methods outlined below were developed to minimize cell damage in order to obtain long-term primary cultures of three somatic cell types in the testis: Leydig cells, Sertoli cells, and peritubular myoid cells. The first method, which uses successive collagenase/dispase digestion, yields both an interstitial cell preparation and a Sertoli cell-enriched preparation. The myoid cells are found primarily in the supernate from the second collagenase digestion of the tubular tissue. Residual interstitial tissue and some Sertoli and germ cells can be found in this fraction, and the myoid cells are thus heavily contaminated with these cell types. The lack of good biochemical or histochemical markers for myoid cells makes quantification of this cell type in a culture particularly difficult.

The glycine/collagenase method is an adaptation of that used by Dziadek [1981] to separate germ layers of mouse embryos. In this case the interstitial tissue is destroyed by the glycine treatment. Clean tubules result that contain Sertoli cells, the basal lamina, peritubular myoid cells, and the basal lamina external to the myoid cells (Fig. 1). These tubules can then be digested briefly with collagenase/dispase to remove myoid cells and give highly homogenous myoid-enriched and Sertoli-enriched cell populations.

Soybean trypsin inhibitor has been included in all enzymatic digestion steps to avoid or decrease tryptic digestion of cell surface receptors. The relatively low enzyme concentrations and large medium-to-tissue volume ratios also help decrease cell damage during disassociation. The first procedure has been successfully used to prepare Sertoli and/or interstitial cell cultures from the testis of human, rat, mouse, dog, rabbit, and pig. The second method has, to date, only been used on testis from immature rats and mice (10-30 days of age).

Method I: Successive Collagenase/Dispase Digestion for Preparation of Sertoli- and Leydig-Enriched Primary Cultures

After removal of testis by sterile procedures, the following protocol is used.

1. Decapsulate testis (SF-F12/DME).

2. Tease apart tubules in 0.05% collagenase/dispase + 0.005% soy trypsin inhibitor (STI) in SF F12/DME (10 min, 25°C).

3. Wash tubules 3 times by ⟶ 9. Collect supernate
unit gravity. Mince tubules with containing free cells.
scissors.

4. Incubate with 0.05% collagenase/dispase + 0.005% STI in SF-F12/DME s(10-20 min, 25°C).

10. Wash and spin 1 time, SF-F12/DME.

5. Wash 2 times by unit gravity, discard supernate.

11. Filter through small Nitex (10μm opening) for single cells.

6. Filter through medium-sized Nitex (102μm opening).

7. Wash by centrifugation 3-5 times.

8. Plate in SF-F12/DME supplemented with indicated hormones (Sertoli-enriched preparation).

12. Wash 2-3 times, SF-F12/DME.

13. Plate in SF-F12/DME supplemented with indicated hormones (Leydig-enriched preparation).

This procedure is a mild enzymatic digestion that yields relative pure preparations of interstitial (Leydig + connective tissue) and tubular cells. The conditions and times shown are chosen for use with immature (10- to 20-day) rat testis.

These preparations have been used with good results to perform the following types of studies: 1) long-term cultures including establishment of cell lines and growth studies; 2) peptide binding to cell surface receptors, immediate and in culture; 3) measurement of secreted products—steroids/proteins; 4) hormone response of 1, 2, and 3 above.

Critical points of procedure

Digestion. While the amount of collagenase digestion is one of the most critical steps of the procedure, it is also one of the hardest to control. 1) This protocol calls for room temperature digestion. Since room temperature can vary from lab to lab and from time to time, this should be taken into consideration and the digestion time adjusted accordingly. 2) The amount of tissue in relation to the amount of collagenase solution is important. For digesting larger amounts of tissue more solution should be used; a 1:10-20 volume ratio is good. 3) The age of the animals used can affect digestion time. Tissue from younger animals will dissociate faster. 4) The species of animal from which the testes are taken will affect digestion time. Rodent testes have less fibrous connective tissue and disassociate faster than bovine or porcine testes. Also, the tubules in other species cannot be teased apart as easily as rodent tissues and one must start with a testicular mince. Here digestion time is critical, as the separation technique depends on the interstitial cells dispersing first as single cells, which can be separated from the less readily digested tubular clumps with various sized mesh Nitex cloth (swiss monofilament nylon, Nitex screening fabrics, Tetko, Inc.).

Excessively long digestion at step 2 will decrease the purity and viability of the interstitial cell preparation. Too short a digestion will decrease yield.

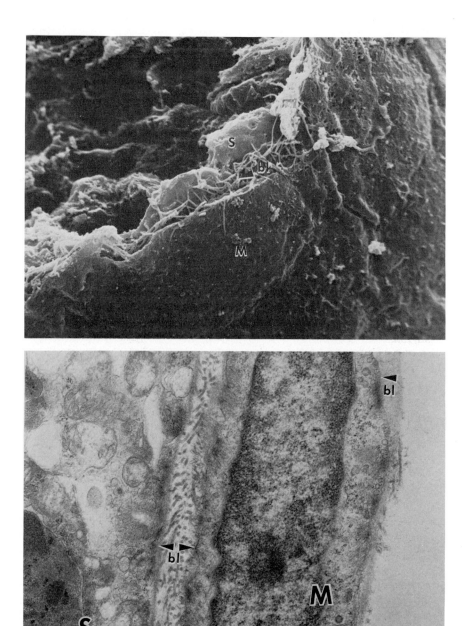

Fig. 1. Scanning and transmission electron micrograph of seminiferous tubule segments from a 20-day-old rat. The tubules were treated with glycine-PBS solution for 8 min and washed in medium. The peritubular myoid cells (M), Sertoli cells (S), and basal lamina (bl) are visible. Upper panel, ×2,000; lower panel, ×14,000.

Similarly, at step 4 digestion for too *short* a time will decrease the yield and purity of the Sertoli cell preparation and too *long* a digestion might injure cells. Visual monitoring of the digestion process (by eye and microscopically) will, with experience, yield consistent results.

Washing. The first wash (step 3) is to remove contaminating cell types and increase the purity of the Sertoli-enriched preparation. Tubules should be thoroughly but gently resuspended and a large excess volume (10-20 ×) of medium should be used. The final washes (steps 7 and 12) remove debris, fat, and any proteases that may have been released by damaged tissue. Incomplete washing will decrease cell adhesion to the substrate and cell viability. While it is important to perform all of the cell preparation as rapidly as possible, decreasing washing time does not pay! The cells are adequately washed when the medium is clear to the eye after centrifugation. Medium with hormones can be prepared, put in plates, and placed in the incubator for equilibration, and cell numbers can be determined during the washing steps so that the cells can be inoculated immediately after the final wash.

Inoculum density. An ideal inoculum density is $(1-3) \times 10^5$ cells per cm^2 culture dish area. This can be varied depending on whether one wishes to study growth (lower) or secretion (higher) and depending on the amount of tissue available.

Collagenase. Varying the type of collagenase as well as the collagenase concentration and digestion time, has proven to be of prime importance in cell survival after plating. We prefer (and this protocol is written for) Collagenase/Dispase #269-638, produced by Boehringer Mannheim and supplied in sterile lyophilized form (100 mg per vial). The collagenase should be solubilized in sterile phosphate-buffered saline (PBS) or water and diluted to the required concentration in medium. This method has also been used to obtain cell suspensions from kidney, pituitary, and adrenals.

Method II: Glycine/Collagenase for Preparation of Primary Cultures Enriched for Peritubular Myoid and Sertoli Cells

After removal of testis, the second method proceeds according to the following protocol.

1. Decapsulate testis.

2. Carefully disperse tubules with forceps in 20 ml of solution A: 1 M glycine; 2 mM EDTA; 20 IU/ml DNase I (purified) + STI (0.002%) in Ca^{+2}, Mg^{+2}-free PBS: pH to 7.2.

3. Gently pipette through large-bore pipette (3-mm diam) while incubating 8-10 min (room temperature). Testis will "unravel" to form a cloudy mass of tubules. Interstitial tissue is released (and destroyed, as the free cell fraction will not attach and grow in culture; DNase is added to prevent clumping of tissue due to "stickiness" of released DNA).

4. Pipette tubules into SF- F12/DME medium (@ 50 ml). Wash 3 times in medium, letting tubules settle at unit gravity.

5. Place tubules (without chopping) in solution B (0.05% collagenase/dispase and 0.005% soy trypsin inhibitor in F12/DME).

6. Incubate 15 min (room temperature) with gentle pipetting through a large-bore pipette at the end of the incubation.

7. Let tubules settle. Collect single cells and filter through fine-mesh (10 μm) Nitex. This is the myoid fraction and will contain some germ cells when older animals are used. Wash 3-5 times (800 × g). Culture cells.

8. Second collagenase: Chop tubules with scissors and treat again as above (with solution B) until small cell clumps result (10-20 min). Let clumps settle and discard supernate.

9. Filter tubular fragments through medium-mesh Nitex (102 μm).

10. Wash 3-5 times in F12/DME by centrifugation (800 × g).

11. Culture "Sertoli" or "Sertoli and Germ."

If myoid cells are not needed, tubules can be chopped immediately after the first wash and treated once with collagenase (solution B) (15-20 min). The first wash should then be at unit gravity to allow tubule clumps to settle. Discard supernate containing myoid and free germ cells.

The importance of the choice of collagenase, washing steps, digestion times, etc. is the same as discussed above for method I.

This procedure gives us high yields of Sertoli cells, good purity, and much better myoid cell preparations than procedure I. Most of the vascular tissue seem to digest more slowly and is filtered out as large clumps during the second Nitex filtration.

SELECTION OF CULTURE CONDITIONS

After the cell population to be studied has been isolated, the proper culture conditions must be chosen. The pertinent conditions include the choice of medium, medium supplements, substrate, inoculum density, and incubation conditions (time, temperature, pH, pO_2, etc.).

As with established cell lines, the choice and preparation of media for primary culture become more critical as the serum supplementation is decreased or eliminated. Minimal essential medium has been successfully used to culture Sertoli cells [Steinberger et al., 1964; Steinberger, 1975; Tung and Fritz, 1977]. However, improved viability and function are obtained with more complex media such as Ham's F12 [Gianetto and Griswold, 1979] or F12/DME [Mather and Sato, 1979]. Leydig cells have been successfully cultured in F12/DME [Mather et al., 1981], a modification of Medium 199 [Murphy and Moger, 1982], MEM with serum supplementation [Cooke et al., 1982], and McCoy's 5A medium [Hseuh, 1980]. Medium should be prepared from powdered media preparations (or individual components, if desired), filter-sterilized immediately, stored in the dark, and used within 2 weeks of preparation. Organic buffers such as HEPES (10-15 mM) are usually added to media for serum-free cultures. There is some variability between different batches of the same medium from different companies (or even the same company). We test several batches and purchase, in powdered form, a sufficient quantity of the best media to last for 6-9 months. Medium is prepared, stored in the dark, and used within 2 weeks. The quality of the water used to prepare media for serum-free culture is of importance. High-purity water such as that used for high-performance liquid chromatography is ideal.

The culture substrate used is usually polystyrene dishes treated for tissue culture. However, the addition of various attachment factors such as collagen, fibronectin, laminin, serum-spreading factor, or cell-produced extracellular matrix may significantly improve cell attachment, survival, and/or function. Fibronectin and polylysine coating of culture dishes has been shown to increase androgen production in cultured mouse Leydig cells [Murphy and Moger, 1982]. The ABP secretion of primary Sertoli cells is slightly stimulated by precoating dishes with laminin or fibronectin and stimulated to a greater extent by precoating with serum-spreading factor. The maximal ABP secretion is seen when cells are plated on the extracellular matrix produced by the rat TR-M (peritubular myoid) cell line (Table I). We use an incubation temperature of 35°C for somatic cell types and 32°C if germ cell survival is desired.

The plating density can also affect cell growth and function. Mouse Leydig cells produce more testosterone per cell when plated at high densities [Murphy

**TABLE I. Androgen-Binding Protein Secretion by Sertoli
Cell Cultures Plated on Various Substrates**

Substrate	ABP (μl equiv/72 h)
Plastic	75
Laminin precoat	90
Fibronectin precoat	105
Collagen precoat	51
Serum-spreading factor precoat	160
Extracellular matrix	290

Sertoli cells were prepared from 20-day-old rats and cultured in F12/
DME medium supplemented with insulin (10 μg/ml), transferrin (5
μg/ml), EGF (1.0 ng/ml), and oFSH (200 ng/ml). Dishes were
precoated by incubating the attachment factor in F12/DME medium
for 4 h at 35°C. Serum-spreading factor was a gift of Dr. David
Barnes (see Barnes et al. [1981]). Plates were then washed twice with
medium. Extracellular matrix was prepared by growing TR-M cells for
2 weeks, removing them from the plate with base (0.02 N NH_4OH),
and then washing the plates.

and Moger, 1982]. Rat Sertoli cells produce 10 times more transferrin and
ABP per cell as the plating density is increased from 0.3×10^5 to 1.2×10^5
cells/cm^2 (Perez-Infante and Mather, unpublished data). On the other hand,
cells plated at confluent densities will undergo little, if any, cell division, so
low-density culture should be used if cell division is desired. In addition,
conditioning of the medium by the cells is concentration-dependent, so the
effects of added factors may be more marked in low-density cultures. Finally,
supplementation of the medium with hormones, growth factors, transport
proteins, vitamins, and/or serum can affect cell survival and function. Recent
work has shown that high levels of serum (10%) can suppress some functions
of primary cultures of granulosa cells [Orly et al., 1980]. This is also true for
Leydig cells [Mather et al., 1983; Murphy and Moger, 1982; Hseuh, 1980]
and Sertoli cells (Fig. 2).

However, in some cases serum supplementation may be desirable. Low
levels (0.01-1%) or fractions (e.g., fetuin or BSA) of serum may be used with
hormone supplementation if a complete definition of the medium components
is not required. In these instances the serum or serum fraction may provide
hormones, attachment factors, or growth factors not added separately or
stabilize added factors. Where serum is used, there is frequently a large
variation between the effects of serum from different animals (equine or
bovine), different ages (fetal vs. adult), or different lots. The serum used
should be tested for its effect on all parameters to be measured.

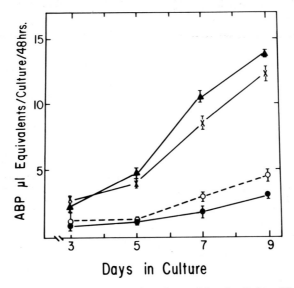

Fig. 2. Androgen-binding protein secretion by cultures of Sertoli cells from 10-day-old rats in serum-free medium (O--O) or medium supplemented with 10% fetal calf serum (●--●); insulin, transferrin and epidermal growth factor (×--×); or insulin, transferrin, epidermal growth factor, and FSH (▲--▲).

The improvements outlined above in cell isolation and media preparation and the appropriate choice of substrate and hormone supplementation have led to more than a tenfold increase in the secretion of androgen-binding protein per cell in primary cultures of Sertoli cells prepared in our laboratory. Each of these factors plays a role in maintaining the optimal viability and hormone response of these cultures.

Hormone-supplemented serum-free media have been reported for mouse [Murphy and Moger, 1982; Mather and Sato, 1979; Mather et al., 1981], rat [Hseuh, 1980], and porcine [Mather et al., 1981, 1982a,b] Leydig cell cultures. Hormone-supplemented media for primary Sertoli cell culture have also been reported [Gianetto and Griswold, 1979; Skinner and Griswold, 1982; Rich et al., 1983]. Most cultures of peritubular myoid cells are carried in medium supplemented with 10–30% fetal calf serum (Table II). While there are reports of culture of myoid cells in serum-free unsupplemented media [Krester et al., 1971], these cultures contained Sertoli cells as well. It is our experience (unpublished observation) that peritubular myoid cells do not survive well in unsupplemented serum-free media in the absence of Sertoli cells, although they will survive in cocultures of the two cell types. This would suggest that the Sertoli cells are producing a substance(s) required for myoid

TABLE II. Media and Supplements Used for Primary Culture of Testicular Somatic Cells

Cell type	Reference	Medium	Supplements[a]
Leydig			
Mouse	Mather and Sato [1979]	F12/DME	Ins, TF, EGF, 0.01% FCS
Mouse	Murphy and Moger [1982]	M199	Ins, TF, EGF, α-tocopherol, poly-l-lysine (or fbn), DMSO (1% O2)
Mouse	Hunter et al. [1982]	MEM	1%–10% FCS
Pig	Mather et al. [1981]	F12/DME	Ins, TF, EGF, α-tocopherol, ± 0.1% CS, RA, Rol, lipids,
	Mather et al. [1982a,b]		lipoproteins
Hypophysectomized rat (coculture with Sertoli)	Hseuh [1980]	McCoy's 5A	None
Seminiferous tubules			
Rat	Steinberger et al. [1964]	MEM	Vitamins A, E, C, glutamine
	Steinberger [1975]		
Sertoli			
Rat	Dorrington and Fritz [1974]	MEM	FSH
Rat	Rich et al. [1983]	F12/DME	Ins, TF, EGF, FSH, Testo, HC, Prog, α-tocopherol, RA
Rat	Gianetto and Griswold [1979]	F12	Ins, TF, EGF, Testo, FSH, smC
Rat	Skinner and Griswold [1982]	F12	Ins, Rol, FSH, Testo
Mouse	Mather and Sato [1979]	F12/DME	Ins, TF, EGF, FSH, smC, GH
Peritubular myoid			
Mouse	Bressler and Ross [1973]	McCoy's 5A	30% FCS
Rat	Tung and Fritz [1977]	MEM	10% FCS

[a]Abbreviations used: Eagle's minimal essential medium (MEM), Dulbecco's modified Eagle's medium (DME) and Ham's nutrient mixture F12 (1:1)(F12/DME), modified medium 199 (M199), insulin (Ins), transferrin (TF), epidermal growth factor (EGF), growth hormone (GH), follicle-stimulating hormone (FSH), somatomedin C (smC), testosterone (Testo), progesterone (Prog), hydrocortisone (HC), retinoic acid (RA), retinol (Rol), fibronectin (fbn), dimethyl sulfoxide (DMSO), fetal calf serum (FCS), calf serum (CS).

cell survival. This suggestion is supported by evidence that conditioned medium from an established Sertoli cell line (TR-ST) will stimulate the growth of a second cell line presumed to originate from myoid cells [Mather and Haour, 1981]. The various media supplements used for culturing Leydig, Sertoli, and myoid cells from several species are summarized in Table II.

Hormone-supplemented media used for the growth of established Sertoli and Leydig cell lines have been reported and are similar to those required for primary culture [Mather, 1980; Mather et al., 1982c]. Proper selection of the experimental system characteristics, including cell dissociation, culture media, substrate, and hormone supplementation, now allow the study of testicular somatic cells such as Sertoli, peritubular myoid, and Leydig cells for several weeks in primary culture. The availability of these primary cultures and cell lines established from these cell types [Mather et al., 1982c; Ascoli, 1981] should do much to contribute to our understanding of testicular physiology.

ACKNOWLEDGMENTS

This work was supported by NIH grants HD 13541 and HD 16149. We would like to thank Alicia L. Byer, Florence Kaczorowski, and Karen Pierce for expert technical assistance.

REFERENCES

Aldred LF, Cooke BA (1980): The deleterious effect of mechanical dissociation of rat testis on the functional activity and purification of Leydig cells using Percoll gradients. Int J Androl 5:191-195.

Ambesi-Impiombato FS, Parks LAM, Coon HG (1980): Culture of hormone dependent functional endothelial cells from rat thyroids. Proc Natl Acad Sci USA 77:3455-3459.

Ascoli M (1981): Regulation of gonadotropin receptors and gonadotropin responses in a clonal strain of Leydig tumor cells by epidermal growth factor. J Biol Chem 256:179-183.

Auerbach R, Alby L, Grieves J, Joseph J, Lindgren C, Morrissey LW, Sidky YA, Watt SL (1982): Monoclonal antibody against angiotensin-converting enzyme: Its use as a marker for murene bovine and human endothelial cells. Proc Natl Acad Sci USA 79:7891-7895.

Barnes D, van der Bosch J, Masui H, Miyazaki K, Sato G (1981): The culture of human tumor cells in serum-free medium. Methods Enzymol 79:368-390.

Bilinska B (1979): Histochemical demonstration of Δ^5, 3β-hydroxy-steroid dehydrogenase activity in cultured Leydig cells under the influence of gonadotropic hormones and testosterone. Int J Androl 2:385-394.

Bottenstein JE, Skaper SD, Varon SS, Sato GH (1980): Selective survival of neurons from chick embryo sensory ganglionic dissociates utilizing serum-free supplemented medium. Exp Cell Res 125:183-190.

Bressler RS, Ross MH (1973): On the character of the monolayer outgrowth and the fate of the peritubular myoid cells in cultured mouse testis. Exp Cell Res 78:295-302.

Cooke BA, Golding M, Dix CJ, Hunter MG (1982): Catecholamine stimulation of testosterone production via cAMP in mouse Leydig cells in monolayer culture. Mol Cell Endocrinol 27:221-231.

Crivello JF, Hornsby PH, Gill GN (1982): Metyrapone and antioxidants are required to maintain aldosterone synthesis by cultured bovine adrenocortical zona glomerulosa cell. Endocrinology 111:469-479.

Dorrington JH, Fritz IB (1974): Cell types influenced by FSH in the rat testis. In Moudgal (ed): "Gonadotropins and Gonadal Functions." New York: Academic, pp 500-512.

Dufau ML, Horner KA, Hayashi K, Tsuruhara T, Conn PM, Catt KJ (1978): Actions of choleragen and gonadotropin in isolated Leydig cells. J Biol Chem 253:3721-3729.

Dziadek MA (1981): Use of glycine as a non-enzymatic procedure for separation of mouse embryonic tissues and dissociation of cells. Exp Cell Res 133:383-393.

Elsdale T, Bard J (1972): Collagen substrate for studies on cell behavior. J Cell Biol 54:626-637.

Emerman JT, Enami J, Pitelka DR, Nandi S (1977): Hormonal effects on intracellular and secreted casein in cultures of mouse mammary epithelial cells on floating collagen membranes. Proc Natl Acad Sci USA 74:4466-4470.

Gianetto BO, Griswold MD (1979): Hormone-supplemented medium enhances androgen binding protein secretion in Sertoli cell cultures. Horm Metab Res 11:1-84.

Gospodarowicz D, Ill C (1980): Extracellular matrix and control of proliferation of vascular endothelial cells. J Clin Invest 65:1351-1364.

Hornsby P (1980): Regulation of cytochrome P-450 supported 11β-hydroxylation of deoxycortisol by steroids, oxygen, and antioxidants in adrenocortical cell cultures. J Biol Chem 255:4020-4027.

Hseuh AJW (1980): Gonadotropin stimulation of testosterone production in primary culture of adult rat testis cells. Biochem Biophys Res Commun 97:506-512.

Hunter MG, Magee-Brown R, Dix CJ, Cooke BA (1982): The functional activity of adult mouse Leydig cells in monolayer culture. Mol Cell Endocrinol 25:35-47.

Krester DM de, Catt KJ, Dufau ML, Hudson B (1971): Studies on rat testicular cells in tissue culture. J Reprod Fertil 24:311-318.

Mather JP (1980): The establishment and characterization of two distinct mouse testicular epithelial cell lines. Biol Reprod 23:243-250.

Mather JP, Sato GH (1979): The use of hormone-supplemented serum-free media in primary cultures. Exp Cell Res 124:215-221.

Mather JP, Haour F (1981): Hormone response of testicular cells in culture: Established cell lines and primary cultures. In Sato G (ed): "Functionally Differentiated Cell Lines." New York: Alan R. Liss, pp 93-108.

Mather JP, Saez JM, Haour F (1981): Primary cultures of Leydig cells from rat, mouse and pig: Advantages of porcine cells for the study of gonadotropin regulation of Leydig cell function. Steroids 38:35-44.

Mather JP, Saez JM, Haour F (1982a): Regulation of gonadotropin receptors and steroidogenesis in cultured porcine Leydig cells. Endocrinology 110:933-940.

Mather JP, Saez JM, Dray F, Haour F (1982b): Hormone-hormone and hormone-vitamin interactions in the control of growth and function of Leydig cells in vitro. Cold Spring Harbor Conferences on Cell Proliferation 9:1117-1128.

Mather JP, Zhuang LZ, Perez-Infante V, Phillips DM (1982c): Culture of testicular cells in hormone-supplemented serum-free medium. Ann NY Acad Sci 383:44-68.

Mather JP, Saez JM, Dray F, Haour F (1983): Vitamin E prolongs survival and function of porcine Leydig cells in culture. Acta Endocrinol 102:470-475.

Mori H, Christensen AK (1980): Morphometric analysis of Leydig cells in the normal rat testis. J Cell Biol 84:340-354.

Murphy PR, Moger WH (1982): Short-term primary culture of mouse interstitial cells: Effects of culture conditions on androgen production. Biol Reprod 27:38-47.

Orly J, Sato G, Erickson GH (1980): Serum suppresses the expression of hormonally induced functions in cultured granulosa cells. Cell 20:817-827.

Parvinen M, Vanha-Perttula T (1972): Identification and enzyme quantitation of the stages of the seminiferous epithelial wave in the rat. Anat Rec 174:435-449.

Purvi EC, Turner DC (1978): Serum-free medium allows chicken myogenic cells to be cultivated in suspension and separated from attached fibroblasts. Exp Cell Res 115:159-173.

Reid L (1982): Regulation of growth and differentiation of mammalian cells by hormones and extracellular matrix. In Ahmad F, Schultz J, Smith E, Whelan W (eds): "From Gene to Protein: Translation into Biotechnology." New York: Academic, pp 53-73.

Rich KA, Bardin CW, Gunsalus GL, Mather JP (1983): Age-dependent pattern of androgen binding protein (ABP) secretion from rat Sertoli cells in primary culture. Endocrinology 113:2284-2293.

Setchell PP (1978): "The Mammalian Testis." Ithaca, New York: Cornell University Press.

Skinner MK, Griswold MD (1982): Secretion of testicular transferrin by cultured Sertoli cells is regulated by hormones and retinoids. Biol Reprod 27:211-221.

Solari AJ, Fritz IB (1978): The ultrastructure of immature Sertoli cells. Maturation-like changes during culture and the maintenance of mitotic potentiality. Biol Reprod 18:329-345.

Steinberger A (1975): Studies on spermatogenesis and steroidogenesis in culture. Am Zool 15:273-278.

Steinberger A, Steinberger E, Perloff WH (1964): Mammalian testis in organ culture. Exp Cell Res 36:19-27.

Taub M, Sato GH (1979): Growth of kidney epithelial cells in hormone-supplemented serum-free medium. J. Supramol Struct 11:207.

Tung PS, Fritz IB (1977): Isolation and culture of testicular cells: A morphological characterization. In Hafez ESE (ed): "Techniques of Human Andrology." Amsterdam: North-Holland, pp 125-146.

Wysocki LJ, Sato VL (1978): 'Panning' for lymphocytes: A method for cell selection. Proc Natl Acad Sci USA 75:2844-2848.

Methods for Serum-Free Culture of Cells of the Endocrine System,
pages 47–61
© 1984 Alan R. Liss, Inc., 150 Fifth Avenue, New York, NY 10011

4
Isolation and Growth of Adult Human Prostatic Epithelium in Serum-Free, Defined Medium

Mukta M. Webber, Donna M. Chaproniere-Rickenberg,
and Robert E. Donohue

Cancer of the prostate is one of the three leading causes of death in the adult male cancer patient. The number of deaths from prostate cancer in the United States in 1983 is estimated to be 24,100, and 75,000 new cases are estimated during the same period [American Cancer Society, 1983]. At least 30% of men over the age of 50 and 50% of men over the age of 70 may have histologic carcinoma of the prostate [Franks, 1976]. Yet very little is known about its etiology. The incidence of benign tumors of the prostate may be as high as 80% in men over the age of 40 [Walsh, 1976]. Therefore, our long-term objective for developing an in vitro cell model system using human prostatic epithelium has been to use this system for studies on the etiology and growth of prostatic neoplasia. Of particular interest are studies on differentiation, carcinogenesis, and the actions and interactions of hormones and other growth factors in the regulation of growth of normal and neoplastic cells.

The importance of establishing an in vitro model system using human cells is based on the following: 1) In an isolated cell system, one is more likely to be able to pinpoint the specific growth effects of agents to be tested; 2) specific changes involved in the early steps in carcinogenesis can be examined by using in vitro systems; 3) until recently, long-term experiments with animals provided the only means for detecting the potential of various agents as carcinogens. The bioassay of compounds by in vivo testing seems to be an insurmountable task. Therefore, in vitro models have proved to be very useful

Division of Urology, Department of Surgery, School of Medicine, University of Colorado Health Sciences Center, Denver, Colorado 80262 for screening potential carcinogens for man. Also, such in vitro procedures can provide results in a shorter time, and they are less costly and are reliable, sensitive, and practical; 4) cultures are also convenient tools for correlating morphologic with biochemical changes, e.g., in cell differentiation; 5) the most common criticism against the use of in vitro systems is that results obtained from in vitro studies may not be easily extrapolated to the human situation. A similar criticism is made just as often of the animal, in vivo studies on the basis that results may not be applicable to man owing to species differences. Both systems have certain advantages; thus, the use of more than one system is advisable. Animal systems provide data based on the whole organism, where complex actions and interactions operate. In vivo, however, it is not always possible to isolate specific hormonal effects because of complicated feedback mechanisms. The cell systems, on the other hand, provide the opportunity to dissect and separate the various actions and interactions of substances influencing growth and differentiation. In the isolated cell system, the complicated in vivo situations can be broken down into their elements, and the problem of whether the effect of a given agent is due to a direct or indirect effect on the cells can be analyzed. Cytologic and biochemical changes can be detected and followed from an early stage and the interactions of several different substances studied in detail; 6) the use of the human cell system is justified because the ultimate answer to the question of human cancer etiology can be provided only by testing various agents on human cells. Also, this is the closest one can get to human experimentation and it eliminates the problems created by species differences [Webber, 1980].

For these reasons, it is necessary to develop an in vitro model system using human prostatic epithelium. In order to develop such a system, it is necessary to meet certain basic requirements and these are: 1) to isolate epithelial cells; 2) to establish their growth and maintenance requirements in vitro; and 3) to characterize them to establish their prostatic epithelial origin.

Our earlier studies established methods for suspension and explant cultures for the growth of prostatic epithelium [Webber and Stonington, 1975; Webber et al., 1974]. Explant cultures have since been frequently used for studies on the prostate [Clarke and Merchant, 1980; Jacobs and Lawson, 1981]. Lechner et al. [1978, 1980] have reported successful cultivation of neonatal human prostatic epithelium. These cultures were initiated from cells spilled after mincing of the tissue. No work, other than that done in our laboratory, has been reported on the successful isolation, cultivation, and maintenance of normal and benign, postpubertal human prostate epithelium in a defined medium. The significance of using postpubertal prostate must be emphasized. Since prostatic carcinomas arise from adult androgen-responsive epithelium, it is important to use such epithelium for developing an in vitro model system.

In the past, it has generally been difficult to isolate, grow, and maintain normal and benign human epithelial cells in vitro. This is paradoxical when one realizes that the majority of human cancers are of epithelial origin. One of the reasons for this failure has been the general dependence on standard, commercially available media and the failure to recognize that prostatic epithelial cells are specialized secretory cells whose growth, maintenance, and differentiation in vivo are controlled by several hormones, vitamins, and other growth-controlling factors. It is therefore logical to assume that these cells would have certain specific requirements for their growth and maintenance in vitro. Our earlier investigations, using cell and organ cultures of normal and benign human prostatic epithelium, showed that a high-serum medium supports good growth of prostatic epithelium and that the growth is further enhanced by a supplement of epidermal growth factor (EGF), insulin, and vitamin A [Webber, 1974, 1980]. These studies also resulted in the selection of RPMI-1640 medium from five media tested, because it supported the best growth [Webber, 1980]. Our further studies were designed to replace the serum with known components and to establish specific growth requirements for prostatic epithelium. In this chapter, we will describe methods for isolation and culture of human prostatic epithelium in a serum-free, chemically defined medium.

ISOLATION OF PROSTATIC EPITHELIUM FROM FRESH TISSUE SPECIMENS
Introduction

One of the major problems in culturing human epithelial cells has been contamination with fibroblasts. When care is not taken to isolate acini free of stroma, prostatic epithelial cultures are generally contaminated with stromal fibroblasts [Clarke and Merchant, 1980; Jacobs and Lawson, 1981; Jones et al., 1976; Rose et al., 1975]. For establishing pure cultures of prostatic epithelium, Webber [1979] has developed a method for the isolation of prostatic epithelial cells, involving digestion of tissue with collagenase. This method is described in a subsequent section of this chapter.

Physiological breakdown of collagen in many mammals and amphibians is accomplished by the action of specific collagenases, produced in very small amounts as needed. These are apparently not stored in vivo [Gross, 1972; Mandl, 1972]. Collagenase activity has been detected in normal and diseased human skin, in the edges of healing wounds, in growing bone, in involuting uterus, in inflamed human tissue (e.g., rheumatoid arthritis), and in regenerating newt limbs [Gross, 1972]. On the basis of these observations, it is logical to conclude that the same enzyme might be used for isolation of cells from tissues after digestion with collagenase. Collagenases by definition are enzymes capable of dissolving fibrous collagen by peptide bond cleavage under physiological conditions of pH and temperature. The specific substrate, collagen, represents 33% of the total protein in mammalian organisms [Mandl, 1972].

Lasfargues [1957] pioneered the use of collagenase for digestion of tissue for cell dispersal in the preparation of primary cultures of mouse mammary epithelium. Since prostate has a histologic composition similar to that of the mammary glands, Webber [1979] used collagenase for the isolation of prostatic epithelium. Collagenase has been used in recent years for dissociation of animal tissues and for isolation of epithelial cells of various types, i.e., aortic endothelium [Schwartz, 1978], liver [Acosta et al., 1978], endocrine pancreas [Leiter et al., 1974], and mammary epithelium [Lasfargues, 1957; White et al., 1978]. In the majority of these cultures some fibroblasts did get carried over into the cultures.

Collagenase is nontoxic at a neutral pH, is active within a pH range of 6.5–7.8, and requires Ca^{2+} ions for its activity and stability. It can therefore be dissolved in complete tissue culture medium. Since collagenase specifically breaks down collagen, it is active even in medium containing 5–10% serum. Thus, minced tissue can be placed in a complete culture medium enriched with serum and still be exposed to the dissociating activity of collagenase. This results in improved cell viability compared to serum-free dissociating media containing proteolytic enzymes.

Stromal elements form a major part of prostatic tissue. Separation of epithelial cells from the stroma, by means of collagenase, is an interesting phenomenon. Electron microscopy was used to pinpoint the site of action of collagenase, which facilitated isolation of acini [Webber, 1979].

Source of Cells

Cells are isolated from prostatic chips of benign tissue obtained from patients undergoing transurethral resection of the prostate (TURP) and from patients undergoing total prostatectomy. Tissue is collected in cold (4°C) transport medium consisting of saline G containing 500 units penicillin, 500 μg streptomycin, 100 μg gentamycin, and 100 μg mycostatin per ml of medium. The tissue is brought to the laboratory and washed several times with fresh transport medium before further processing.

Method for Isolation of Prostatic Epithelial Cells

Collagenases of bacterial origin (*Clostridium histolyticum* and *Clostridium perfringens*) have been found to be the most efficient agents for cell dispersal.

The impure enzyme preparations are more effective for tissue digestion, and their stability is excellent even at room temperature [Mandl, 1972]. Stock solutions should, however, be kept frozen, and media containing collagenase should be refrigerated (4°C). Temperatures above 56°C inactivate the enzyme rapidly and completely [Mandl, 1961]. All antibiotics are compatible with collagenase. Gibco collagenase (Clostridiopeptidase A from *Clostridium histolyticum*) was found to be the best for digestion of prostatic tissue [Webber, 1979].

Superficial connective tissue is removed from the tissue specimen and discarded, and the remaining tissue is minced and digested with collagenase. The volume of the cut tissue is measured and the tissue is divided into 100-mm petri dishes, each dish containing 2 ml of tissue. To each dish 15 ml of medium containing collagenase is added.

The medium used for dissociating the tissue consists of RPMI-1640 with 5% fetal bovine serum (FBS) and 100 units penicillin, 100 μg/ml streptomycin, and 10 μg/ml gentamycin per ml of medium. To this medium collagenase is added at a level of 200 units/ml or 400 units/ml. Collagenase is freely soluble in tissue culture media. It should be pointed out that the concentration of collagenase must be expressed in units/ml rather than μg/ml because the activity of collagenase (i.e., units/μg) varies from lot to lot. Tissue can be incubated at 37°C, in 400 units/ml collagenase medium for 24–48 h and in 200 units/ml collagenase for up to 60 h without loss of epithelial cell viability. After this time, the tissue is pipetted vigorously to break it up and placed in the incubator for further digestion for 1–2 h. The digested tissue is again pipetted vigorously and centrifuged at 1,200 rpm for 10 min in 10-ml sterile centrifuge tubes, the supernatant is discarded, and the sediment is resuspended in Puck's saline G and again centrifuged. This is followed by washing the sediment 2–3 times with saline G and settling by gravity in 50-ml conical centrifuge tubes. All supernatants from washings can be saved, and fibroblasts can be recovered from these by centrifugation. Although these cells have low viability, sufficient cells can be collected for studies requiring fibroblasts. The last sediment consists of acini of various sizes. The volume of these is measured, which for tissue with normal histology is 1/20th the original volume of the tissue digested.

The cleaned acini are finally resuspended (generally, 1 ml of sediment per 50 ml suspension) in RPMI-1640 containing 2% FBS with a supplement of 0.03 IU/ml zinc-stabilized insulin, 1 μg/ml transferrin, 10^{-8} M dexamethasone, 0.05 IU/ml vitamin A, and 2 μg/ml spermine and then are refrigerated for 2–3 days. We have earlier shown [Webber and Chaproniere-Rickenberg, 1980] that spermine oxidation products are selectively toxic to fibroblasts in cultures of normal human prostatic epithelium. In the above culture medium, in which the acini are refrigerated, the spermine oxidase in the serum apparently oxidizes the spermine to oxidation products that are cytotoxic to any remaining fibroblasts but do not affect the epithelium. The plating efficiency of the acini stored in this medium is maintained or it increases for up to 5 days, beyond which it begins to decline.

Estimation of Viable Acini

The number of viable acini per ml of suspension (plating efficiency) varies with each tissue sample. The plating efficiency of acini derived from radical prostatectomy tissue specimens is much greater than that of acini derived from TURP specimens, which contain cauterized tissue. It is therefore necessary to determine the number of viable acini present in the suspension.

Before refrigerating the final acinar suspension, a few milliliters are removed and diluted by 1/2, 1/4, and 1/8 (for TURP tissue specimens) or 1/20, 1/40, and 1/80 (for prostatectomy tissue specimens) in plating medium (see below). Into 35-mm culture dishes 1 ml of each dilution is seeded and allowed to settle for 2 days to obtain maximal adhesion. After 2 days, the number of adhering acini, including acini surrounded by a halo of epithelium, are counted and the concentration of these viable acini in the original suspension is determined.

SEEDING THE ACINI
Seeding

When seeding acini into culture dishes for experiments using defined medium and testing the effect of growth factors, the following points should be considered: 1) Acini should be seeded in serum-free medium to avoid contamination with serum components that readily adhere to cells and culture dishes; and 2) acini should be seeded at a low concentration (< 15 acini per ml) to avoid mutual cooperative growth stimulation or conditioning of medium.

Serum-Free Plating Medium

Insulin and EGF increase the adhesion of prostatic acini to the substrate, whereas dexamethasone appears to have little effect (Chaproniere-Rickenberg and Webber, manuscript in preparation). The best plating medium therefore consists of 10 ng/ml EGF, 1 μg/ml transferrin, and 0.3 IU/ml zinc-free insulin. The use of zinc-free insulin is essential, since the concentration of zinc in 0.3 IU/ml zinc-stabilized insulin is toxic to prostatic epithelium in the absence of serum [Chaproniere-Rickenberg and Webber, 1982a, 1983].

Dispensing Acini

Acini should be centrifuged out of the serum-containing medium and then resuspended in the plating medium. The acini should be kept in suspension by means of a magnetic stirrer for even distribution. Acini rapidly settle when not stirred. It is also essential, to ensure even distribution of acini in the culture dishes, to take into the dispensing pipette only that volume of suspension sufficient for one culture at a time. For our experiments on growth factors, generally 10 viable acini per 1.5 ml medium were plated per 60-mm culture dish.

ADHESION AND GROWTH OF PROSTATIC EPITHELIUM IN DEFINED MEDIUM
Adhesion

A period of at least 48 h is required for adhesion of the maximum number of acini. After 24 h, only about half this number settle and adhere tightly. By the second or third day after seeding, a halo of large epithelial cells surrounds the original acinus. These are cells that have migrated from the acinus. Between the fifth and seventh day, groups of small, cuboidal cells appear among the large cells. These are proliferating cells probably derived from basal cells in the acinus. They grow as a monolayer, eventually constituting the total outgrowth adhering to the culture dish. As the central area of the outgrowth becomes densely packed with small cuboidal cells, a second layer of cells forms. This layer consists of larger cells that eventually die, are sloughed, and are continuously replaced by other cells.

Chemically Defined Medium

Using RPMI-1640 as a basal medium, optimal growth of prostatic epithelium is obtained by supplementing this medium with 10 ng/ml EGF, 0.3 IU/ml zinc-free insulin, 1 μg/ml transferrin, 10^{-8} M dexamethasone, and 10^{-8} M $ZnCl_2$ (Table I). The insulin and EGF are the main growth-stimulating hormones and transferrin is essential for maximal activity of insulin and EGF. Thus, in our chemically defined medium consisting of RPMI-1640 containing EGF, insulin, transferrin, dexamethasone, and $ZnCl_2$, doubling of the area of cell outgrowth occurs every 2 days [Chaproniere-Rickenberg and Webber, 1982b].

Preparation of Defined Medium

The following stock solutions are made up and stored frozen at $-20°C$. They are then used to make a stock medium supplement at 100 $\times$ the final

TABLE I. Composition of Different Media Used

	Concentration in medium		
Components	Storage medium	Plating medium	Growth medium
EGF	—	10 ng/ml	10 ng/ml
Insulin	0.03 IU/ml (Zn-stabilized)	0.3 IU/ml (Zn-free)	0.3 IU/ml (Zn-free)
Transferrin	1 μg/ml	1 μg/ml	1 μg/ml
Dexamethasone	10^{-8} M	—	10^{-8} M
Vitamin A	0.05 IU/ml	—	—
Spermine	2 μg/ml	—	—
Zinc chloride	—	—	10^{-8} M
Fetal bovine serum (FBS)	2%	—	—

TABLE II. Amounts of Individual Component Stocks Used to Make 100 × Stock of the Medium Supplement, the Volume Being Made Up to 10 ml With Saline G

Component	Concentration in stock solution used to make 100 × stock	100 × storage medium, 10 ml	100 × plating medium, 10 ml	100 × growth medium, 10 ml
EGF	10,000 ng/ml	—	1 ml	1 ml
Insulin (zinc-free)	300 IU/ml	—	1 ml	1 ml
Insulin (zinc-stabilized)	30 IU/ml	1 ml	—	—
Transferrin	1,000 μg/ml	1 ml	1 ml	1 ml
Dexamethasone	10^{-5} M	1 ml	—	1 ml
Vitamin A	50 IU/ml	1 ml	—	—
Spermine	200 μg/ml	[a]	—	—
Zinc chloride	10^{-5} M	—	—	1 ml
Fetal bovine serum (FBS)	—	[b]	—	—

[a]Add directly to the final medium. 1 ml in 100 ml storage medium to get a concentration of 2 μg/ml.
[b]Added directly to the final medium at 2%.

concentration, which can be stored frozen also at $-20°$C or refrigerated at 4°C for up to 2 weeks before use. The stock medium supplement is diluted 1/100 in RPMI-1640 for use (Table II). Tissue culture grade water is used.

Dexamethasone. Stock solution is prepared at 10^{-2} M concentration in absolute ethyl alcohol and stored frozen at $-20°C$ for up to 4 months. After 6 months, activity diminishes significantly.

EGF. Stock solution at 10,000 ng/ml concentration is made by dissolving sterile EGF (provided as 100 μg per bottle) in sterile water. This stock is stored frozen at $-20°C$ in 1-ml aliquots for up to 3 months. We have not tested its activity after storage for longer than 3 months.

Spermine tetrahydrochloride. Stock solution at 2 mg/ml (1,000 $\times$ the final concentration) is prepared in water, millipore-filtered, and stored at $-20°C$ for up to 6 months.

Transferrin. Stock solution is prepared at 1,000 μg/ml concentration in water and millipore-filtered. Stock solution is stored frozen at $-20°C$ for up to 6 months. We have not tested its activity after storage for longer than 6 months.

Zinc chloride (ZnCl₂). Stock solution is prepared at 10^{-4} M concentration in water, millipore-filtered to sterilize, and stored at $4°C$.

Zinc-free insulin. Stock solution is prepared at 300 IU/ml concentration by dissolving unsterile powder in water. The solution is sterilized by filtration and stored frozen at $-20°C$ in 1-ml aliquots for up to 2 months. We have not tested insulin activity after longer storage time. Insulin adsorbs to glass more than it does to plastic. To minimize loss, it should not be pipetted to dissolve and should be filtered and transferred to new vessels as little as possible.

Zinc-stabilized insulin. Stock solution is prepared at 300 IU/ml concentration in water acidified with 5 ml 0.1 N HCl per 100 ml solution and filtered. Sometimes the insulin comes out of solution on dilution with saline G. Addition of 1-2 drops of 0.1 N HCl redissolves the insulin. Stock solution is stored at $-20°C$.

Vitamin A/retinol acetate. Vitamin A activity is destroyed by light; therefore all manipulations must be carried out in dim light. A stock solution is made up as 1,000 IU/ml solution in absolute ethyl alcohol and stored in the dark at $-70°C$ for up to 1 year. More dilute solutions (500 IU/ml in alcohol) may be stored at $-20°C$ in the dark for up to 4 weeks.

Further dilutions should be made immediately before use and discarded after use.

Sources of Materials

Catalog numbers are given in parentheses.

1. Medium RPMI-1640 (330-2511), saline G (310-4100), fetal bovine serum (240-6290), collagenase (840-7018), tissue culture grade sterile water (670-5230)—Gibco (Grand Island Biological Company).

2. EGF (40001), zinc-free insulin (40305)—Collaborative Research.

3. Dexamethasone (D1756), putrescine dihydrochloride (P7505), spermine tetrahydrochloride (S2876), transferrin (T2252), vitamin A (retinol acetate, type 1, R3000)—Sigma.

4. Zinc-stabilized insulin (812633)—Schwartz-Mann.

5. To sterilize stock solutions of medium supplements use 0.22 μm Millex-GV, low-binding, filter unit (SLGV025LS)—Millipore.

6. Culture dishes—Falcon Plastics.

QUANTITATION OF GROWTH IN PRIMARY CULTURES OF PROSTATIC EPITHELIUM

Quantitation of cell growth in vitro is necessary to establish the growth-enhancing effects or toxicity of the test substances. When using cells that can be easily dissociated and dispersed into single-cell suspension, it is easy to determine the extent of growth on the basis of cell number. However, many epithelial cells in primary culture do not dissociate easily into single cells but remain as sheets or clumps after enzymatic treatment. Assessment of growth on the basis of cell counts in these cases therefore may not be reliable.

Densitometry

Growth measurements with a Datacolor Scanning Densitometer [Webber, 1980] are based on the measurement of the dish area covered with cells. This system is generally used in the interpretation of aerial photographs and other remote sensing images. It is used to locate areas of similar density within the same image and to measure the extent of their area. Details of the use of this system for quantitation of growth in cultures are described elsewhere (Webber et al., in preparation).

The Datacolor Scanning Densitometer (made by Spatial Data Systems, Inc., 132 Aero Camino, Goleta, CA 93017) is designed to slice the tone-continuum of an image into as many as 32 discrete segments and then assign a color to each segment. This instrument then displays the color-enhanced image on a television monitor. The components of the system include: 1) a light system, consisting of a lightbox to illuminate an image, usually a photographic transparency or, in this case, a petri dish culture; 2) a Vidicon, which is a precision monochrome TV camera that converts the transmitted light to an electrical video signal; 3) an electronic analyzer that separates the voltage levels of the video signal into as many as 32 levels and encodes color to each level; 4) a color TV monitor; 5) an electronic planimeter that measures the percentage area of colors displayed on the monitor; and 6) a control keyboard for controlling the colors and the electronic planimeter.

Growth measurements are based on the measurement of the dish area covered with cells. Cultures are stained with Giemsa [Poché et al., 1974] and examined with the Datacolor system. A mask to fit over the lightbox was carefully machined to fit around standard petri dishes. Colors are assigned to all areas where there is cell growth and the computer is instructed to measure the area of these colors. Area of the blank portions of the dish is also measured as a check. The area figures are read off as percentages on a panel on the keyboard. The image can be continuously visualized on the TV screen and photographed. Once the system has been calibrated, it takes only a few minutes to measure each dish. When the cell sheet is double-layered, the area of each layer can be measured separately.

The system was calibrated by making several models of cell cultures in petri dishes. The models consisted of various shapes such as disks, dots, and rectangles of known area fixed to the bottom of petri dishes to simulate cell cultures. Each model provided a series from 1% to 100% cell coverage in intervals of a few percent. A nomogram of the calibration curve was constructed of actual area against measured area. The curve was close to a 1:1 slope except above 70% actual cover. Above this value, the departure from a 1:1 slope followed a consistent and predictable pattern.

This method correlates well with cell counts, provided the cultures contain cells of uniform size. This system can also distinguish between areas occupied by the large, thin cells and the small dense, cuboidal cells resembling basal cells. The size of the colonies derived from individual acini can be measured by placing the dish over graph paper or by planimetry of enlarged photographs of the dish. Various methods for quantitation of cell growth are compared elsewhere (Webber et al., in preparation).

Our studies on growth regulation have all been based on primary cultures. Since cells, when placed in culture, have a tendency to deviate sometimes from their in vivo physiological behavior and genetic composition, we have elected to use short-term primary cultures, which are relatively close, in this regard, to their cells of origin in vivo.

CHARACTERIZATION OF PROSTATIC EPITHELIAL CELLS AND THEIR DIFFERENTIATED CELL FUNCTION

We have characterized the cultured prostatic epithelial cells on the basis of morphologic characteristics by means of light, transmission, and scanning electron microscopy [Webber 1975, 1981a; Webber and Bouldin, 1977] and on the basis of their biochemical characteristics, e.g., the presence of prostatic acid phosphatase and plasminogen activator, and the secretion of spermine oxidase [Hughes et al., 1981; Stonington et al., 1975, 1978; Webber, 1979].

Morphologic Characterization

The epithelial cell cultures are initiated from prostatic acini isolated by the method developed by Webber [1979] as described earlier in this chapter. In the chemically defined medium, cells are organized in two layers. The superficial layer, farthest from the substrate continuously sloughs, and the culture is maintained by the multiplication of cells in the layer in contact with the petri dish surface [Chaproniere-Rickenberg and Webber, 1982b]. This bilayer formation is similar to the in vivo architecture of prostatic acini [Webber, 1979]. This kind of spatial organization and sloughing are characteristic of epithelial cells in culture. These cultures also show hemicyst or dome formation, which in epithelial cultures has been interpreted as the retention of an in vivo epithelial characteristic (unpublished observations). The pumping or secretion of fluids across the cell sheet may be a general characteristic of secretory epithelia.

The ultrastructure of isolated prostatic acini has been described earlier [Webber, 1979]. The double layer of epithelial cells (basal and secretory) remains intact around a lumen in these acini. On plating, these cells spread out and multiply to form a monolayer. The ultrastructure of the cells in monolayer has also been examined [Webber, 1975; Webber and Bouldin, 1977]. Specialization of the cell surface for cell-to-cell attachment in the form of junctional complexes and desmosomes is a characteristic feature of epithelial cells. We have studied these extensively in preparations for transmission electron microscopy. The presence of desmosomes establishes the epithelial nature of these cells [Webber, 1981a]. The gross morphologies of fibroblasts and prostatic epithelial cells have been compared (unpublished observations) and the cell surface architecture of isolated prostatic acini has been examined by scanning electron microscopy [Webber, 1979, 1981a]. These observations further support the transmission electron microscopy findings, thus establishing the epithelial nature of our cells being grown in vitro.

Biochemical Characterization

Earlier studies by Webber and collaborators have demonstrated the presence of prostatic acid phosphatase in these cells by cytochemical [Stonington et al., 1975; Webber, 1979] and by immunologic methods [Stonington et al., 1978]. Other secretory proteins, such as plasminogen activator, have also been used as markers for prostatic cell function [Hughes et al., 1981]. On the basis of the presence of the various morphologic and cytochemical markers, the prostatic epithelial origin of these cells has been established.

SUMMARY AND CONCLUSIONS

Because of the large variety of differentiated functions expressed by different cells, it is reasonable to expect that each cell type may require a unique combination of factors for its growth and for the expression of its differentiated functions. There are, however, certain common factors that appear to be required for growth by many different epithelial cells [Chaproniere-Rickenberg and Webber, 1982b; Webber, 1981b; Webber et al., 1982]. These are EGF, insulin, transferrin, and glucocorticoid, such as hydrocortisone or dexamethasone. We have established the requirement by human prostatic epithelium of these factors. In conclusion, it can be stated that we have developed a method for the isolation of prostatic epithelium from fresh human adult tissue and we have also developed a serum-free, chemically defined medium for the growth of these cells in vitro. A detailed discussion of the use and action of collagenase for dissociation of prostatic tissue and the isolation of acini from it is given elsewhere [Webber, 1979]. Further modification of the present medium [Chaproniere-Rickenberg and Webber, 1982b] will occur as it is altered for long-term maintenance and for the expression of other differentiated functions. An in vitro cell model system using adult human prostatic epithelium has thus become available for studies on the etiology and growth of prostatic neoplasia, on the mechanism of carcinogenesis, and on initiation and promotion by intrinsic and extrinsic factors. This cell system may also be used for screening suspected carcinogenic agents; for studies on cell nutrition, metabolism, growth, and aging; and for examining the actions and interactions of hormones and other growth regulators on normal and benign prostatic epithelium.

ACKNOWLEDGMENTS

The authors wish to thank Lucy Jankowsky for her technical assistance in accomplishing this work and Jeanne Nozawa and Rose Marie Vukovich for their help in the preparation of this manuscript. The authors thank their colleagues Drs. L. Blitstein, J. Clark, H. Dovey, G. Miller, R. Pfister, S. Pfister, J.N. Wettlaufer, and C. White for their help in the acquisition of tissue for this work. This work was supported by the Division of Cancer Cause and Prevention, National Cancer Institute, DHHS grant No. CA-28279 to M.M.W.

REFERENCES

Acosta D, Anuforo DC, Smith RV (1978): Primary monolayer cultures of postnatal rat liver cells with extended differentiated functions. In Vitro 14:428-436.

American Cancer Society (1983): Cancer Statistics 1983, Ca—A Cancer Journal for Clinicians 33:2-25.

Chaproniere-Rickenberg DM, Webber MM (1982a): Toxicity of zinc present in zinc-stabilized insulin in defined culture media. In Vitro 18:286.

Chaproniere-Rickenberg DM, Webber MM (1982b): A chemically defined medium for the growth of adult human prostatic epithelium. In Sato GH, Pardee AB, Sirbasku DA (eds): "Cold Spring Harbor Symposium on Growth of Cells in Hormonally Defined Media," Vol 9: "Hormones and Cell Culture." Cold Spring Harbor, New York: Cold Spring Harbor Laboratory, Book B, pp 1109-1115.

Chaproniere-Rickenberg DM, Webber MM (1983): Zinc levels in zinc-stabilized insulin are inhibitory to the growth of cells in vitro. In Vitro 19:373-375.

Clarke SM, Merchant DJ (1980): Primary cultures of human prostatic epithelial cells from transurethral resection specimens. Prostate 1:87-94.

Franks LM (1976): History of prostatic cancer. Prog Clin Biol Res 6:103-109.

Gross J (1972): Collagenases of animal origin. In Mandl I (ed): "Collagenase: First Interdisciplinary Symposium on Collagenase." New York: Gordon & Breach, pp 33-36.

Hughes B, Webber MM, James G, Lucero L, Van Buskirk JJ, Wettlaufer JN (1981): Plasminogen activator: A marker for human prostatic epithelium and prostate cancer. In Vitro 17:244.

Jacobs SC, Lawson RK (1981): Tissue culture of normal human post-pubertal prostate. Urol Int 36:196-198.

Jones RE, Sanford EJ, Rohner TJ, Rapp F (1976): In vitro viral transformation of human prostatic carcinoma. J Urol 115:82-85.

Lasfargues EY (1957): Cultivation and behavior in vitro of the normal mammary epithelium of the adult mouse. Anat Rec 127:117-129.

Lechner JF, Narayan KS, Ohnuki Y, Babcock MS, Jones LW, Kaighn ME (1978): Replicative epithelial cell cultures from normal human prostate gland: Brief communication. J Natl Cancer Inst 60:797-801.

Lechner JF, Babcock MS, Marnell M, Narayan KS, Kaighn E (1980): Normal human prostate epithelial cell cultures. Methods Cell Biol 21:195-225.

Leiter EH, Coleman DL, Waymouth C (1974): Cell culture of the endocrine pancreas of the mouse in chemically defined media. In Vitro 9:421-433.

Mandl I (1961): Collagenases and elastases. Adv Enzymol 23:163-264.

Mandl I (1972): Collagenase comes of age. In Mandl I (ed): "Collagenase: First Interdisciplinary Symposium on Collagenase." New York: Gordon & Breach, pp 1-15.

Poché PA, Webber MM, Janowsky L (1974): A rapid method for in situ staining of prostatic and other tissue culture cells. Stain Technol 49:229-233.

Rose NR, Choe BK, Pontes JE (1975): Cultivation of epithelial cells from the prostate. Cancer Chemother Rep 59:147-149.

Schwartz SM (1978): Selection and characterization of bovine aortic endothelial cells. In Vitro 14:966-980.

Stonington OG, Szwec N, Webber MM (1975): Isolation and identification of the human malignant prostatic epithelial cells in pure monolayer culture. J Urol 114:903-908.

Stonington OG, Szwec N, Webber MM (1978): Identification of cultured human malignant prostatic epithelial cells. In "Workshop on Genito-urinary Cancer Immunology." Natl Cancer Inst Monogr 49:31-33.

Walsh PC (1976): Benign prostatic hyperplasia: Etiological considerations. Prog Clin Biol Res 6:1-8.

Webber MM (1974): Effects of serum on the growth of prostatic cells in vitro. J Urol 112:798-801.

Webber MM (1975): Ultrastructural changes in human prostatic epithelium grown in vitro. J Ultrastruct Res 50:89-102.

Webber MM (1979): Normal and benign human prostatic epithelium in culture. I. Isolation. In Vitro 15:967-982.

Webber MM (1980): Growth and maintenance of normal prostatic epithelium in vitro—A human cell model. Prog Clin Biol Res 37:181-216.

Webber MM (1981a): In vitro models. In Hafez EE, Spring-Mills E (eds): "Clinics in Andrology, Prostatic Carcinoma, Biology, and Diagnosis." The Hague: Martinus Nijhoff, Vol 6, pp 145-159.

Webber MM (1981b): Polypeptide hormones and the prostate. In Murphy GP, Sandberg AA, Karr JP (eds): "The Prostatic Cell: Structure and Function. Part B. Prolactin, Carcinogenesis and Clinical Aspects." New York: Alan R. Liss, pp 63-88.

Webber MM, Bouldin TR (1977): Ultrastructure of human prostatic epithelium: Secretion granules or virus particles? Invest Urol 14:482-487.

Webber MM, Chaproniere-Rickenberg DM (1980): Spermine oxidation products are selectively toxic to fibroblasts in cultures of normal human prostatic epithelium. Cell Biol Int Rep 4:185-193.

Webber MM, Stonington OG (1975): Stromal hypocellularity and encapsulation in organ cultures of human prostate—Application in epithelial cell isolation. J Urol 114:246-248.

Webber MM, Stonington OG, Poché PA (1974): Epithelial outgrowth from suspension cultures of human prostatic tissue. In Vitro 10:196-205.

Webber MM, Chaproniere-Rickenberg DM, Donohue RE (1982): Effects of insulin on the growth of normal, benign and malignant human prostatic epithelium. Proc Am Assoc Cancer Res 23:29.

White MT, Hu ASL, Hammamoto ST, Nandi S (1978): In vitro analysis of proliferating epithelial cell populations from the mouse mammary gland: Fibroblast-free growth and serial passage. In Vitro 14:271-281.

Methods for Serum-Free Culture of Cells of the Endocrine System,
pages 63–87
© 1984 Alan R. Liss, Inc., 150 Fifth Avenue, New York, NY 10011

5

Growth of Functional Primary and Established Rat Ovary Cell Cultures in Serum-Free Medium

Joseph Orly

Many in vitro studies with various cultured cell types have suggested that the expression of the differentiated phenotype was markedly influenced by the culture milieu, mainly by the presence or absence of serum in the culture medium [Coon, 1966; Seeds et al., 1970; Bottenstein and Sato, 1979; Darmon et al., 1981]. Similarly, the present chapter demonstrates the absolute necessity of serum-free medium for the study of ovarian cell functions in vitro. We were preferentially interested in the follicular granulosa cells because of their major physiologic role throughout the maturation process of the gonad follicle, which eventually leads to ovulation.

The cytodifferentiation process of the granulosa cells is regulated by a concerted action of various hormones, including gonadotropins (follicle-stimulating hormone [FSH] and luteinizing hormone [LH]), prolactin, prostaglandins, and steroids. While the principal roles of these hormones have been elucidated [Richards et al., 1976; Zeleznik et al., 1974; Channing, 1970; Armstrong and Papkoff, 1976; Erickson and Ryan, 1975; McNatty et al., 1974; Dorrington and Armstrong, 1979; Lindner et al., 1980; Wang et al., 1979; Sala et al., 1979] in both in vivo and in vitro systems, a variety of aspects of the mode of action of these hormones still await further analysis. For this purpose, there is a need to isolate the desired ovarian cell type from the multitude of systemic influences to which it is normally subjected in vivo,

Department of Biological Chemistry, Institute of Life Sciences, The Hebrew University of Jerusalem, 91904 Jerusalem, Israel and to examine its hormonally controlled differentiation under totally defined culture conditions.

MATERIALS AND METHODS
Culture Media

The basic nutrient culture medium consisted of a 1:1 (v/v) mixture of Dulbecco modified Eagle's medium (DME) (Gibco, Grand Island, NY) and Ham's nutrient mixture F12 (Gibco). The two media were freshly prepared every 7-14 days and stored separately in 200-ml aliquots at 4°C (DME) or −20°C (Ham's F12). HEPES buffer (15 mM, pH 7.9) and $NaHCO_3$ (1.2 gm/liter) were added to the media at the time of preparation. Only sealed moisture barrier pouches, containing dry powdered media, ready to prepare 1-liter quantities of medium, were used. Penicillin (200 units/ml) and streptomycin (200 μg/ml) were prepared as 200 × stock solutions in H_2O, filter-sterilized, and stored at −20°C in small aliquots. The antibiotics were added when the two media were mixed and the mixtures were then stored at 4°C and consumed within 7 days. The quality of the water used to prepare the culture media is extremely important for the serum-free culture of the ovarian cells. High-quality distilled water was obtained by means of a High-Q Model 102SC All Glass Water Still (Ultrascience Inc., Wilmette, IL), which also removes organic and inorganic contaminants from the distilled water.

The serum-free, hormone-supplemented medium (4F medium) used to culture both the ovarian cell line (RF-1) and the primary rat ovarian cells [Orly and Sato, 1979; Orly et al., 1980] contained insulin (2 μg/ml), transferrin (5 μg/ml), hydrocortisone (40 ng/ml), and fibronectin (3 μg/cm^2). Dishes (35 × 10 mm; Falcon) were used for culture of RF-1 cells and multiwell plates (24 wells, 16 mm diameter; Nunc, Denmark) were used for the studies of primary granulosa cells. Human fibronectin was added to each culture well already containing 0.5 ml of medium, and incubated for 30-60 min at 37°C prior to inoculation of cells. In contrast, the hormones, i.e., insulin, transferrin, and hydrocortisone, were added into each well from 100 × stock solutions immediately after inoculation of cells. Stock solution of hormones (100 ×) were prepared every week from concentrated solutions (1,000 ×), which were stored as follows: insulin (2 mg/ml) in 0.01 M HCl (stored for no longer than 4 weeks at 4°C); transferrin (5 mg/ml) in phosphate-buffered saline (PBS) (stored at −20°C for unlimited time); and hydrocortisone (1 mg/ml) in ethanol (stored at −20°C to minimize ethanol evaporation).

Purification of Fibronectin

Human fibronectin was purified from plasma of freshly drawn blood of healthy individuals. To avoid coagulation, the blood was collected into phosphate-buffered saline containing Na^+ citrate (10 mM final concentration, pH 7.4) or heparin (0.25 units/ml blood). The blood cells were removed by centrifugation, and fibronectin was isolated in one step by affinity chromatography on a gelatin-Sepharose column as previously described by Ruoslahti et al. [1978]. Plasma (150 ml) was applied to a gelatin-Sepharose column (0.8 gm gelatin/1 ml swollen Sepharose, 120 ml packed bed volume, 25 × 250 mm), and equilibrated with PBS containing 10 mM Na^+ citrate, pH 7.4. The plasma was eluted through the column at a flow rate of 1.25 ml/min at room temperature. Serum proteins were washed with five bed volumes of PBS containing citrate. Bound fibronectin was eluted by 8 M urea solution in 50 mM Tris-HCl, pH 7.4. Fractions (5 ml each) were manually collected into polypropylene tubes kept at 4°C. A short length of Tygon tubing was connected at the column effluent, so that the eluting urea drops carefully slid along the tube walls. It should be noted that from this point onwards, all manipulations (pipetting, storage, etc.) with purified fibronectin should be carried out only with polypropylene labware. It is also recommended that vigorous shaking of fibronectin solutions by vortex be avoided. The fibronectin content in each fraction was determined by a standard protein assay, and pooled fractions were diluted before dialysis so that the final fibronectin concentration did not exceed 0.8 mg/ml. The pooled fractions were dialyzed at 4°C against PBS containing 1 M urea (pH 7.4) and stored after filter-sterilization at 4°C. Urea was needed to maintain the plasma fibronectin soluble at neutral pH. In our experience, the presence of up to 30 mM urea in the culture medium does not harm the cell monolayer. Alternatively, urea can be removed from the culture medium before inoculation of the cells, by washing from the dish after fibronectin has already coated the plastic substratum within 30–60 min of incubation at 37°C (see Culture Media above).

Rat Follicular RF-1 Cell Line

Both serum containing and serum-free media consisted of a 1:1 mixture of DME:F12 nutrient media prepared as described above. Stock cultures were grown in 100-mm tissue culture dishes (Falcon) and maintained in the medium supplemented with 5% (v/v) horse serum (Gibco) and 2.5% (v/v) fetal calf serum (Reheis). Serum-free medium consisted of 4F medium as described above. All cultures were incubated at 37°C and 100% humidity with 5% CO_2 and 95% air. The rat ovary cell line was kindly donated by Dr. H. Masui [Orly and Sato, 1979]. Frozen RF-1 cells from early passage were thawed every 3–4 weeks, and for routine subculture (1:20 split), subconfluent cultures were trypsinized every 3 days with 0.1% crude trypsin (ICN 1-300) and 0.7 mM EDTA in Ca^{2+}- Mg^{2+}-free PBS.

Cells were prepared for experiments in SF medium as follows: About 10^5 cells were plated and grown for 2 days in 100-mm dishes containing 10 ml of serum-supplemented medium. At the time of trypsinization, the cells were no more than 40% confluent (10^6 cells per dish) and in logarithmic growth. The cells were washed three times with warm SF medium and then once with PBS containing 0.7 mM EDTA. One milliliter of 0.01% crystallized trypsin (Sigma), 0.01% chymotrypsin (Sigma), and 0.7 mM EDTA in PBS [Schramm et al., 1977] was added to the dish, and after a few seconds, was aspirated off. After 2–3 min at room temperature, the trypsinization was terminated by addition of 10 ml of SF medium containing 0.25 mg/ml soybean trypsin inhibitor (Sigma), and the cells were removed from the dish by gentle pipetting of the medium over the cells. After two washes with SF medium, the cells were resuspended and plated into 35×10-mm dishes (9.6 cm^2) that already contained 2 ml medium and fibronectin. Hormones were added immediately after inoculation of the cells.

Animals

Immature female rats (Wistar-derived strain, 22–25 days old) were not hypophysectomized or treated with diethylstilbestrol (DES). The animals were sacrificed by cervical dislocation.

Granulosa Cell Culture

Granulosa cells were collected as previously described [Orly et al., 1982]. Immature, intact rats (22–25 days old) were killed by cervical dislocation, and the ovaries were then removed and dissected free of nonovarian tissue. The intercellular gap junctions of the granulosa cells were disrupted [Campbell, 1979] by incubation of the intact ovaries in 4F medium containing 10 mM EGTA and 0.5 M sucrose. After 45 min at 37°C, the ovaries were transferred to 4F medium for a second 45-min incubation at room temperature. The granulosa cells were expressed into warm 4F medium by puncturing the follicles with a 22-gauge sterile needle. The cells were washed twice in the above medium and counted in a hemocytometer, after trypan blue staining. About 5×10^4 viable cells were plated into each well (2 cm^2) of a 24-well plate containing 0.5 ml of medium. As mentioned above, insulin, transferrin, and hydrocortisone were added immediately after inoculation of the cells, whereas purified human fibronectin (6 μg per well) was added to the wells 30 min before inoculation of the cells. A standard preparation of granulosa cells obtained from immature, intact rats yielded approximately 2×10^5 cells per ovary. A five-fold higher yield of cells was obtained when the rats were primed with diethylstilbestrol.

Cell Count

Number of cells was determined after trypsinization by means of a Coulter counter. The medium was removed from the well and 0.2 ml of 0.3% trypsin (Difco, 1:300) in PBS, also containing 0.7 mM EDTA, was added to the cell monolayer. The trypsin solution was aspirated from the monolayer and, within 1-3 min of incubation at room temperature, the cells' detachment from the substratum was checked microscopically. Trypsinization was terminated by addition of 10 ml of PBS to suspend the cells. The Coulter counter (Industrial D, 140-μ orifice tube) threshold was increased to exclude counting of dead cells, cell debris, or red blood cells, which interfere with the granulosa cell count.

Steroid Measurements

The 20α-hydroxypregn-4-ene-3-one (20αOH-P), which is the main progesterone metabolite secreted into the culture medium by the responding granulosa cells, was measured by radioimmunoassay (RIA) as previously described [Orly et al., 1980]. Anti-20α-OH-P antibody was a generous gift from Dr. F. Kohen of the Weizmann Institute of Science, Rehovot, Israel.

Cyclic AMP Determinations

Accumulation of cAMP in the intact cells was measured, after some modifications, as previously described [Orly et al., 1982]. Prior to the addition of agonists, the cell monolayers were incubated in 0.2 ml of 4F medium containing 2 μCi of [^{3}H]adenine (2 μM). After 2 h of incubation at 37°C, the monolayers were washed twice with warm 4F medium and agonists were added at zero time. About 25% of the added [^{3}H]adenine was incorporated into the cells ($\sim 10^5$ per well), most of it being converted to [^{3}H]ATP [Schulster et al., 1978; Clark and Menon, 1976]. After 40-50 min with agonist, the cells were lysed by addition of 0.3 ml ethanol solution (70%) and 0.2 ml "stop solution." The content of the stop solution and the procedure for the determination of [^{3}H]cAMP, by means of chromatography on Dowex (Bio-Rad Laboratories, Richmond, CA) AG 50W-X4 and aluminum oxide columns, were described in a previous report [Schulster et al., 1978].

The counts corresponding to purified [^{3}H]cAMP were normalized when expressed as percentage of conversion of tritium cpm to [^{3}H]cAMP (percentage of conversion). This radioactive measurement of cAMP accumulation of intact granulosa cells was the method of our choice because it is more accurate, highly sensitive, inexpensive, and much less tedious than the one using RIA for cAMP determinations.

Agonist

Ovine FSH (NIAMDD-oFSH-13) was a generous gift from the National Institute of Arthritis, Metabolism, and Digestive Diseases. If not otherwise stated, FSH was used at a concentrate of 100 ng/ml.

Reagents

α-Amanitin (A-2263), cycloheximide (C-6255), and 3-isobutyl-1-methylxanthine (I-5879), as well as insulin (I-5500), transferrin (T-4515), and hydrocortisone (H-4001), were obtained from Sigma Chemicals (St. Louis, MO).

Radiochemicals

All radiochemicals were purchased from New England Nuclear (Boston).

RESULTS
Growth of Established Ovarian Cell Line in Culture

It is now clear that the serum requirement for growth of cells in culture can be successfully replaced by appropriate, defined hormones and growth factors (reviewed by Barnes and Sato [1980a,b]). An additional concept that originated from the pioneering work of Sato and his collaborators predicted that a serum-free medium, designed for a particular cell line, will probably also support the survival of that specific cell type in primary culture [Mather and Sato, 1979; Bottenstein et al., 1980; Rizzino and Sherman, 1979; Taub and Sato, 1979]. We, therefore, paved the road for the study of cultured primary ovarian granulosa cells by adopting the hormone-supplemented serum-free formulation that we tailored to meet the growth requirements of a rat follicular normal cell line, namely, RF-1 cells.

The rat follicular (RF-1) cell line was established in our laboratory by H. Masui [Bottenstein et al., 1978] from ovaries of normal Fisher rats. It is a cloned line of epithelioid cells that grow indefinitely in culture. These cells do not produce tumors in Fisher rats or nude mice [Bottenstein et al., 1978] and exhibit so-called "normal" behavior in culture. The cells attach firmly and are well spread on the dish substratum and, upon confluency, they show density inhibition of growth. The cells are routinely maintained in a 1:1 mixture of DME:F12 media supplemented with serum (see Materials and Methods).

Table I shows that in the DME:F12 mixture, insulin (2 μg/ml), transferrin (5 μg/ml), hydrocortisone (40 ng/ml), and a fibronectin-coated (3 μg/cm^2) substratum (4F medium) were the defined factors needed to support the growth of RF-1 cells at a rate comparable to that achieved in 7.5% serum.

TABLE I. RF-1 Cell Line: Defined Growth Factors Substituted for Growth-Promoting Activity of Serum

Incubation medium	Number of cells per dish $\times 10^{-4}$ (inoculum size $= 1.2$)	Relative number of cells (inoculum size $=1$)
Serum[a]	32.8 ± 1.7	27.3
No growth factors added	Cell death	—
Ins, Tf, HC	4.0 ± 0.4	3.3
Fibronectin + Ins, Tf, HC	15.3 ± 0.6	12.7
Fibronectin + Ins	8.1 ± 0.2	6.7
Fibronectin + Tf	2.1 ± 0.03	1.8
Fibronectin + HC	1.3 ± 0.1	1.0
Fibronectin + Ins, Tf	15.4 ± 0.4	12.8
Fibronectin + Ins, HC	8.0 ± 0.3	6.6
Fibronectin + Tf, HC	2.7 ± 0.1	2.2
Fibronectin only	3.1 ± 0.06	2.6

RF-1 cells were plated into dishes (35 × 10 mm) containing serum-free medium (see Materials and Methods) supplemented with 16 μg of fibronectin and various combinations of three growth factors: insulin (Ins), transferrin (Tf), and hydrocortisone (HC). The cells were counted after 3 days of culturing.
[a]Cells were plated into serum-containing medium.

Fibronectin-mediated adhesion of the cells to the dish substratum was found obligatory for the cytokinesis process of RF-1 cells inoculated into this serum-free medium [Orly and Sato, 1979]. Studies by time-lapse photography of RF-1 cells in mitosis clearly indicated that when this cell type was inoculated on bare plastic, the progressive advance of the cleavage furrow was normal until midtelophase. However, for as yet unknown reasons, at later stages of telophase the division furrow regressed (Fig. 1m) and eventually disappeared (Fig. 1n). Consequently, lack of cytokinesis produced a single binucleated cell instead of two daughter cells, the normal product. In contrast, normal cytokinesis was made possible if the cells were plated on a fibronectin-coated substratum, where each round of mitosis gave rise to a typical daughter cell doublet (Fig. 1a–g). Since 70-80% of the freshly inoculated cells became binucleated after the first round of division, the cell growth in the absence of fibronectin was practically arrested.

It should be noted here that the lack of cytokinesis leading to binucleation of cells plated on bare plastic in serum-free medium was not restricted to RF-1 cells only. Figure 2A shows that baby hamster kidney (BHK) cells, which are commonly used to assay adhesive properties of fibronectins [Grinnell and Minter, 1978], also became binucleated when inoculated onto bare plastic in 4F medium without fibronectin. Coating the culture dish with fibronectin

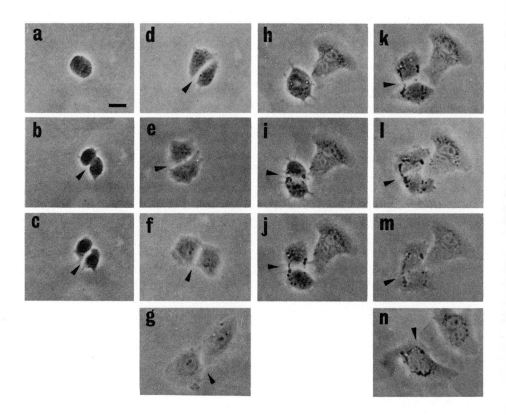

Fig. 1. Time lapse, phase-contrast photomicrographs of mitotic RF-1 cells on a fibronectin-coated substratum (a-g) or bare plastic (h-n). Progress of cell division on a fibronectin-coated substratum. a) Six hours following plating in 4F medium (see Materials and Methods), a typical rounded-up mitotic cell was selected at anaphase (zero time); b) at 20 min, arrow indicates the cleavage furrow; c) at 30 min, cytokinesis has been completed; d) at 50 min, the two daughter cells begin respreading; e) at 65 min, the nuclei membrane is first seen; f) at 120 min, a normal doublet of the daughter cells; g) after 24 h, the two daughter cells are still in close proximity. Progress of cell division on bare plastic. h) A rounded-up mitotic cell was selected in anaphase (zero time). Note the neighboring well-spread cell, which is already binucelated; i) at 15 min, telophase; the arrow indicates the brighter area of the cleavage furrow; j) at 30 min, late telophase, the daughter cells are apparently separated but black intracellular cholesterol-ester droplets (arrow) indicate that intercellular bridges are still in existence; k) at 45 min, the daughter cells respread but the cleavage furrow zone is still visible; l) at 75 min, the cleavage furrow regresses and can hardly be seen; m) at 120 min, the daughter cells are fully respread, although the nuclei membranes are not yet detectable; n) at 5 h, the cleavage furrow has completely regressed. The two daughter nuclei indicate successful karyokinesis but failure of cytokinesis, which has resulted in a single binucleated cell. Bar = 20 μM.

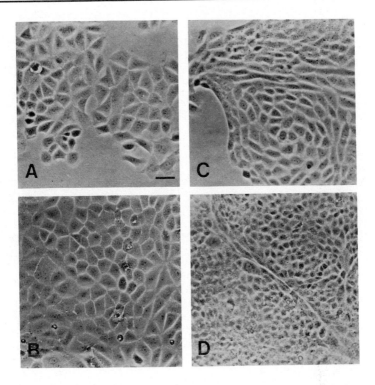

Fig. 2. Phase-contrast micrographs of RF-1 cells grown in serum-free or serum-containing medium. Cells (1.3×10^4) were plated into 4F medium (A,B) or into medium containing 5% horse serum and 2.5% fetal calf serum (C,D). Phase-contrast micrographs were taken on the third (A,C) and the fifth (B,D) day after plating. Note that confluent monolayers in 4F medium (B) contained fewer cells than those in serum-containing medium (D). In 4F medium, the epithelioid cells were spread and thinner, whereas in serum the crowded cells acquired a more columnar appearance (D). Bar = 40 μM.

allowed physiologically compatible adhesion of the BHK cells to the substratum, which consequently completed several normal cell divisions, as seen in Figure 3A,B. However, in contrast to RF-1 cells, BHK cells did not spread in 4F medium and stayed rounded-up, probably owing to lack of an appropriate spreading protein other than fibronectin. Serum-spreading factor [Barnes et al., 1982, 1983] might have been a reasonable candidate for this matter.

Regarding the rat follicular cells, we could therefore ascribe fibronectin as a permissive factor for the other growth-stimulating substances in 4F medium, since fibronectin alone could not support the growth of RF-1 cells (Table I). In the presence of fibronectin, insulin was the most stringently required hormone.

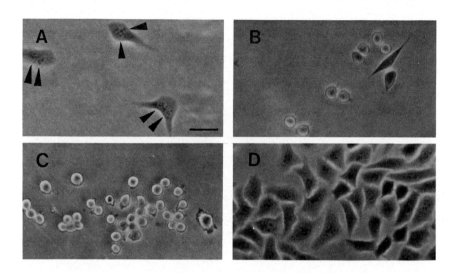

Fig. 3. Effect of fibronectin on cytokinesis of baby hamster kidney (BHK) cells in 4F medium. Cells (2×10^4 per 35-mm dish) were inoculated into DME:F12 medium containing insulin, transferrin, and hydrocortisone in the absence (A) or the presence of fibronectin (B,C). Control cells were inoculated into serum-containing medium (D). A. At 24 h after plating on bare plastic, 75% of the cells were binucleated as indicated by the arrows. B. At 24 h after plating on fibronectin-coated substratum, typical doublets of postmitotic daughter cells can be observed. Note that BHK cells did not spread on the fibronectin carpet, which, however, did not alter the normal doubling time of the cells (18 h). C. After 3 days of growth in 4F medium, the cells underwent 3-4 cell cycles but remained rounded-up. D. Control monolayers of well-spread cells grown in serum-containing medium. Bar = 60 μM.

Insulin acted synergistically with transferrin to produce the maximal growth rate in SF medium. Although hydrocortisone did not have any additional effect on cell proliferation, we included it in our medium because of its effect on cell morphology. In the absence of hydrocortisone, cells were less spread as well as morphologically heterogeneous [Orly and Sato, 1979]. Figure 3 shows the epithelioid morphology of RF-1 cells grown in 4F medium (A,B) or serum-containing medium (C,D). The latter contained two to three times more cells at confluent densities than the former. In 4F medium, the cells formed typical rosettes of hexagonal cells (Fig. 3B), which spread and acquired a more flattened morphology when compared with the crowded columnar appearance of cells grown in serum-containing medium (Fig. 3D).

Growth and Function of Primary Ovarian Granulosa Cells in Culture

For obvious reasons, the gonads have always been an attractive object for fundamental and applied research. Indeed, many investigators applied tissue culture techniques to isolate specific gonadal cell types to study their cellular differentiation under defined environments. In particular, follicular granulosa cells from ovaries of various mammalian species became a most suitable cell system to study in vitro owing to the simple procedure necessary for the isolation of this cell type from the entire ovary. Syringe aspiration of granulosa cells from follicles of pig, cow, sheep, or rabbit ovaries or, alternatively, needle-puncturing into the ovaries of the rat or mouse, is all it takes to achieve a pure and homogeneous population of this physiologically important cell type. Lack of the enzymatic treatment (trypsin, collagenase) that usually is required for the dissociation of the desired cells from the surrounding tissue preserves the surface of the cell membrane intact and maintains the receptor-mediated cellular response unaltered. However, the first attempts to study the hormonal control of granulosa cell cytodifferentiation in culture encountered serious difficulties in demonstrating FSH-induced functions when serum was tradition-ally included in the culture medium. Consequently, studies were initiated by Erickson [1983] and his colleagues, who employed serum-free medium as a tool for examining functional ovarian cells in culture. These investigators studied granulosa cells cultured in McCoy's 5a medium without serum or any other supplement. With SF medium, FSH was shown to successfully induce aromatase enzyme as well as receptors for LH and prolactin [Gore-Langton et al., 1980; Adashi and Hsueh, 1982; Erickson et al., 1979; Wang et al., 1979], which had previously been shown to appear in response to FSH administered in vivo [Armstrong and Papkoff, 1976; Richards and Williams, 1976; Zeleznik et al., 1974]. Most of these in vitro studies, however, have been concerned primarily with short-term cultures of follicular cells, and little was known about the long-term survival and functionality of these cells in SF medium.

In this chapter we summarize some of our findings, showing that 4F medium, originally designed for growth of the RF-1 cell line, also supports long-term growth and maintenance of functional primary granulosa cells. We shall also demonstrate how severely serum suppresses the hormonally in-duced functions of these cells in culture.

When ovarian granulosa cells from immature rats were inoculated into DME:F12 media containing insulin, transferrin, hydrocortisone, and fibronec-tin, most of the cells were alive (75% as determined by trypan blue staining) and survived for 60 days or more in culture. In a previous publication, we have described the role of the individual supplements for the maintenance of the granulosa cells in 4F medium [Orly et al., 1980]. Again, fibronectin and insulin were vital to the survival of the plated cells, whereas, in contrast to the response of RF-1 cell line, transferrin and hydrocortisone had no significant effect on the cells' viability and growth. Nevertheless, hydrocortisone was required for the steroidogenic activity of the follicular cells. Figure 4 demonstrates the FSH-induced 20α-OH-P (the main progestin metabolite in the rat granulosa cells) production in the presence of graded doses of hydrocortisone. Lack of hydrocortisone resulted in a 70% inhibition of steroidogenesis, and 20 ng/ml ($\sim 10^{-7}$ M) was the glucocorticoid concentration that maximally restored the steroidogenic activity.

The proliferative activity of the granulosa cells in culture was found to be rather limited. No more than one round of cell doubling occurred within the first 4 days in culture (Fig. 5C). The mitotic activity of the cells in 4F medium was easily detected by autoradiograms of [³H]thymidine-labeled nuclei (Fig. 6B). However, growth of the cultured cells was not expressed by hyperplasia alone but also by hypertrophy. Figure 5 shows that the granulosa cell mass in a given dish increased five times within 7 days in culture (Fig. 5A), at which time the rate of protein synthesis increased concomitantly until it reached a plateau at day 8 (Fig. 5B). Interestingly enough, we noticed that the response of the granulosa cells to FSH in steroid production was temporarily lost during days 2-7, when intensive growth activity was observed in the culture monolayers. After 8 days in culture, however, the cells regained their responsiveness to gonadotropin hormone at a time that correlated with the entry of the confluent monolayers into the stationary phase of growth (Fig. 5A).

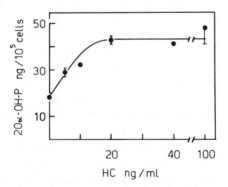

Fig. 4. FSH-induced progestin production in the presence of graded doses of hydrocortisone. Cells (4 × 10⁵ per well) were incubated into DME:F12 medium containing insulin, transferrin, fibronectin, and graded doses of hydrocortisone. After 18 h in culture, 100 ng/ml of FSH was added into duplicate wells, and 48 h later the culture medium was assayed for 20α-OH-P content by RIA.

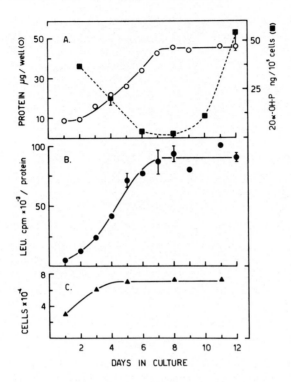

Fig. 5. Growth and function of cultured granulosa cells. Cell proliferation, rate of [³H]leucine incorporation into cellular proteins, increase in cellular proteins, and steroidogenic responsiveness to FSH were simultaneously monitored throughout 12 days in culture. A. FSH-induced progestin production (■ — — ■). Cells (3 × 10⁴ per well) were exposed for 2 days to 100 ng/ ml FSH. After 48 h of incubation with FSH, the 20α-OH-P content was assayed by RIA. Cellular protein (○ — ○). Duplicate wells were lysed by 1.0 N NaOH solution and the protein content of the well was determined daily by the Lowry assay. B. Incorporation of [³H]leucine into cellular proteins. [³H]leucine (1 µCi/ml, 1 µCi/mmole) was added to duplicate wells containing 0.5 ml medium. After 24 h, the cells were washed twice and dissolved in 0.2 ml solution of 1.0 N NaOH. Duplicate aliquots (50 µl) were placed on Whatman 3 filter paper, and TCA-precipitable radioactivity was determined after several washes in hot and cold 5% TCA solutions. C. Cell proliferation. Trypsinized cells were counted with a Coulter counter.

Moreover, Figure 6A clearly demonstrates that the incorporation of [³H]thymidine into the cells' nuclei was restricted to areas of the monolayer containing only sparse cells. In contrast, we recently provided histochemical evidence showing that the high-cell-density areas of the monolayer, which did not show proliferative activity, were exclusively responsive to the FSH stimulus (not shown). We therefore postulated that the granulosa cells may present an

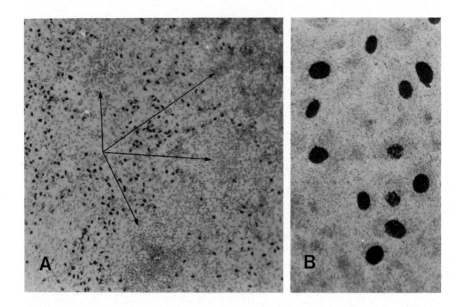

Fig. 6. Incorporation of [^{3}H]thymidine into nuclei of cultured granulosa cells. Cells (5 × 10^4 per 16-mm-diameter well) were inoculated into 4F medium. After 3 days in culture, [methyl-^{3}H]thymidine was added (5 μCi/ml, 5μCi/mmole) to label the cells for 18 h of incubation at 37°C. The cells were then rinsed, fixed with methanol:acetic acid solution, dehydrated with ethanol, and exposed for 3 days to Kodak nucelar track emulsion (type NTB2). After developing, the monolayers were counterstained with toluidine blue O [Orly et al., 1982]. A. Note the areas of high cell density (arrows) in which no labeled nuceli can be observed. Magnification = 40×. B. Higher magnification of labeled nuceli. Magnification = 200×.

additional example of a well-known concept regarding the inverse relationship between growth and differentiation. In other words, it may very well be that growth-related processes occurring in the granulosa cell monolayers negatively regulate the hormonally induced functions of this cell type in culture.

Figure 7 summarizes the morphologic features of our long-term granulosa cell monolayers in 4F medium. After 10 days in culture, the confluent monolayers shown in Figure 5B underwent dramatic morphologic changes within 30 min of incubation with FSH (Fig. 7C). These FSH-induced cell shape changes have already been described by Lawrence et al. [1979] and we applied it as a sensitive and easy assay to detect various substances that can stimulate steroidogenesis [Orly et al., 1982; Weinberger-Ohana et al., 1983]. In addition, the granulosa cells underwent profound cytologic changes after an exposure to gonadotropin for several days (Fig. 7D). The cells acquired an epithelioid morphology, a round nucleus with prominent nucleolus, and the

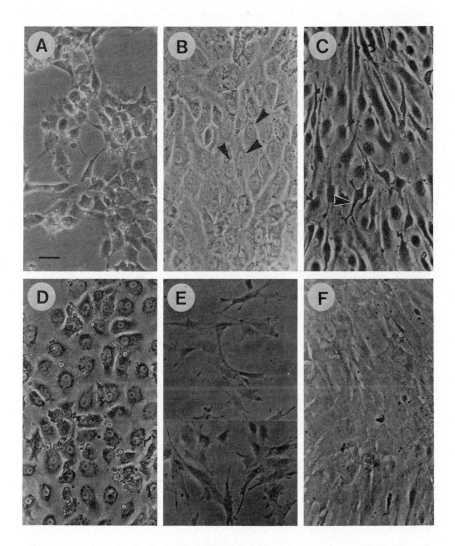

Fig. 7. Long-term culture of granulosa cells in 4F medium (A–E) or serum-containing medium (F). A. Cells (4×10^4 per well) were photographed (phase-contrast) after 48 h in 4F medium. B. Confluent monolayers were photographed after 10 days in 4F medium. Note the large oval nuclei (arrowheads) containing one faint nucleolus or more. C. After 10 days in 4F medium, 100 ng/ml FSH was added to the monolayer. Phase-contrast micrographs were taken subsequent to 30 min of incubation at 37°C. Note the dramatic cell shape changes that have resulted in contraction of the cytoplasm (arrow). D. After 6 days in culture in the continuous presence of 100 ng/ml FSH and 100 ng/ml LH, the cells underwent morphologic cytodifferentiation to become lutein cells. Note the epithelioid morphology, round nucleus, and prominent nucleolus as well as the cholesterol-ester droplets in the cytoplasm. E. Cells were photographed after 6 days in 4F medium without fibronectin. Note the sparse monolayer with fibroblastic-shaped cells. F. Cells were photographed after 8 days in serum-containing medium. Bar = 40 μM.

cytoplasm filled with cholesterol-ester droplets. These long-term morphologic changes are typical for granulosa cells that have been terminally differentiated to become lutein cells in culture. When the cells were plated in 4F medium without fibronectin, fewer cells (5%) survived after 7 days in culture (Fig. 7E). It should be noted that these cells responded well to FSH stimulus (not shown) in spite of their "sick" fibroblastic appearance. If serum was included in the culture medium (Fig. 7F), none of the above FSH-induced phenomena could be observed.

Serum suppression of FSH-induced functions. We shall briefly demonstrate that serum impairs the FSH-induced functions that are associated with the differentiation of the follicular cells.

a. Progestin production. The primary response of the granulosa cells to FSH is expressed in progestin production. Serum remarkably inhibited FSH-induced progestin production, compared with cell responsiveness in 4F medium (Fig. 8). When cells were incubated in culture medium containing graded doses of serum, as little as 0.3% of serum was sufficient to block 95% of the inducible 20α-OH-P biosynthesis. Since decreasing the serum concentration in the medium below 0.5%, reduced the plating efficiency of the inoculated granulosa cells (Fig. 8), we conducted an additional experiment in which the cells were inoculated also onto a plastic substratum that had been pretreated with fibronectin. On such a fibronectin "carpet," the cells exhibited improved growth properties and high cell counts uniformly independent of the serum concentration. Nevertheless, the presence of fibronectin did not alter the inhibitory effect of serum on cell functioning, hence ruling out the possibility that the weak responsiveness of the cells at low serum concentrations results from physiologically incompatible growth conditions.

b. Serum inhibition of FSH induction of LH receptors. Following the FSH induction of LH receptors, the granulosa cells acquire competence to undergo their last step of differentiation in response the preovulatory surge of LH. However, attempts to mimic FSH induction of LH receptors in isolated granulosa cells failed, apparently because of the presence of serum in the culture medium [Nimrod et al., 1977; Hiller et al., 1978].

As it is accepted that both FSH and LH trigger steroidogenesis via cAMP as a second messenger, we chose to demonstrate the serum inhibitory effect on the induction of LH receptors by measuring the ability of newly appeared LH receptors to activate the adenylate cyclase in the intact cells. By so doing, we studied functioning and, therefore, the physiologically relevant receptors, rather than estimating the number of LH receptors by a direct [125I]hCG-binding assay. For the study of adenylate cyclase in intact cells, we incubated the cell monolayers with [3H]adenine, which was rapidly incorporated into

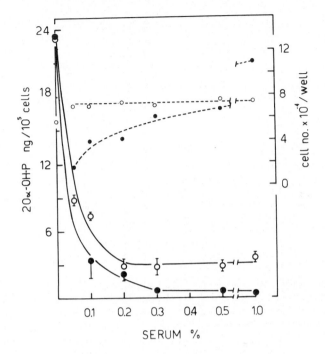

Fig. 8. Dose-dependent inhibition of serum on FSH-induced steroidogeneisis. Cells (7 × 10⁴) were inoculated into duplicate wells (d = 1.6 cm, 24 wells per plate) containing graded doses of serum (horse serum:fetal calf serum, 2:1). A similar inoculation was also performed into wells that had been precoated with 6 μg of human fibronectin. After 24 h in culture, the cells were challenged with FSH (100 ng/ml), and 48 h later the culture media were collected for steroid RIA (●—● and ○—○ symbols represent naked or fibronectin coated substrate, respectively), and number of cells was determined after trypsinization (●———● and ○———○ symbols represent without or with fibronectin, respectively).

intracellular [³H]ATP [Schulster et al., 1978; Humes et al., 1969]. Consequently, in the presence of adenylate cyclase agonist, the cellular [³H]ATP was readily converted into [³H]cAMP, the content of which was assessed as described in Materials and Methods. This technique was found to be more accurate, highly sensitive, inexpensive, and much less tedious than the one using RIA for cAMP determinations. Figure 9 demonstrates a time-dependent accumulation of cAMP in granulosa cells responding to FSH. Maximal cAMP production is obviously monitored in the presence of phosphodiesterase (PDE) inhibitor, 3-isobutyl-1-methyl-xanthine (IBMX). This experiment also indicates that within the first 30–40 min of incubation, the majority of the generated cAMP remains within the cell and does not leak out.

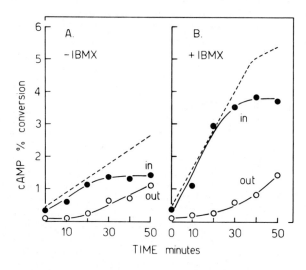

Fig. 9. Time-dependent accumulation of cAMP in response to FSH. One-day-old granulosa cell monolayers (8×10^4 cells per well) were incubated in 0.2 ml of 4F medium containing 2 μCi of [^{3}H]adenine (8 Ci/mmole). After 2 h of incubation, the monolayers, in duplicate wells, were washed and further incubated in 4F medium containing FSH (100 ng/ml) with (A) or without (B) 0.5 mM IBMX. At the indicated times, the culture media were removed from duplicate wells and the cells were lysed by addition of 0.3 ml ethanol solution (70%) and 0.2 ml "stop solution" (see Materials and Methods). The [^{3}H]cAMP content released from the lysed cells (in) and the cyclic nucleotide that spontaneously leaked into the culture medium during the incubation periods (out) were determined as described in Materials and Methods. The counts corresponding to purified [^{3}H]cAMP were normalized when expressed as percentage of conversion of total intracellular tritium cpm to [^{3}H]cAMP (% conversion).

We now studied the inhibitory effect of serum on the formation of functional LH receptors. For that purpose, we primed the cells for 2 days with (or without) FSH, prior to the adenylate cyclase assay itself. The latter was carried out in 4F medium and in the presence of IBMX to reflect maximal adenylate cyclase capacity. Figure 10 shows that in 4F medium a small but significant amount of cAMP was generated in the presence of LH (four times the basal level), even without priming with FSH. However, after 2 days of priming with FSH in 4F medium, LH caused a dramatic 32-fold increase in intracellular cAMP levels accumulated during 40 min of incubation with the gonadotropin. In striking contrast, when the priming period with FSH was conducted in the presence of serum, LH totally failed to cause any significant rise in cAMP formation, thus reflecting the severe serum impairment of the hormonally induced expression of LH receptors.

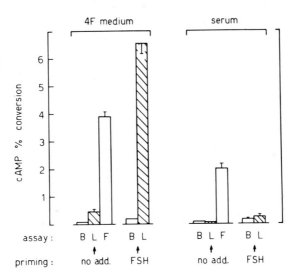

Fig. 10. Failure of FSH to induce LH receptor in the presence of serum. One-day-old granulosa cells (~8 × 10^4 cells per well) were primed for 2 days in either 4F medium or medium containing 5% serum (horse:fetal calf sera, 2:1) in the absence (no add.) or presence (FSH) of FSH. Prior to an adenylate cyclase assay, the cells were labeled with [^{3}H]adenine in duplicate wells. After thorough washings, all the cells were further incubated in 4F medium without additions (B, basal) or in the presence of 100 ng/ml LH (L) or 100 ng/ml FSH (F). After 40 min of incubation at 37°C, the content of [^{3}H]cAMP was assessed and expressed as percentage of conversion, as described in the legend to Figure 9.

c. FSH-induced estrogen formation. An additional biochemical marker that characterizes the differentiation process in granulosa cells involves the FSH induction of estrogen production. Although it is well established that FSH induces aromatase activity in granulosa cells cultured in serum-free medium [Dorrington et al., 1975; Erickson and Hsueh, 1978], the effect of serum on the induction of this enzyme complex has not been examined. We have shown [Orly et al., 1980] that after priming of the cells for 2 days in 4F medium containing FSH, the cells converted substantial amounts of exogenously added androgen into estrogen. On the other hand, when cells were primed with FSH in the presence of serum, little, if any, of the estrogen was produced during the subsequent incubation of the cells with androgen.

d. Serum inhibition of hormonal response: Search for mechanism of action. In recent years, a large body of evidence has been presented to support the general concept that cAMP regulates the entire differentiation process of ovarian granulosa cells. Thus, it has been shown that progestin production [Marsh, 1975], induction of LH receptors [Nimrod, 1981; Knecht and Catt, 1981], and expression of aromatase activity [Hsueh et al., 1980] are all FSH-induced responses mediated by cAMP. Therefore, it seemed reasonable to test whether serum impairs the accumulation of intracellular cAMP triggered by FSH. Figure 11 depicts a typical experiment in which two groups of granulosa cells were grown for 36 h in the presence or absence of serum. After labeling with [³H]adenine, the cells were challenged with graded doses of FSH, while bathing in either 4F medium or serum-containing medium, in the presence or absence of IBMX. It is evident that in the absence of IBMX, cells grown and challenged with FSH in 4F medium accumulated levels of cAMP up to 15 times higher than did cells maintained in serum-containing medium. However, addition of IBMX to these very cells held in serum remarkably caused a sixfold increment in the cyclic nucleotide levels

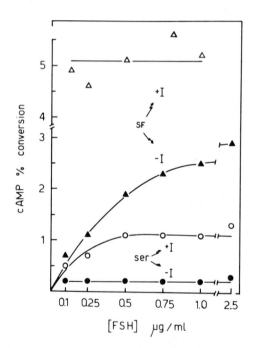

Fig. 11. Effect of serum on cAMP accumulation in response to graded doses of FSH. Cells (~5 × 10⁴ per well) were inoculated into serum-containing medium (ser) or serum-free 4F medium (SF). After 24 h in culture, the cells, in duplicate wells, were preincubated with [³H]adenine, and graded doses of FSH were added to the cells in the presence or absence of 0.5 mM IBMX (+I and −I, respectively). After 45 min, the cells were lysed by addition of 0.3 ml of ethanol solution (70%) and 0.2 ml "stop solution." [³H]cAMP was determined and expressed as percentage of conversion of total intracellular cpm to [³H]cAMP (% conversion).

produced in response to FSH. This clearly ruled out the possibility that serum severely alters the gonadotropin binding to its receptors.

Furthermore, our recent findings indicate that serum also inhibits prostaglandin-induced cAMP accumulation (not shown). Therefore, serum inhibition is probably not exclusive to the FSH-induced phenomenon. Alternatively, these experiments suggest that putative serum components either uncouple the hormone receptor interaction with the adenylate cyclase catalytic unit, or activate an intracellular phosphodiesterase (PDE) that rapidly degrades the inducible accumulation of the cyclic nucleotide in the granulosa cells. At present, we are seeking a direct assay of PDE activity in intact cells that, hopefully, will help us to assess the possible role of this enzyme in the regulation of the ovarian cell responsiveness to hormones. In addition, we have identified a serum protein that may prove to be the source of the serum inhibitory effects on cell function.

DISCUSSION

Three different culture media are currently used for in vitro studies of ovarian and testicular cells in serum-free cultures. Except for our mixture of DME:F12 media and a modification of Eagle's minimum essential medium used by Gore-Langton and Dorrington [Gore-Langton et al., 1980, 1981], the most frequently used medium is McCoy's 5a (modified). Since the purpose of this study was to culture primary granulosa cells in synthetic medium, we avoided the use of McCoy's 5a formula, which contains undefined components such as 600 mg/liter bactopeptone. Moreover, as a fibronectin-coated substratum was found to be so crucial for cell viability in long-term cultures of the granulosa cells, the presence of partially hydrolized proteins in McCoy's 5a medium may compete with fibronectin for binding to the plastic substratum. However, it should be noted that, at least for short-term cultures of follicular cells, McCoy's 5a medium was found quite satisfactory for most studies concerning FSH-induced responses [Erickson, 1983; Amsterdam et al., 1981].

Sanders and Midgley [1982] recently conducted a thorough comparative study of functional rat granulosa cells in serum-free medium. Their findings indicate that FSH treatment of granulosa cells, cultured in DME-F12 media, yielded twice as many LH receptors per cell as similar incubation in McCoy's 5a medium. In addition, when FSH-induced LH receptors were monitored in DME:F12 supplemented with various combinations of insulin, transferrin, and hydrocortisone, these supplements had inhibitory effects on the number of LH-inducible receptors. The number of LH receptors determined by binding assay of [^{125}I]iodo-hCG appeared to be independent, however, of the LH-mediated induction of progesterone accumulation; on the contrary, the medium supplements such as transferrin and hydrocortisone were *obligatory* for the gonadotropin stimulation of steroidogenesis [Sanders and Midgley, 1982]. It, therefore, seems that the culture medium's composition and any substances added to it should be carefully tested for the effects they might exert on the multitudinous biochemical responses that are included under the term "cellular responsiveness." By the same token, maximal expression of FSH-induced LH receptors may indeed occur in DME:F12 mixture without any additions. However, such a medium composition does not allow either the optimal functioning of the LH receptor or the long-term viability of the cells in this medium's formula. In light of the goals pursued, the decision should be made whether to choose culture conditions supporting a maximal *number* of receptors, or preferably, to select the culture combinations that are more physiologically suited to allowing the *optimal functioning* of the receptor under study.

In summary, the successful application of cell culture techniques in the study of reproduction clearly indicates that the day is not far off when culture techniques will provide the means of maintaining pure populations of all the cell types constituting the gonads. It should then be possible to design an in vitro ovary reconstitution to finally allow the study of the mutual relationship between the different cell types in the gonads.

ACKNOWLEDGMENTS

We wish to thank Dr. F. Kohen from the Department of Hormone Research, The Weizmann Institute of Science, Rehovot, Israel, for providing us with the anti-20α-OH-P antibody. We are also grateful to Mrs. E. Dicker for her excellent editorial and secretarial assistance.

This work was supported by the United States–Israel Binational Science Foundation, grant #2656/81, and by the Bat-Sheva de Rothschild Fund for Advancement of Science and Technology.

J.O. is an incumbent for the Charles H. Revson Career Development Chair.

REFERENCES

Adashi EH, Hsueh AJ (1982): Estrogen augment of stimulation of ovarian aromatase activity by follicle stimulating hormone in cultured rat granulosa cells. J Biol Chem 257:6077–6083.
Amsterdam A, Knecht M, Catt KJ (1981): Hormonal regulation of cytodifferentiation and intercellular communication in cultured granulosa cells. Proc Natl Acad Sci USA 78:3000–3004.

Armstrong DT, Papkoff H (1976): Stimulation of aromatization of exogenous androgens in ovaries of hypophysectomized rats in vivo by follicle stimulating hormone. Endocrinology 99:1144-1151.

Barnes D, Sato G (1980a): Methods for growth of cultured cells in serum-free medium. Anal Biochem 102:255-270.

Barnes D, Sato G (1980b): Serum-free cell culture: A unifying approach. Cell 22:649-655.

Barnes DW, Darmon M, Orly J (1982): Serum spreading factor: Effects on RF-1 rat ovary cells and 1003 mouse embryonal carcinoma cells in serum free medium. In Sato GH, Pardee AB, Sirbasku DA (eds): "Cold Spring Harbor Conferences on Cell Proliferation: Growth of Cells in Hormonally Defined Media." Cold Spring Harbor Laboratory, Vol 9, pp 155-167.

Barnes DW, Silnutzer J, See C, Shaffer M (1983): Characterization of human serum spreading factor with monoclonal antibody. Proc Natl Acad Sci USA 80:1362-1366.

Bottenstein JE, Sato GH (1979): Growth of rat neuroblastoma cell line in serum-free supplemented medium. Proc Natl Acad Sci USA 76:514-517.

Bottenstein J, Hayashi I, Hutchings S, Masui H, Mather J, McClure DB, Ohasa S, Rizzino A, Sato G, Serrero G, Wolfe R, Wu R (1978): The growth of cells in serum-free hormone supplemented media. In Jakoby W, Pastan I (eds): "Methods in Enzymology." New York: Academic, Vol 58, pp 94-109.

Bottenstein JE, Skaper SD, Varon SS, Sato GH (1980): Selective survival of neurons from chick embryo sensory ganglionic dissociates utilizing serum-free supplemented medium. Exp Cell Res 125:183-190.

Campbell KL (1979): Ovarian granulosa cells isolated with EGTA and hypertonic sucrose: Cellular integrity and function. Biol Rep 21:733-786.

Channing CP (1970): Influence of the in vivo and in vitro hormonal environment upon luteinization of granulosa cells in tissue culture. Recent Prog Horm Res 26:589-622.

Clark MR, Menon KMJ (1976): Regulation of ovarian steroidogenesis. Biochim Biophys Acta 444:23-32.

Coon HG (1966): Clonal stability and phenotypic expression of chick cartilage cells in vitro. Proc Natl Acad Sci USA 55:66-73.

Darmon M, Bottenstein JE, Sato GH (1981): Neural differentiation following culture of embryonal carcinoma cells in serum-free defined medium. Dev Biol 85:463-473.

Dorrington JH, Armstrong DT (1979): Effects of FSH on gonadal functions. Recent Prog Horm Res 35:301-342.

Dorrington JH, Moon YS, Armstrong DT (1975): Estradiol-17β biosynthesis in cultured granulosa cells from hypophysectomized immature rats: Stimulation by follicle stimulating hormone. Endocrinology 97:1328-1331.

Erickson GF (1983): Primary cultures of ovarian cells in serum-free medium as models for homone-dependent differentiation. Mol Cell Endocrinol 29:21-49.

Erickson GF, Hsueh AJW (1978): Stimulation of aromatase activity by follicle stimulating hormone in rat granulosa cells in vivo and in vitro. Endocrinology 102:1275-1282.

Erickson GF, Ryan KJ (1975): The effect of LH/FSH dibutyryl cyclic AMP and prostaglandins on the production of estrogens by rabbit granulosa cells in vitro. Endocrinology 97:108-116.

Erickson GF, Wang C, Hsueh AJW (1979): FSH induction of functional LH receptors in granulosa cells cultured in chemically defined medium. Nature 279:336-338.

Gore-Langton RE, McKreracher H, Dorrington JH (1980): An alternative method for the study of follicle stimulating hormone effects on aromatase activity in Sertoli cell culture. Endocrinology 107:464-471.

Gore-Langton RE, Lacroix M, Dorrington JH (1981): Differential effects of luteinizing hormone releasing hormone on follicle stimulating hormone dependent responses in rat granulosa and Sertoli cells in vitro. Endocrinology 108:812-819.

Grinnell F, Minter D (1978): Attachment and spreading of baby hamster kidney cells to collagen substrata: Effects of cold insoluble globulin. Proc Natl Acad Sci USA 75:4408-4412.

Hiller SG, Zeleznik AJ, Ross GT (1978): Independence of steroidogenic capacity and luteinizing hormone receptor induction in developing granulosa cells. Endocrinology 102:937-946.

Hsueh AJW, Wang C, Erickson GF (1980): Direct inhibitory effect of gonadotropin-releasing hormone upon follicle stimulating hormone induction of luteinizing hormone receptor and aromatase activity in rat granulosa cells. Endocrinology 106:1697-1705.

Humes JL, Rounbehler M, Kuehl F (1969): A new assay for measuring adenylate cyclase activity in intact cells. Anal Biochem 32:210-217.

Knecht M, Catt KJ (1982): Induction of luteinizing hormone receptors by adenosine-3', 5'-monophosphate in cultured granulosa cells. Endocrinology 111:1192-1200.

Lawrence TS, Ginzberg RD, Gilula NB, Beers WH (1979): Hormonally induced cell shape changes in cultured rat ovarian granulosa cells. J Cell Biol 80:21-36.

Lindner HR, Zor U, Kohen F, Bauminger S, Amsterdam A, Lahav M, Salomon Y (1980): Significance of protaglandins in the regulation of cyclic events in the ovary and uterus. In Samuelson B, Ramwel PW, Paoletti R (eds): "Advances in Protaglandin and Thromboxane Research." New York: Raven, Vol 8, pp 1371-1390.

Marsh JM (1975): The role of cyclic AMP in gonadal function. Adv Cyclic Nucleotide Res 6:137-199.

Mather J, Sato GH (1979): The use of hormone supplemented serum-free media in primary culture. Exp Cell Res 124:215-221.

McNatty KP, Sawers RS, McNeilly AS (1974): A possible role for prolactin in control of steroid secretion by the human Graafian follicle. Nature 250:653-655.

Nimrod A (1981): The induction of ovarian LH-receptors by FSH is mediated by cyclic AMP. FEBS Lett 131:31-33.

Nimrod A, Tsafriri A, Lindner HR (1977): In vitro induction of binding sites for hCG in rat granulosa cells by FSH. Nature 267:632-633.

Orly J, Sato GH (1979): Fibronectin mediates cytokinesis and growth of rat follicular cells in serum-free medium. Cell 17:295-305.

Orly J, Sato GH, Erickson GF (1980): Serum suppresses the expression of hormonally induced functions in cultured granulosa cells. Cell 20:817-827.

Orly J, Farkash Y, Hershkovits N, Mizrahi L, Weinberger P (1982): Ovarian substance induces steroid production in cultured granulosa cells. In Vitro 18:980-989.

Richards JS, Williams JJ (1976): Luteal cell receptor content for prolactin (PRL) and luteinizing hormone (LH): Regulation by LH and PRL. Endocrinology 99:1571-1581.

Richards JS, Ireland JJ, Rao MC, Bernath GA, Midgley AR Jr, Reichert LH Jr (1976): Ovarian follicular development in the rat: Hormone receptor regulation by estradiol, follicle stimulating hormone, and luteinizing hormone. Endocrinology 99:1562-1570.

Rizzino A, Sherman MI (1979): Development and differentiation of mouse blastocysts in serum-free medium. Exp Cell Res 121:221-233.

Ruoslahti E, Vuento M, Engvall E (1978): Interaction of antibodies and collagen in radioimmunoassay. Biochim Biophys Act 534:210-218.

Sala GB, Dufau ML, Catt KJ (1979): Gonadotropin action of isolated ovarian luteal cells: The intermediate role of adenosine 3', 5'-monophosphate in hormonal stimulation of progesterone synthesis. J Biol Chem 254:2077-2083.

Sanders MM, Midgley AR Jr (1982): Rat granulosa cell differentiation: An in vitro model. Endocrinology 111:614-625.

Schramm M, Orly J, Eimerl S, Korner M (1977): Coupling of hormone receptor to adenylate cyclase of different cells by fusion. Nature 268:310-313.

Schulster D, Orly J, Seidel G, Schramm M (1978): Intracellular cyclic AMP production enhanced by a hormone receptor transferred from a different cell. J Biol Chem 253:1201-1206.

Seeds N, Gilman A, Amano T, Nirnberg M (1970): Regulation of axon formation by clonal lines of neural tumor. Proc Natl Acad Sci USA 66:160-167.

Taub M, Sato GH (1979): Growth of kidney epithelial cells in hormone-supplemented serum-free medium. J Supramol Struct 11:207-216.

Wang C, Hsueh AJW, Erickson GF (1979): Induction of functional prolactin receptors by follicle stimulating hormone in rat granulosa in vitro and in vivo. J Biol Chem 254:11330-11336.

Weinberger-Ohana P, Farkash Y, Hershkovits N, Goldring N, Epstein-Almog R, Shoshani R, Orly J (1984): Low molecular weight substance from rat ovary induces steroidogenesis in cultured granulosa cells. Mol Cell Endocrinol (in press).

Zeleznik AJ, Midgley AR Jr, Reichert LE Jr (1974): Granulosa cell maturation in the rat: Increased binding of human chorionic gonadotropin following treatment with follicle stimulating hormone in vivo. Endocrinology 95:818-826.

Methods for Serum-Free Culture of Cells of the Endocrine System,
pages 89–104
© 1984 Alan R. Liss, Inc., 150 Fifth Avenue, New York, NY 10011

6
Growth of Rat Mammary Tumor Cells in Serum-Free Hormone-Supplemented Medium

Tamiko Kano-Sueoka

Serum-free defined culture medium has been devised for a number of different cell lines representing widely divergent cell types [Barnes and Sato, 1980; Ham, 1981]. As for mammary carcinoma cells, serum-free media have been developed for human breast carcinoma cell lines [Allegra and Lippman, 1978; Barnes and Sato, 1979], mouse mammary carcinoma lines [Bauer et al., 1976], and a rat mammary carcinoma cell line [Kano-Sueoka et al., 1979b].

In this chapter, we will describe a serum-free medium for a rat mammary carcinoma cell line, 64-24, and also describe the effects of some of the key components of the medium on these cells.

Our purpose of formulating a serum-free medium for the 64-24 cell line was to develop a prolactin-responsive cell culture system. Although these cells were isolated from a prolactin-dependent tumor, they did not show any growth stimulation by prolactin in serum-containing media [Kano-Sueoka and Hsieh, 1973]. As has been suggested by G. Sato and his colleagues [Barnes and Sato, 1979], it is very likely that serum in culture medium either contains hormones that mask the stimulatory effect of added hormones, or contains some agent that interferes with the action of hormones. The medium thus devised can support growth of 64-24 cells and, most importantly, a distinct mitogenic effect of prolactin has been shown in the cells grown in this medium. Moreover, the use of serum-free medium aided in discovering a novel growth-promoting agent, ethanolamine (Etn) or phosphoethanolamine (PEtn), which

Department of Molecular, Cellular, and Developmental Biology, University of Colorado, Boulder, Colorado 80309

stimulates the growth of not only 64-24 cells, but also a number of different cell lines of diverse origin [Kano-Sueoka et al., 1979b; Kano-Sueoka and Errick, 1982]. Since our sole purpose in obtaining a serum-free medium has been to find a condition in which a clear hormone response of the cells can be exhibited, optimization of the medium described below has not been achieved as yet.

CELLS AND THEIR MAINTENANCE

Studies described in this article were carried out mainly with a clonal cell line, 64-24, that was isolated from a transplantable, prolactin-estrogen-dependent rat mammary carcinoma MCCLX of an A × C rat [Kano-Sueoka and Hsieh, 1973]. The cells are of typical secretory epithelial cell morphology and grow as a multi-cell-layer sheet on the plastic surface of tissue culture plates. Under optimum growth conditions their generation time is about 8-9 h. The cells are normally maintained in high-glucose Dulbecco's modified Eagle's medium (DME) with penicillin (50 units/ml), streptomycin (50 μg/ml), 5% (vol/vol) horse serum, and 2.5% (vol/vol) fetal calf serum. This particular cell line does not grow at all or grows poorly in a medium supplemented with calf serum at any concentration. The cells are grown in plastic tissue culture dishes at 37°C in a humidified atmosphere of air containing 5% CO_2 and are subcultured every 4-5 days.

HEPES buffer (15 mM, pH 7.2) was added to the serum-free medium to improve the buffering capacity. Previous to plating the cells in serum-free HEPES buffer-containing medium, it was necessary to adapt the cells to the presence of the buffer. The adaptation took about three subculturings in HEPES- and serum-containing medium. Upon adaptation, the cells maintained their original growth characteristics. When the CO_2 content in the incubator was carefully controlled and the culture dishes were allowed to be out of the incubator for a minimum length of time, we found it unnecessary to have HEPES buffer in the serum-free medium.

MATERIALS

DME and Ham's F12 nutrient mixture were obtained from Gibco (Grand Island, NY) or Flow Laboratories (McLean, VA). All supplements, unless otherwise specified, were obtained from Sigma (St. Louis, MO). Bovine serum albumin (BSA) is Cohn fraction V. Growth-stimulating activity of BSA for 64-24 cells has been variable from lot to lot. Therefore, it is advisable to use the same lot of BSA to obtain reproducible results. Ovine prolactin was obtained from NIAMDD. According to our experience, purity and potency of the NIAMDD prolactin have also been variable. Ovine prolactin NIAMDD-oPRL-14 was used for most of the experiments described in this article. Epidermal growth factor (EGF) was from Collaborative Research (Waltham, MA).

Prolactin (1 mg/ml) was dissolved in 0.01 M $NaHCO_3$ (pH 9.0) and stored at 4°C. The prolactin solution was used within 7 days after preparation. Porcine insulin (1 mg/ml) was dissolved in 0.005 N HCl. Triiodothyronine (T3) (1 μg/ml) was prepared in saline solution with a trace amount of 0.1 N NaOH. Hydrocortisone (10 μg/ml) and 17β-estradiol (1 μg/ml) were dissolved in 95% ethanol. BSA (100 mg/ml) and human transferrin (1 mg/ml) were dissolved in saline. All of the above, except prolactin, were aliquoted and stored at -20°C.

The medium was made by using deionized and further glass-distilled water. Prior to plating the cells in serum-free medium, trypsinized cells (0.025% trypsin with 10^{-3} M EDTA) were treated with serum-free medium containing 0.05% soybean trypsin inhibitor. Although the serum-free medium we used contains 1 mg/ml BSA, trypsin inhibitor considerably improved the survival of the cells after plating.

COMPOSITION OF THE SERUM-FREE MEDIUM

The MCCLX tumor, from which the 64-24 cell line was isolated, has been shown to be prolactin-dependent for growth [Horn and Kano-Sueoka, 1979]. Therefore, we expected 64-24 cells to be growth-responsive to prolactin in culture as well. The cells plated in serum-containing media prepared with serum from various sources, however, did not exhibit any growth stimulation with prolactin [Kano-Sueoka and Hsieh, 1973]. There are two possible explanations of the cells' lack of response to prolactin: 1) The effect of prolactin observed in vivo is not due to the direct action of prolactin, but rather a secondary effect; and 2) the serum-containing medium either contains enough prolactin to support the growth or contains some factor that interferes with the prolactin action. Accordingly, a serum-free medium was devised to test the above possibilities. When 64-24 cells were grown in this medium (the composition shown in Table I), the growth-stimulating activity of prolactin was clearly demonstrated.

A DME/F12 mixture has been used as recommended by Sato and his colleagues (see review by Bottenstein et al. [1979]; see also Barnes and Sato [1980]). Indeed, when used with the hormone mixture as listed in Table I, DME/F12 is better in supporting the growth of 64-24 cells than DME alone,

TABLE I. Composition of Serum-Free Medium

DME/F12	1:1
HEPES buffer, pH 7.2	15 mM
Penicillin	50 units/ml
Streptomycin	50 μg/ml
Porcine insulin	5 μg/ml
Hydrocortisone	0.1 μg/ml
Triiodothyronine	10^{-10} M
17β-Estradiol	10^{-8} M
Human transferrin	5 μg/ml
Bovine serum albumin	1 mg/ml
Ovine prolactin	1 μg/ml

as shown in Figure 1. In most experiments the generation time in this serum-free medium was almost two times longer than that in a serum-containing medium, and the plating efficiency also was poorer in serum-free conditions than in serum-containing medium. In this regard, we found that when serum-free medium was used, the plating efficiency varied considerably depending on which brand of plastic dishes the cells were plated in. For example, a lot of Lux plastic dishes gave better and more consistent plating efficiency than a lot of Falcon plastic dishes. Therefore, one should be aware that the plating efficiency may improve just by selecting the right kind of plastic plate in which to seed the cells in a serum-free medium.

GROWTH-PROMOTING EFFECT OF PROLACTIN

Involvement of prolactin in the proliferation of many rodent mammary carcinomas has clearly been indicated [Welsch and Nagasawa, 1977; Welsch and Meites, 1978]. Using a clonal cell line of a rat mammary carcinoma grown in a serum-free medium, we were also able to demonstrate a clear mitogenic effect of prolactin. As shown in Figure 2, amounts of ovine prolactin varying from 50 ng to 5 μg/ml are equally growth-stimulating. In another experiment, even 30 ng/ml prolactin was shown to be clearly growth-stimulating (data not shown). These concentrations of prolactin are normal circulating levels in female animals. The parent tumor in vivo is absolutely dependent on prolactin to grow. However, prolactin is not obligatory for growth of the isolated cells, as can be seen in Figure 2.

The degree of purity of hormones or growth factors has to be considered important, since many growth-promoting factors can be active at very low concentrations, in the range of 1 or 2 ng/ml or even less. Thus, even if a given hormone is contaminated by a potent growth factor at one-thousandth

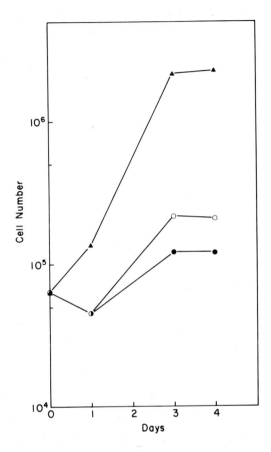

Fig. 1. Effects of different media on cell growth. 64-24 cells (6.4×10^4) were plated in duplicate in a 60-mm × 10-mm plate with various media. The number of cells was determined 1, 3, and 4 days after plating by releasing the cells with trypsin and counting in a Coulter counter. The media tested were DME supplemented with 10% horse and 2.5% fetal calf serum (▲); the serum-free medium described in Table I (○); and essentially the same serum-free medium except that only DME was used instead of the DME/F12 mixture (●).

of the hormone level, 1 μg/ml of the hormone should contain enough contaminant to show an effect. The ovine prolactin preparation we have used (NIAMDD-oPRL-14) for the above experiment is relatively pure. Sodium dodecylsulfate-acrylamide gel electrophoresis (SDS-PAGE) of the prolactin preparation up to 40 μg gave distinctly a single protein band corresponding to the molecular weight of prolactin. Since our limit in detecting a distinct protein band was about 0.1 μg, it is possible that the prolactin preparation provided

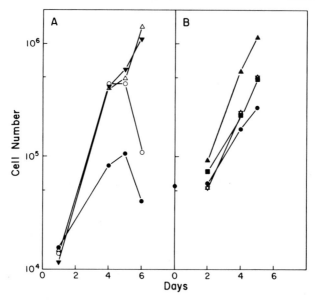

Fig. 2. The growth-promoting effect of ovine prolactin on 64-24 cells was examined in the serum-free medium with varied concentrations of prolactin. For the experiment shown in panel A, 5.4×10^4 cells per plate were plated and for the experiment in panel B, 5.5×10^4 cells per plate were plated in duplicate. The doses of prolactin tested were as follows: no prolactin (●); 0.05 μg/ml (✿); 0.1 μg/ml (○); 0.3 μg/ml (▼); 1 μg/ml (△); and 5 μg/ml (■). The growth of cells in a serum-containing medium (5% horse and 2.5% fetal calf serum) was also included as a comparison (▲).

some protein contaminant at 2.5 ng/ml or less when the medium contained 1 μg/ml prolactin. However, since 50 ng/ml prolactin was clearly mitogenic, we can conclude rather safely that the growth-promoting activity we observed was due to prolactin per se. The possibility of having a low molecular-weight contaminant with growth-promoting activity was also eliminated by examining extensively dialyzed prolactin preparations [Kano-Sueoka and Errick, 1982]. Prolactin has been known to be contaminated with vasopressin [Waters, 1977], which is growth-stimulating to 3T3 cells [Rosengurt et al., 1979]. Also, as shown in Figure 2, prolactin seems to affect the growth rate rather than the plating efficiency.

The growth response of 64-24 cells to prolactin is not always reproducible. Possible reasons for this are as follows. First, nonreproducibility may result from the state of the cells before prolactin is given. This seems not to be the case, since whether the cells were previously grown in the serum-free medium with or without 1 μg/ml prolactin or in a medium containing serum, we obtained similar degrees of nonreproducibility. Second, the plating density of the cells may cause the variability, since the cells may carry a certain amount of prolactin or some other factors that affect prolactin action. However, a tenfold different plating density (6×10^3 to 6×10^4 cells per plate) does not systematically influence the prolactin effect. Third, washing of the cells before plating may have been variable. However, systematic washings of the cells did not yield reproducible results either. Irrespective of the fact that maintenance of the cells, preparations of hormones and medium, and plating of the cells have been carried out with the utmost care to reproduce the same conditions, there seems to be an element or elements which is unknown to us that affects the ability of the cells to respond to prolactin. In contrast to prolactin the cells always respond to insulin and most other hormones in a reproducible manner.

GROWTH-PROMOTING EFFECT OF ETHANOLAMINE AND PHOSPHOETHANOLAMINE

Bovine pituitary extract contained a potent growth-promoting activity to 64-24 cells [Kano-Sueoka et al., 1979b]. The active material was purified and identified as phosphoethanolamine (PEtn) [Kano-Sueoka et al., 1979a]. Subsequently, ethanolamine (Etn) was found to be an equally potent growth-stimulator [Kano-Sueoka and Errick, 1981]. Originally, this discovery was made by using the cells grown in a medium (DME) containing 5-10% calf serum. In this medium Etn or PEtn was required for growth of 64-24 cells. These agents are also growth-stimulating to 64-24 cells when tested in a serum-free medium. As has been shown in Figures 1 and 2, the cells can grow without Etn or PEtn, but at a slower rate, at least in the first cycle of growth in a serum-free medium. The magnitude of growth stimulation by Etn gets larger as subculturing of the cells is repeated in the serum-free medium. Figure 3 shows an example of the growth-promoting effect of Etn in the serum-free medium. A $0.1~\mu M$ concentration of Etn is quite effective and, in this particular experiment, this concentration exerts the maximum growth stimulation. Concentrations higher than 5-10 μM are often growth-inhibitory.

Commercially available cell culture media such as Eagle's medium, modified Eagle's media, RPMI media, or Ham's nutrient mixtures contain all polar head groups of major phospholipids, choline, inositol, and serine, but not Etn, which is a structural component of the second most abundant phospholipid, phosphatidylethanolamine. Obviously, when serum-supplemented medium was used, none of the cells needed the supplement of Etn to grow. Since our discovery, serum-free medium for many types of cells, particularly

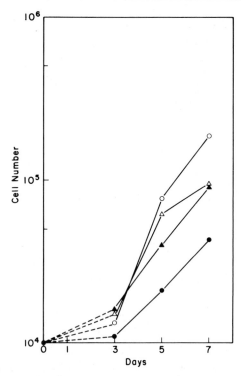

Fig. 3. Growth-promoting effect of Etn. 64-24 cells (10^4 cells per plate) were plated in duplicate in serum-free medium with various amounts of Etn, but without prolactin. Cells were counted 3, 5, and 7 days after plating. No Etn (●); 0.1 μM Etn (○); 1 μM Etn (▲); and 5 μM Etn (△).

epithelial cells, have been shown to include Etn as a necessary component. A compilation of cell lines that are responsive and nonresponsive to Etn is given in Table II (this may not be exhaustive).

Mouse plasmacytoma cells and hybridoma cells (hybrid between mouse plasmacytoma and mouse or rat splenocytes) require Etn to grow continuously in a serum-free medium [Murakami et al., 1982]. Human epidermal keratinocytes and lung and bronchial epithelial cells also require Etn to grow optimally [Tsao et al., 1982; Lechner et al., 1982; Minna et al., 1982]. As for the Etn response of rat mammary carcinoma cells (other than the 64-24 cell), WRK-1 cells and 22-1 cells [Kano-Sueoka and Hsieh, 1973] were unresponsive, whereas growth of MTW9 cells was stimulated by Etn (D. Sirbasku, personal communication). Among several human breast carcinoma cells so far tested in my laboratory, only the T-47D line was found to be responsive

TABLE II. Growth Response to Etn and PEtn

Etn-responsive cell types
  Normal rat mammary epithelial cells
  Rat mammary carcinoma cell lines (64-24, MTW9/PL)
  Human breast carcinoma cell lines (T-47D)
  Human epidermal keratinocytes
  Human bronchial epithelial cells
  Human small lung carcinoma cells
  Mouse hybridomas
  Mouse plasmacytomas

Etn-nonresponsive cell types
  Rat mammary carcinoma cell lines (22-1, WRK-1)
  Human breast carcinoma cell lines (MCF-7, MDA-MB-231,
    Hs0578T)
  Human breast cell line (HBL-100)
  Mouse fibroblast cell line (3T3)
  Chinese hamster fibroblast cell line (V9)
  Rat neuronal tumor cell lines (RT4 family)
  Rat glial tumor cell line (RT4-D)

[Kano-Sueoka and Errick, 1982]. Therefore, mammary carcinoma cells in general seem to fall into responsive and nonresponsive types. Furthermore, there seems to be a correlation between the Etn responsiveness of a given mammary cell line and its hormone responsiveness. If a given mammary carcinoma cell type grows poorly in a serum-free medium, the effect of Etn should definitely be tested.

Compared to other Etn-responsive cell types, 64-24 cells seem to have lower optimum concentrations for Etn (20 μM for keratinocytes or hybridoma vs. 1–5 μM for 64-24 cells). Since higher concentrations of Etn ($> 10~\mu$M) are growth-inhibiting to the 64-24 cell, a wide range of Etn concentrations should be tested when a new cell line is examined. Another fact to be pointed out is that Etn and PEtn are equally effective on 64-24 cells, but Etn is far more effective than PEtn on hybridoma cells.

GROWTH-PROMOTING EFFECT OF BOVINE SERUM ALBUMIN

BSA is one of the essential components of 64-24 cells' serum-free medium. Serum albumin is known to carry fatty acids. Beside fatty acids, BSA preparations (Cohn fraction V) contain various protein contaminants, as indicated by SDS-acrylamide gel electrophoresis (unpublished observations). Therefore, BSA may be supplying essential fatty acids or some unknown protein factors to 64-24 cells. Furthermore, since the growth-promoting activity of BSA varies in different batches, it is more likely that something other than BSA itself is growth-stimulating.

Since growth of dimethylbenzanthracine-induced (DMBA-induced) tumor cells in culture was found to be stimulated by unsaturated fatty acids such as oleic acid or linoleic acid [Wicha et al., 1979], we tested whether the requirement for BSA by 64-24 cells is due to fatty acids included in BSA preparations. Fatty acids were removed from BSA by charcoal treatment at low pH according to the method described by Chen [1967]. When the serum-free medium contained 1 mg/ml of the delipidized BSA, the number of cells obtained after 4 days growth was significantly reduced compared to that grown with untreated BSA. Delipidized BSA was then reassociated with known amounts of known unsaturated fatty acids [Spector and Hoak, 1969], and their growth-promoting effect was tested. The fatty acid-conjugated BSA and delipidized BSA were mixed to yield a desired amount of fatty acid per mg of BSA before being added to the medium. As shown in Table III, 0.1–5 μg/ml oleic acid or linoleic acid showed a significant growth-stimulating activity. Moreover, growth attained by adding reconjugated BSA was near that of untreated BSA. These results suggest strongly that the supply of one or more unsaturated fatty acids is important in growth of 64-24 cells, and the growth-promoting effect of BSA is largely due to the undefined amount and kind of fatty acids bound to BSA.

As mentioned above, BSA contains a considerable amount of contaminating proteins, some of which may possess growth-promoting or growth-inhibiting activity. Recently, Yamane and Kan [1982] sucessfully used α-cyclodextrin as a vehicle to carry fatty acids in place of BSA. Liposomes are another way to carry fatty acids [Hosick, 1979]. However, phospholipids that are constituents of liposomes might obscure the effect of fatty acids, since the cells can take up phospholipids and utilize them.

TABLE III. Growth-Promoting Effect of Fatty Acids (number of cells per plate × 10^{-5})

	Untreated BSA	Delipidized BSA with fatty acid (μg/ml)				
		0	0.1	1.0	3.0	5.0
Oleic acid	2.3	0.5	1.4	1.2	—	2.1
Linoleic acid	3.0	2.2	3.3	3.3	3.6	2.8

BSA concentration was adjusted to 1 mg/ml with delipidized BSA. Fatty acid concentration was estimated on the assumption that the efficiency of association of free fatty acid and BSA was 100%. Cells (6 × 10^4)were plated in duplicate in serum-free medium and the number of cells was determined 4 days later.

GROWTH-PROMOTING EFFECT OF OTHER HORMONES AND GROWTH FACTORS

The serum-free medium (Table I) with 2.5 μM Etn is sufficient to support growth of 64-24 cells with a generation time of 14-15 h. In order to improve the medium further and also to examine the effect on 64-24 cells, additional growth factors known to stimulate mammary cells have been tested in the serum-free medium as described below.

Epidermal Growth Factor (EGF)

EGF is known to stimulate growth of many epithelial cells. Indeed, EGF has been shown to be growth-stimulating to human breast epithelial cells when the cells were plated with feeder cells [Stoker et al., 1976]. Growth of secondary cultures of DMBA-induced rat mammary carcinoma is stimulated by EGF [Rudland et al., 1977]. EGF (TC grade, obtained from Collaborative Research, Waltham, MA) has also shown to stimulate growth in 64-24 cells in the serum-free medium. As shown in Figure 4, at 1 ng/ml the activity of EGF reached a plateau when the regular serum-free medium (without Etn) was used. When the concentration of insulin was reduced to 1/10 the regular amount (i.e. 0.5 μg/ml), the stimulatory activity of EGF plateaued at 5 ng/ml. Concentrations of EGF higher than 20 ng/ml were often growth-inhibitory to 64-24 cells.

Cholera Toxin (CT)

CT raises intracellular cAMP levels [Green, 1978] and a growth-promoting effect of CT on normal human mammary epithelial cells has clearly been shown [Taylor-Papadimitriou et al., 1980]. However, neoplastic mammary cells seem to respond variably to CT [Yang et al., 1980]. CT (obtained from Sigma) is growth-stimulatory to 64-24 cells. When DME/F12 medium was

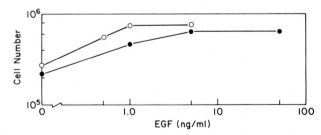

Fig. 4. Growth-promoting effect of EGF. Cells (1×10^5) were plated in duplicate in serum-free medium with various amounts of EGF. Number of cells was determined 4 days after plating. Standard serum-free medium ($\bigcirc$); serum-free medium containing 1/10 the standard amount of insulin ($\bullet$).

supplemented with 5 μg/ml insulin, 5 μg/ml transferrin, and 1 mg/ml BSA, 1-10 ng/ml CT caused a 1.5-fold to threefold increase in cell number after 5 days growth. Prolactin and CT have also shown synergistic effects. The effect of CT in the regular serum-free medium has not been tested.

Other Factors Tested With No Effect

Human cold insoluble globulin does not seem to improve plating efficiency or growth rate of 64-24 cells in serum-free medium. Vasopressin and prostaglandin, F2α and E1 did not have any growth-stimulating activity within the concentrations tested.

SUMMARY AND DISCUSSION

This chapter has described a serum-free hormone-supplemented medium for a rat mammary carcinoma cell line, 64-24. It is composed of the ingredients shown in Table I plus 2.5 μM Etn. We have not included EGF or CT in routine culture. Also described are the growth-promoting effects of key factors included in the medium. As mentioned previously, the medium we formulated has not been ideally optimized. However, the cells grow reasonably well in this medium with a cellular morphology similar to that in a serum-containing medium. The serum-free medium, as it is, therefore can be useful for many studies.

Insulin is the most important hormone for growth of 64-24 cells as in many examples of serum-free growth of various cell types. The most important finding in our study was that 64-24 cells are prolactin-responsive in this medium, a phenomenon not to be seen in serum-containing medium. Although the role of prolactin on induction and proliferation of human breast tumors has not been clearly demonstrated, the crucial role of this hormone in development of mammary carcinoma in rodents has been well established [Welsch and Nagasawa, 1977; Welsch and Meites, 1978]. This is, then, a good model system for studying prolactin action on mammary tumor cells under controlled conditions. For example, there is a question regarding prolactin receptors in 64-24 cells. These cells possess a rather limited number of prolactin-binding sites when the binding assay is carried out with the cells grown in fetal calf serum-containing medium (R. Shiu, personal communications). It would be of interest to determine if prolactin receptors are induced in response to prolactin, and, if so, whether there is any correlation between the growth rate of the cells and the number of prolactin-binding sites per cell.

The necessity of Etn for growth of 64-24 cells in culture was first discovered when cells grown in serum-containing medium were used. Subsequently, Etn was also shown to be necessary to achieve an optimum growth in the serum-free medium. Our surveys of various cell lines of diverse origin, as well as the compositions of serum-free media for various cell lines recently published by other investigators, indicate that the requirement of Etn by 64-24 cells is not a peculiar exception, but rather a widely distributed phenomenon, and therefore the cells can be classified as either Etn-responsive or Etn-nonresponsive. Both types include normal and neoplastic cells. Rat mammary carcinoma cells seem to be classified in two types, also. It will be interesting to find out why some cells require Etn to grow optimally. A sufficient amount of Etn is certainly circulated in the blood to support the growth of Etn-responsive cells. These cells must utilize circulating Etn to synthesize sufficient amounts of phosphatidylethanolamine to support growth, while others seem to be capable of synthesizing de novo the necessary amount of phosphatidylethanolamine [Kano-Sueoka and Errick, 1982].

It now seems certain that fatty acids, such as oleic acid or linoleic acid, are important for growth of rat mammary carcinoma cells in general. Moreover, involvement of prolactin in selective uptake of fatty acids has been indicated [Kidwell et al., 1982]. Since 64-24 cells grown in serum-free medium are both prolactin- and fatty acid-responsive, studies on interrelations between prolactin and fatty acids can be facilitated.

The parent tumor of 64-24 cells produces milk components in a hormone-dependent manner [Horn and Kano-Sueoka, 1979]. And 64-24 cells produce a considerable amount of triglycerides accumulated in the form of fat droplets under certain growth conditions [Kano-Sueoka et al., 1979b]. Differentiating mammary epithelial cells contain a large number of such fat droplets. Hormonal control of milk fat synthesis and accumulation can now be studied under defined conditions. These cells do not produce a measureable amount of α-lactalbumin, as determined by radioimmunoassay. This may be because the ability of these cells to produce α-lactalbumin may have been lost permanently in the process of establishing the clonal cell line or because the culture conditions currently employed may not be suitable for 64-24 cells to produce α-lactalbumin. These possibilities can be examined. The parent tumor cells, which are transplantable, do not have a basement membrane typical of normal mammary epithelial cells or primary tumors (W. Kidwell, personal communications), and yet they are able to grow and differentiate in a hormone-dependent manner. This is then a hormone-responsive differentiating system less complicated than the normal situations. The possible requirement of cell-cell interactions, tertiary structures of cells, or hormonal activity can be studied by combining the use of serum-free medium and collagen gel matrix or suspension culture conditions.

Clonal growth of 64-24 cells has also been attained in a serum-free medium (B. Van der Haegen and R. G. Ham, personal communications). This medium consists of MCDB 202 [Ham and McKeehan, 1978] with 10 μg/ml insulin, 10 ng/ml EGF, 1 μg/ml hydrocortisone, 5 μg/ml prolactin, and 10.26 μg/ml of a lipid mixture in the form of liposomes (58.47% soybean lecithin, 29.23% cholesterol, 9.74% sphingomyelin, 1.94% vitamin E, and 0.58% vitamin acetate). The growth rate of 64-24 cells in the MCDB 202-hormone-supplemented medium has not been compared to that in the serum-free medium used in our laboratory, however.

ACKNOWLEDGMENTS

The author is grateful to Dorothy Cohen for technical assistance and to Beverly Rice for carrying out experiments on the effects of bovine serum albumin and fatty acids. Data shown in Figure 2 were also obtained by Beverly Rice. This work was supported by grants from the American Cancer Society (BC-178) and National Science Foundation (PCM-8104480).

REFERENCES

Allegra JC, Lippman ME (1978): Growth of a human breast cancer cell line in serum-free hormone-supplemented medium. Cancer Res 38:3823–3829.

Barnes D, Sato G (1979): Growth of a human mammary tumor cell line in a serum-free medium. Nature 281:388–389.

Barnes D, Sato G (1980): Methods for growth of cultured cells in serum-free medium. Anal Biochem 102:255–270.

Bauer RF, Arthur LO, Fine DL (1976): Propagation of mouse mammary tumor cell lines and production of mouse mammary tumor virus in a serum-free medium. In Vitro 12:558–563.

Bottenstein, J, Hayashi I, Hutchings S, Masui H, Mather J, McClure DB, Ohasa S, Rizzino A, Sato G, Serrero G, Wolfe R, Wu R (1979): The growth of cells in serum-free hormone-supplemented media. Methods Enzymol 58:94–109.

Chen RF (1967): Removal of fatty acids from serum albumin by charcoal treatment. J Biol Chem 242:173–181.

Green H (1978): Cyclic AMP in relation to proliferation of the epidermal cell, a new view. Cell 15:801–811.

Ham RG (1981): Survival and growth requirements of nontransformed cells. In Baserga R (ed): "Handbook of Experimental Pharmacology." New York: Springer-Verlag, Vol 57, pp 13–88.

Ham RG, McKeehan WL (1978): Nutritional requirements for clonal growth of non-transformed cells. In Katsuta H (ed): "Nutritional Requirements of Cultured Cells." Tokyo: Jpn Sci Soc Press, pp 63–115.

Horn TM, Kano-Sueoka T (1979): Effects of hormones on growth and α-lactalbumin activity in the transplantable rat mammary tumor MCCLX. Cancer Res 39:5028–5035.

Hosick HL (1979): Uptake and utilization of free fatty acids supplied by liposomes to mammary tumor cells in culture. Exp Cell Res 122:127-136.

Kano-Sueoka T, Errick JE (1981): Effects of phosphoethanolamine and ethanolamine on growth of mammary carcinoma cells in culture. J Exp Cell Res 136:137-145.

Kano-Sueoka T, Errick JE (1982): Roles of phosphoethanolamine, ethanolamine, and prolactin on mammary cell growth. Cold Spring Harbor Conf Cell Prolif 9:729-740.

Kano-Sueoka T, Hsieh P (1973): A rat mammary carcinoma in vivo and in vitro: Establishment of clonal lines of the tumor. Proc Natl Acad Sci USA 70:1922-1926.

Kano-Sueoka T, Cohen DM, Yamaizumi Z, Nishimura S, Mori M, Fujiki H (1979a): Phosphoethanolamine as a growth factor of a mammary carcinoma cell line of rat. Proc Natl Acad Sci USA 76:5741-5744.

Kano-Sueoka T, Errick JE, Cohen DM (1979b): Effects of hormones and a novel mammary growth factor on a rat mammary carcinoma in culture. Cold Spring Harbor Conf Cell Prolif 6:499-512.

Kidwell WR, Knazek RA, Vonderhaar BK, Losonczy I (1982): Effects of unsaturated fatty acids on the development and proliferation of normal and neoplastic breast epithelium. In Arnott MS, Van Iys J, Wang YM (eds): "Molecular Interrelations in Nutrition in Cancer." New York: Raven, pp 219-236.

Lechner JF, Haugen A, McClendon IA, Pettis EW (1982): Clonal growth of normal adult human bronchial epithelial cells in a serum-free medium. In Vitro 18:633-642.

Minna JD, Carney DN, Oie H, Bunn PA Jr, Gazdar AF (1982): Growth of human small-cell lung cancer in defined medium. Cold Spring Harbor Conf Cell Prolif 9:627-639.

Murakami H, Masui H, Sato GH, Sueoka N, Chow TP, Kano-Sueoka T (1982): Growth of hybridoma cells in serum-free medium: Ethanolamine is an essential component. Proc Natl Acad Sci USA 79:1158-1162.

Rosengurt E, Legg A, Pettican P (1979): Vasopressin stimulation of mouse 3T3 cell growth. Proc Natl Acad Sci USA 76:1284-1287.

Rudland PS, Hallowes RC, Durbin H, Lewis D (1977): Mitogenic activity of pituitary hormones on cell cultures of normal and carcinogen-induced tumor epithelium from rat mammary gland. J Cell Biol 73:561-577.

Spector AA, Hoak JC (1969): An improved method for the addition of long-chain free fatty acid to protein solutions. Anal Biochem 32:297-302.

Stoker MWP, Pigotte D, Taylor-Papadimitriou J (1976): Response to epidermal growth factors of cultured human mammary epithelial cells from benign tumours. Nature 264:764-767.

Taylor-Papadimitriou J, Purkis P, Fentiman IS (1980): Cholera toxin and analogues of cyclic AMP stimulate the growth of cultured human mammary epithelial cells. J Cell Physiol 102:317-321.

Tsao MC, Walthall BJ, Ham RG (1982): Clonal growth of normal human epidermal keratinocytes in a defined medium. J Cell Physiol 110:219-229.

Waters AK (1977): Augmentation of vasopressin antidiuresis by prolactin with a note on the contamination of international standard prolactin. J Endocrinol 75:435-436.

Welsch CW, Meites J (1978): Prolactin and mammary carcinogenesis. In Sharma RK, Criss WE (eds): "Endocrine Control in Neoplasia." New York: Raven, pp 71-92.

Welsch CW, Nagasawa H (1977): Prolactin and murine mammary tumorigenesis: A review. Cancer Res 37:951-963.

Wicha MS, Liotta LA, Kidwell WR (1979): Effects of free fatty acids on the growth of normal and neoplastic rat mammary epithelial cells. Cancer Res 39:426-435.

Yamane I, Kan M (1982): A novel substitute (α-cyclodextrin included with oleic and linoleic acids) for bovine serum albumin in serum-free culture of mammalian cells. In Vitro 18:306-307 (abstract).

Yang J, Guzman R, Richard J, Imagawa W, McCormick K, Nandi S (1980): Growth factor- and cyclic nucleotide-induced proliferation of normal and malignant mammary epithelial cells in primary culture. Endocrinology 107:35-41.

Methods for Serum-Free Culture of Cells of the Endocrine System,
pages 105–125

7
Growth of Normal Mammary Epithelium on Collagen in Serum-Free Medium

William R. Kidwell, Mozeena Bano, and David S. Salomon

Although it has long been recognized that the mammary glandular epithe-lium is completely encased and partitioned from the mammary stroma by a thin layer of matrix material called the basal lamina or basement membrane, it has only recently been recognized that this material is made by the mammary epithelium and in fact appears to be important for the growth and survival of the epithelium [Liotta et al., 1980; Wicha et al., 1979a, 1980].

Our progress in understanding the role of the basal lamina has increased exponentially as a result of the successful separation and identification of the major components of this biological scaffolding. Although it is not yet clear how these components are associated one with another, the major substances of the basal lamina are type IV collagen [Timpl et al., 1978], laminin [Timpl et al., 1979], and heparan sulfate proteoglycan [Hassell et al., 1980]. In cultured mammary epithelium, synthesis of these components has been dem-onstrated [Liotta et al., 1980; Kidwell et al., 1982a, 1982b].

The importance of the lamina in growth and survival of the epithelium has been inferred from the fact that synthesis of one of the components of the lamina, type IV collagen, can be selectively blocked by culturing cells in media containing a proline analog such as cis-hydroxyproline. Cis-hydroxyproline is incorporated into collagen (which is very proline-rich) with a consequent formation of faculty protein, which cannot form a triple helix, thus rendering the protein much more subject to degradation in the cell [Uitto and Prockop,

Laboratory of Pathophysiology (W.R.K., M.B.) and Laboratory of Tumor Immunology and Biology (D.S.S.), National Cancer Institute, National Institutes of Health, Bethesda, Maryland 20205

1977]. Utilizing this analog as well as the four-membered ring analog L-azetidine-5-carboxylate, 3,4-dehydroproline, and 4-thioproline—all selective inhibitors of collagen synthesis—we have shown that blocking formation of a complete lamina causes the death of the mammary epithelium both in vivo and in vitro [Wicha et al., 1980; Lewko et al., 1981; Kidwell et al., 1980a]. In the case of normal mammary epithelium, it appears that synthesis of collagen is important for mammary cell survival since cultured mammary epithelium is selectively rescued from the toxic effects of cis-hydroxyproline if the cells are plated on type IV collagen, the collagen species these cells synthesize. Such a rescue is not produced by plating the cells on stromal collagen, the collagen made by fibroblasts [Wicha, 1979a].

In this chapter we will detail some of these experiments and additionally, utilizing the production of type IV collagen as an index of basement membrane production, show that almost all growth factors that stimulate mammary cell division also differentially stimulate basal lamina biosynthesis or prevent its turnover. The results of these studies conducted in serum-free medium allow an unequivocable identification of a variety of factors that can amplify basement membrane collagen synthesis. But more importantly, these studies allow us to conclude that for mammary cells production of basement membrane is intimately tied to the cells' response to growth factors.

ISOLATION OF MAMMARY EPITHELIUM

The mammary gland is composed of a tree of mammary epithelium that is imbedded in stroma consisting of bundles of collagen fibers, glycosaminoglycans, fibronectin, etc.—components synthesized by the stromal cells. These elements, including the stromal cells, surround the epithelial tree, which is separated from the stroma by a narrow, continuous layer—the basement membrane. Some of the components of the basal lamina have been isolated and characterized and include type IV collagen [Timpl et al., 1978], laminin [Timpl et al., 1979], and sulfated proteoglycan [Hassell et al., 1980]. The basal lamina is in fact produced by the epithelium, a finding that has been demonstrated from in vitro studies, as indicated earlier. Within the mammary tree there are two easily recognized cell types, the epithelial cells and the myoepithelial cells. The tree is itself composed of a series of ducts that decrease in size as a function of distance from the nipple. The ducts terminate in morphologically distinct structures depending on the state of differentiation of the gland. In very immature rats the termination is the so-called terminal end bud, which is a multilayered cuboidal epithelial cell population and scanty myoepithelial cells, primarily seen at the junction of the terminal end bud and the proximal duct. The terminal end bud, like the ducts and alveoli of a more developed gland, appears to be encapsulated by a basal lamina. Terminal end buds appear to be the precursors of alveolar buds and ultimately of mature alveoli [Russo and Russo, 1978]. The latter two structures along with the ductal tree are the most prominent components of the epithelium following puberty in rats. Both the alveolar buds and alveoli consist of myoepithelial cells and epithelial cells in rats and humans, but the former cell type is less abundant in these structures in mice. Usually the alveoli and alveolar buds consist of no more than one or two cell layers, a single layer of epithelial cells either directly lying on the basal lamina or separated from it by a single layer of myoepithelial cells. The major morphological difference between ducts and alveoli is that the epithelial cells are completely separated from the basal lamina by the myoepithelial cell layer. There are reports of different types of epithelial cells within the alveoli and also of differences between the epithelial population of ducts and alveoli, but these differences are not considered in the present report.

The typical isolation procedure for ducts and alveoli is as follows. Sprague Dawley rats (3 months old) are administered perphenazine to initiate glandular proliferation in vivo following the procedure outlined by Rudland et al. [1977], as adapted from Ben-David [1968]. A 0.2-mg amount of the drug is given subcutaneously at 29 and 3 h before animals are sacrificed. This markedly improves the yield of alveolar structures. The inguinal glands are removed from the animals aseptically and gently minced with scissors. Minced tissue is resuspended in 10 ml collagenase solution and the suspension is added to a 50-ml Erlenmeyer flask. The tissue from one rat per flask is digested efficiently by incubation for 1 h at 37°C, followed by a further incubation for 10 min after the addition of 100 μl of DNase I solution per flask. During the incubation with collagenase solution but not during the incubation with DNase solution, the tissue digest is gently agitated with a magnetic stirring bar. Vigorous agitation results in extensive damage to the alveolar and ductal elements that are liberated by the digestion procedure. Following the DNase I digestion step, the digest is filtered through sterile Nitex filters with a pore size of 530 μm. This removes any undigested pieces of tissue that do not pass through the filters. The filtrate contains single cells and ductal and alveolar structures. The latter are conveniently isolated from the single cells by sedimentation through Ficoll gradients [Wicha et al., 1981] or by selective filtration through Nitex filters of the appropriate pore size. Both methods will be described.

The filtrate from the 530 μm filter is centrifuged at 500g and the pellet is recovered and resuspended in 10 ml washing solution and recentrifuged. The

resultant pellet is resuspended in layering solution (5 ml per rat tissue equivalent) and this material is gently layered on a linear gradient of 2–10% Ficoll
that has been solubilized in Earle's balanced salt solution and sterilized by
autoclaving for 6 min. (Longer autoclaving times should be avoided since the
Ficoll tends to decompose, giving rise to toxic substances that kill cells.) The
linear gradients are generated from 42.5 ml each of 2% and 10% Ficoll
solution introduced into 100-ml tubes (3.5 cm × 15.5 cm) into which a 5-ml
cushion of 20% Ficoll has been added. The centrifuge tubes and gradient-
generating device are sterilized in 70% ethanol for 0.5 h. The alcohol solution
is then decanted and the residual alcohol is allowed to evaporate off in a
laminar flow hood. Sedimentation of the ducts and alveoli is performed by
centrifugation for 5 min at 500 rpm in a Sorvall centrifuge, HL8 head, after
the rotor is gradually brought up to speed. The rotor is then allowed to slow
down with the brake off. The ducts and alveoli are recovered in the lower
one-third of the gradient. This portion of the gradient is collected and diluted
with four volumes of Earle's balanced salt solution, and this solution is centrifuged for 5 min at 2,000g to pellet the organoids. These structures are
recovered and resuspended in growth medium and are ready for plating.
Electron micrograph analysis shows the organoids to have survived the isolation procedures with a maintenance of organized structure comparable to that
in the intact gland (Fig. 1).

An alternate procedure for the recovery of ducts and alveoli that works
very well for rat, mouse, and human mammary glandular digests is selective
filtration through Nitex membranes. The procedure is based on techniques
described by Hallowes [Stampfer et al., 1980]. Tissue digests prepared as
described are filtered through 530-μm filters that are sandwiched between two
aluminum sheets each of which has a 5-cm hole cut out of the center.
Organoids pass through this filter and are subsequently collected free of single
cells by passing the filtrate through a second filter sandwich into which a Nitex
filter with a pore size of 60 μm is placed. The organoids are retained by the
filter and can be recovered by inverting the filter and washing. For best results
one filter should be used for each gram of tissue processed. It may be
necessary to repeat filtration for elimination of all single cells.

The digestion and wash solutions needed for the above isolation procedure
are outlined below.

Wash solution: 2% fetal calf serum in Earle's balanced salt solution. Sterilization by filtration through 0.2-μm filters.

Collagenase digestion solution: 1.25 ml fetal calf serum plus 23.5 ml
Medium 199 containing 85 mg collagenase and 25 μl Gentamycin. The
collagenase required for a successful preparation is critical. Best results have

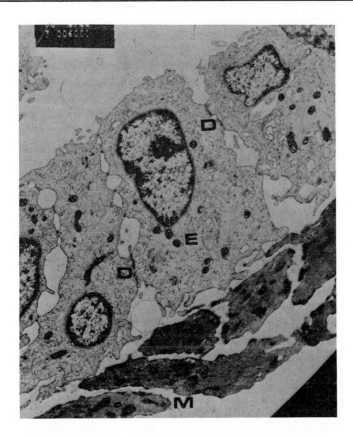

Fig. 1. Electron microscopic appearance of isolated mammary organoids. Organoids were isolated by the Ficoll gradient method. Reproduced from Wicha et al. [1979b], with permission.

been obtained with type II collagenase from Worthington with a specific activity of 160 units per mg or higher. It is best to obtain small amounts of various enzyme preparations and test them for suitability and then purchase a large supply of enzyme that gives good yield. The collagenase solution is sterilized by filtration.

DNase solution: 10,000 units DNase I per ml of Earle's balanced salt solution containing 1% bovine serum albumin. Sterilize by filtration. Can be stored frozen without loss of activity.

Ficoll gradient solutions: 20% Ficoll is made by dissolving the commercial product (Ficoll 400, Pharmacia) at 20 g per 100 ml final solution in Earle's balanced salt solution. The solution is autoclaved for 6 min at 250°C and any water lost during this step is replaced by adding sterile, distilled water. The 2% and 10% Ficoll solutions are prepared by dilution of the 20% stock solution with Earle's balanced salt solution.

Layering solution: Combine 2 ml fetal calf serum plus 1 ml 20% Ficoll solution and 17 ml Earle's balanced salt solution.

As indicated earlier, the viability of the epithelial cells in the isolated organoids is dramatically reduced by dissociating them into single cells. For purposes of determining plating efficiencies, however, an aliquot can be digested with trypsin and counted. Although the single cells exclude trypan blue, the plating efficiency of such cells, even on type IV collagen-coated dishes, is only 5% compared to the 90% plating efficiency of cells plated as organoids on the same substratum.

ISOLATION AND PURIFICATION OF VARIOUS COLLAGEN TYPES

We have utilized techniques and tissue sources thoroughly described by other investigators for the purification of types I, II, III, and IV collagen. Consequently, we will only briefly describe the procedures here.

Type I Collagen

Type I collagen is made by various stromal cells and is readily purified from the skin of young adult rats as demonstrated by Bornstein and Piez [1966]. Recovery of collagen from tissues or cells is greatly facilitated by administration of a lathrogen such as β-aminoproprionitrile, which blocks the generation of collagen cross-links. Following lathrogen treatment, the skin of rats is removed and extensively extracted with 1 M NaCl in 50 mM Tris-HCl, pH 7.5. (We included the protease inhibitors, phenyl methyl sulfonyl fluoride and N-ethyl-maleimide at 50 μg/ml to limit proteolysis.) The collagen in the extract is then precipitated by adjusting the extract, clarified by centrifugation, to 20% NaCl, and after dialysis this precipitate is heat-denatured or acid-denatured to separate the various collagen α_1- and α_2-chains from the triple helix. The denatured collagen is chromatographed on carboxymethylcellulose columns as described by Bornstein and Piez [1966].

Type III Collagen

Type III collagen was shown to be abundant in fetal skin by Epstein [1974]. The procedure of this author was utilized for the isolation and briefly is as follows. Fetal calf or rat skin is first extensively extracted with a NaCl-Tris buffer as described above in order to remove type I collagen. The residual collagen, mainly type III, is liberated from the insoluble residue by digestion with pepsin. The extract is then selectively precipitated by dialysis against increasing salt concentrations and finally is purified on carboxymethylcellulose columns as described by Epstein [1974].

Type II Collagen

Type II collagen was obtained from a chondrosarcoma, a cartilage tumor, according to the procedure of Smith et al. [1975]. The tumor tissue from lathrogenic animals was extracted with molar salt–Tris-HCl, pH 7.4, and the solubilized material was precipitated with 20% NaCl. Proteoglycans were removed by chromatography on DEAE-cellulose. Final purification included chromatography on carboxymethylcellulose as described.

Type IV Collagen

This collagen species was isolated either from the mouse Engelbreth-Holm-Swarm (EHS) sarcoma, which makes basement membranous material in large amounts, or from primary cultures of normal rat mammary epithelium or carcinogen-induced rat mammary tumor cells as described by Timpl et al. [1978] and Wicha et al. [1979a]. The latter preparations proved to be better substrata than the mouse tumor type IV collagen for normal mammary cell attachment [Wicha et al., 1979a]. Extraction of collagen from the cultures included the following steps. Cell cultures were grown in serum-free medium that will be subsequently described or in serum-supplemented medium [Liotta et al., 1980] either with or without ^{14}C-proline (5 μCi/ml) and with β-aminoproprionitrile present at 50 μg/ml and ascorbic acid added at a final concentration of 0.02–0.05 mM. After 3 days, the medium was removed and the cell layer was washed briefly with normal saline. Collagen in the cell layer was solubilized in 0.5 M acetic acid, 8 mM EDTA, and 4 mM N-ethylmaleimide (NEM), the latter two components being present to block any proteolysis [Lewko et al., 1981]. Unlike the case with many studies with fibroblasts and other cell types, more than 90% of the collagen was recovered in the cell layer and not released into the growth medium. The type IV collagen extracted into the acid solution was precipitated by the addition of NaCl to a final concentration of 10% (wt/vol) and the precipitate was redissolved in the acid-EDTA-NEM solution described above. The sample was dialyzed against the same solution and insoluble residue was removed by centrifugation. The soluble fraction was subsequently dialyzed against 50 mM Tris-HCl, pH 7.4. The soluble material from this step was dialyzed against the same buffer containing 1.71 M NaCl, which precipitated the collagen. The precipitate was subsequently dialyzed against 50 mM tris-HCl, pH 8.6, 2 M urea, and the dissolved material was applied to a DEAE-cellulose column in the same buffer.

Type IV collagen was recovered by column elution with a 0-0.2 M NaCl gradient. This step served to remove any type III collagen or laminin contaminants. Finally, the peak representing type IV collagen was extensively dialyzed against 0.1 M acetic acid and lyophilized to dryness.

Gel electrophoresis of the above collagen preparations on modified Laemmli gels [Lewko et al., 1981] with urea and sodium dodecyl sulfate (SDS) showed that the four collagens were homogenous. Collagen coating of the culture dishes was performed by adding sufficient solubilized collagen (in 0.1 M acetic acid) to yield 10 μg of the protein per cm^2 of dish surface. This gave dishes coated with denatured (nontriple helical) collagen. Alternatively, native collagen was coated onto the dishes by neutralizing the acid-solubilized collagen as described by Pearlstein [1976]. In either case, preferential attachment of the mammary cells for type IV collagen was observed with "native" or "denatured" collagen substrata.

GROWTH OF CELLS IN SERUM-FREE MEDIUM

Cultures of rat mammary ducts and alveoli were first conducted in serum-supplemented medium, and from such studies we were able to conclude that the production of basement membrane collagen was important for the growth and survival of mammary epithelium [Liotta et al., 1980; Wicha et al., 1979a; Kidwell et al., 1980b]. It was also clear from such studies that one hormone, hydrocortisone, was promoting mammary cell growth in part by inhibiting the turnover of collagen [Salomon et al., 1981]. However, to define the other types of growth factors that might enhance growth, possibly by facilitating basal lamina production, it was necessary to devise a serum-free growth medium. Fortunately, parallel studies on the growth requirements of an embryonal carcinoma cell line by one of us [Salomon, 1981] provided a growth cocktail that proved, with a few modifications, to be satisfactory for the growth of the normal ductal and alveolar cells [Salomon et al., 1981]. The composition of this medium and optimal concentrations of the additions are listed in Table I. These concentration optima refer only to the growth of the normal cells on tissue culture plastic surfaces. As will be demonstrated in the subsequent section, the hormone and growth factor requirements may vary depending on the type of substratum on which the cells are grown. This is especially true of EGF and hydrocortisone or dexamethasone.

With one exception, the Pedersen fetuin component, all the ingredients of the serum-free medium cocktail listed in Table I are defined. Recently some progress in identifying the active principles in this crude fetuin preparation have also been made. Pedersen fetuin obtained commercially (Sigma, Type

**TABLE I. Composition and Optimal
Concentrations of Media Supplements for
Mammary Cell Growth in Serum-Free Medium**

Factor	Concentration optimum
Dexamethasone	5-10 nM
Epidermal growth factor	10 ng/ml
Insulin	10 μg/ml
Transferrin (rat, human)	10 μg/ml
Fetuin, Pedersen	1-1.5 mg/ml
CaCl$_2$	0.2 mM
Ascorbic acid	0.01-0.005 mM

Isolated ducts and alveoli were plated on tissue culture plastic and the increase in cell number was determined after 4 days of culture. Improved Eagle's medium was the basal medium. At the optimal concentration of factors, the doubling time of the cells was 36 h, which is very comparable to the growth rate seen with serum-supplemented medium [Wicha et al., 1979b].

III) contains a protein that we have named embryonin. Embryonin appears to be the growth-conferring principle in this fetuin preparation and is considerably reduced in amount or absent in the more purified fetuin preparations such as those described by Deutsch [1954] and Spiro [1960]. A much fuller description of embryonin, its molecular weight, amino acid composition, and biological properties is given in Salomon et al. [1982]. For the present purposes, suffice it to say that the protein resembles α_2-macroglobulin in several of its properties. It is very potent in stimulating the proliferation of rat mammary ductal and alveolar cells in culture and dramatically stimulates their production of collagen. In some cases as much as a 10-fold differential labeling of collagen compared to total cell protein is produced by embryonin [Salomon et al., 1982].

MODULATION OF BASEMENT MEMBRANE COLLAGEN PRODUCTION IN VITRO

Using the serum-free medium cocktail formulated as described in Table I, a number of proteins, growth factors, and other substances have been screened for their ability to stimulate rat or mouse mammary ductal and alveolar cell growth. These factors have also been examined for their ability to differentially stimulate collagen production. The results of these studies are summarized in Table II. With no exception except insulin, any factor that is observed to

TABLE II. Correlation Between Medium Supplement Effects on Mammary Epithelium Growth and Differential Stimulation of Collagen Synthesis[a]

Factor added[b]	Concentration tested	Growth stimulation[c]	Differential stimulation[d] of collagen production
Insulin	10 μg/ml	Yes	No
MSA	1-50 ng/ml	Yes	Yes
PDGF	0-100 ng/ml	No	No
FGF	0-100 ng/ml	No	No
EGF	0-50 ng/ml	Yes	Yes
Embryonin	0-25 μg/ml	Yes	Yes
α_2-Macroglobulin (bovine)	0-25 μg/ml	Yes	Yes
α-Fetoprotein (mouse)	0-25 μg/ml	Yes	Yes
MTF	100 μg/ml	Yes	Yes
DB cAMP	1 mM	Yes	Yes
Ascorbic Acid	0.05 mM	Yes	Yes
Estradiol-17β	1 ng/ml	No	No
Progesterone	1-10 ng/ml	No	No
Prolactin	0-200 ng/ml	No	No
Prostaglandins			
E_1	0-5 μg/ml	Yes	Yes
E_2	0-5 μg/ml	No	No
$F_2\alpha$	0-5 μg/ml	No	No

[a]Ducts and alveoli were plated on tissue culture plastic in serum-free basal medium containing the factors listed in Table I. Individually, these medium supplements were omitted and the effects of factor omission were determined by measuring the changes in ^{14}C-proline incorporation into total cell protein and collagenase-digestible protein utilizing the procedure outlined by Lewko et al. [1981]. Cells were allowed to preattach for 24 h, and then unattached cells were removed with a medium change before addition of the labeled proline. The above results, therefore, do not include effects on cell attachment.

[b]Abbreviations: MSA, Multiplication Stimulating Activity; PDGF, Platlet Derived Growth Factor; FGF, Fibroblast Growth Factor; EGF, Epidermal Growth Factor; MTF, Mammary Tumor Factor; DB cAMP, Dibutryl Cyclic AMP.

[c]An increase in cell number by more than 20% after 3 days culture was considered a positive response.

[d]A differential stimulation of labeled collagen formation of more than 20% was considered a positive response.

significantly stimulate mammary cell proliferation is also seen to differentially promote the formation of collagen more than the formation of total cell protein. Although this relationship is obvious from the data in Table II, it should be mentioned that in these experiments with cells on tissue culture plastic, a very large stimulation of cell growth may be obtained with no more than a 30-40% differential stimulation of collagen labeling. Conversely, a very large differential stimulation of collagen synthesis may be reproduced with only a 30-40% stimulation of cell growth rate. Examples of these two phenomena are normal mammary cells stimulated with mammary tumor factor (MTF) [Kidwell et al., 1982a] and the same cells stimulated with α-fetoprotein, respectively (Bano et al., manuscript in preparation).

Several comments regarding the data in Table II are in order. In vivo the mammary cells normally rest on a basal lamina. However, in the process of proliferation, a penetration of the lamina and contact with the underlying stromal elements is a likely event. In fact, in experiments in which the mammary gland has been stimulated to proliferate but the formation of new lamina is blocked (for example by the administration of cis-hydroxyproline), mammary cells have been detected in direct contact with the stromal collagen fibers [Wicha et al., 1980]. Presumably, these are the areas where active mammary epithelial cell proliferation have taken place. An implication of these observations is that growth factor or hormonal responsiveness may be regulated in part by the substratum with which a cell is in contact. Such a possibility is realistic, as shown by the differential responsiveness of mammary cells to dexamethasone and EGF, depending on the substratum of the culture dish [Salomon et al., 1981] and by the differential responsiveness of corneal epithelium and smooth muscle cells on different substrata [Gospodarowicz et al., 1978, 1980]. The substratum effects on mammary cells will be examined subsequently. A second implication is that collagen synthesis (and probably other basal lamina components) is coordinated with mammary cell proliferation.

Also of interest from Table II is the observed responsiveness of mammary epithelium to the growth factor MTF which we have detected in extracts of breast tumor tissue. This factor is a protein of fairly large molecular weight (68,000) with an acidic pI [Bano et al., 1983]. It is present in well-differentiated mammary tumors that produce a basal lamina. Although it markedly stimulates collagen production by normal mammary cells, it has little effect on collagen production by the tumor cells from which the factor is derived. This observation, coupled with the fact that the tumor cells making MTF also do not respond to EGF, a growth factor that also stimulates collagen production by normal mammary epithelium (Table II), suggests that collagen production by mammary tumor cells may be constitutively conferred on such cells by virtue of their production of MTF [Bano et al., 1983].

Although we have yet to detect MTF in extracts of virgin or lactating rat mammary tissue, collagen synthesis-stimulating activity has been found in extracts of normal bovine mammary gland primed to proliferate by treatment of the animal with progesterone and estrogen. Also, some extracts of human breast tumors have been found to be very potent in differentially stimulating collagen synthesis. These results raise the possibility that growth factors might couple the functions of two or more cell types in the gland. For example, the mammary epithelial cells might produce a factor like MTF that promotes the formation of a new basal lamina by the myoepithelial cells, the cells that have been shown to be the major producers of type IV collagen in the adult gland [Wicha et al., 1980]. A model depicting this possibility is presented in Figure 2. Our current knowledge of the mammary tumor factor, the putative cell-coupling factor, is summarized in Table III. Serious consideration of this model will require detection of MTF in normal glandular tissue. Our attempts at detecting the activity in such tissue is severely hampered by the large amount of fat present in the glands.

At first glance the observed stimulation of collagen by α_2-macroglobulin as indicated in Table II might not seem surprising, since this agent is a widely

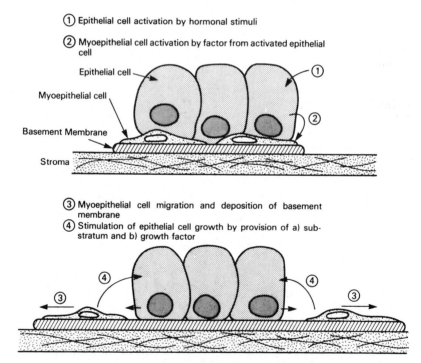

Fig. 2. Model depicting the possible mechanism by which MTF might stimulate mammary glandular epithelium to proliferate. First the epithelial cells would respond to a hormonal stimulus and produce MTF. MTF would then activate the myoepithelial cells to lay down new basement membrane upon which the epithelium could spread and divide.

TABLE III. Collagen Synthesis-Stimulating Activity (MTF):
Properties and Tissue Distribution

Size: 68,000 (minor species, 6,000)

pI: 5.9

Substance: Probably proteinaceous since it is heat-labile and protease-sensitive.

Sources: Activity that differentially stimulates collagen synthesis is extractable into acidified ethanol from the following tissues: normal bovine mammary gland, well-differentiated rat and mouse mammary tumors (primary and some transplatable tumors), some human mammary tumors, some mammary cell lines (weak activity). Activity is not detected in poorly differentiated rat mammary tumors such as transplantable DMBA, NMU, or MTW9a tumors, nor is activity detectable in extracts of normal rat mammary gland or liver.

The activity was extracted from tissues with acidified ethanol, was ether-precipitated, and was further fractionated as described by Bano et al. [1983]. Approximately 100 μg protein/ml was added to cultures of rat or mouse mammary ducts and alveolar cells, and the amounts of incorporation of ^{14}C-proline into total cell protein and collagenase-sensitive protein were determined after 3 days culture in the medium described in Table I.

recognized endopeptidase inhibitor [Barrett and Starkey, 1973] that can potentially block collagenase action either directly or by preventing the conversion of latent collagenase to an active form, which is accomplished by proteolytic cleavage of the enzyme [Werb and Aggeler, 1978; Salomon et al., 1981]. However, in some cells that respond to α_2-macroglobulin with an increased production of collagen, there is good evidence that the effect is not mediated via alterations in the rate of collagen turnover [Bano et al., 1983]. Indirect evidence that the α_2-macroglobulin effect is not via the action of this agent as a protease inhibitor also derives from the fact that soybean trypsin inhibitor, lima bean trypsin inhibitor, and ovomucoid at concentrations up to 100 μg/ml in the serum-free medium cocktail did not affect net collagen production or growth of normal mammary cells (unpublished observations).

Two other points worth noting about the entries in Table II are the responses on the mammary cells to the so-called mammatrophic hormones and the response to ascorbic acid. Thus far we have not observed any significant response of the normal mammary epithelium to estrogen, progesterone, or prolactin—hormones thought to modulate directly or indirectly the growth of mammary epithelium in vivo. This includes a lack of response on cell growth as well as on collagen IV synthesis or turnover. This does not necessarily mean that these hormones do not affect these processes in vivo, but only that our culture conditions may not be appropriate for the responses to occur. Concerning the stimulation of collagen by ascorbic acid, the mammary cells behave differently than fibroblastic cells in two ways. First, mammary cells are much more sensitive to ascorbic acid levels than fibroblasts. While fibroblastic cells are frequently cultivated in medium containing 40-50 μg ascorbic acid per ml [Peterkofsky, 1972], the cultured mammary epithelium suffers a marked reduction of cell growth at this concentration of the vitamin. This appears to be due to the fact that the mammary epithelium contains insufficient peroxidase to break down hydrogen peroxide, which is generated by the spontaneous decomposition of ascorbic acid (unpublished observations). At sufficiently low levels of ascorbate (Table II), there is a clear-cut stimulation of mammary cell growth, and a differential stimulation of collagen production as indicated in Table II.

Not surprising was our observation that dibutryl cyclic AMP stimulated growth in the mammary epithelial cells (Table II). It has been reported by Taylor-Papadimitriou et al. [1979] and by Nandi's group [Yang et al., 1980] that cholera toxin, an agent that activates adenyl cyclase and thus elevates cellular cyclic AMP, stimulates mammary cell growth. Although there are undoubtedly many cellular responses to an elevation in the cellular levels of this nucleotide, our results, which demonstrate that it produces a differential stimulation of collagen production, are consistent with our model (Fig. 2), which proposes that formation of new basal lamina is a part of the growth response of mammary cells to a mitogenic stimulus.

MODIFICATION OF MAMMARY CELL GROWTH FACTOR RESPONSIVENESS BY COLLAGEN SUBSTRATA

In the preceding section we listed a large number of factors we have examined for possible stimulation of mammary cells in cultures in serum-free medium. These experiments were performed on an artificial growth surface, namely tissue culture plastic. As we showed in Table II, there is almost always a differential stimulation of 14C-proline incorporation into collagen compared to proline incorporation into total cell protein in response to growth promoters. In this section we will describe the evidence we have obtained that suggests that this correlation is causally related. Basically our approach has been 1) to examine the growth responses of the cells on different types of substrata, including the various collagen types and tissue culture plastic, and 2) to determine whether cell growth and attachment is differentially blocked by collagen synthesis inhibitors depending on the type of substratum provided. Presently our survey is incomplete, since not all the growth-promoting factors listed in Table II have been compared on the different substrata. However, all the constituents given in Table I have been analyzed for their ability to promote both cell growth and attachment on the different substrata.

A preferential attachment of mammary cells to basement membrane collagen versus other collagen types has been seen both in serum-supplemented as well as serum-free medium (compare Tables IV and V). In serum-supplemented medium about 2.5 to 3 times more cells attach in 15 h onto type IV

TABLE IV. Attachment of Mammary Epithelial Organoids to Various Collagen Types in Serum-Supplemented Medium

Substratum	% Cells attached
Experiment I	
Bacterial plastic petri dishes	6 ± 1
Type I collagen	19 ± 1
Type III collagen	21 ± 2
Type II collagen	19 ± 2
Type IV collagen (EHS)	57 ± 4
Experiment II	
Bacterial plastic	10 ± 2
Type I collagen	28 ± 1
Type IV collagen (EHS sarcoma)	51 ± 2
Type IV collagen (mammary cells)	68 ± 3

Bacterial plastic dishes were coated with purified collagen types and the plates were sterilized by ultraviolet irradiation. The percentage of plated cells attached in 15 h was determined by cell counting. The values are given ± standard errors. The data presented are adapted from Wicha et al. [1979a].

TABLE V. Attachment Efficiency of Mammary Organoids on Various Substrata and Effects of Medium Supplements on Rates of Attachment in Serum-Free Medium

Factor omitted	% Cells attached		
	Type I collagen	Tissue culture plastic	Type IV collagen
EGF	61 ± 12	77 ± 8	102 ± 5
Insulin	60 ± 3	80 ± 5	104 ± 6
Dexamethasone	43 ± 3	81 ± 7	96 ± 3
Transferrin	68 ± 9	76 ± 4	98 ± 5
Ascorbic acid	59 ± 6	74 ± 1	99 ± 5

The percentage of plated cells that attached in 12 h was determined by cell counting. The factors, when present, were at the concentration optimum for cell growth as listed in Table I. As is apparent from the data, any omission reduced cell attachment efficiencies on type I collagen but was somewhat less important for attachment on tissue culture plastic surfaces and was unimportant when the cells were plated on type IV collagen substrate.

collagen substrata than onto types I, III, or II collagens. This preferential attachment is seen whether the collagen is native (triple helical) or denatured [Wicha et al., 1979a]. This preferential attachment to type IV collagen is somewhat amplified when the collagen is derived from the mammary gland itself, suggesting some structural differences between type IV collagen from the mouse EHS sarcoma and the rat mammary gland (Table IV).

In serum-free medium, the mammary ductal and alveolar cells attach to type IV collagen with 100% efficiency in 24 h, regardless of whether EGF, insulin, dexamethasone, transferrin, or ascorbic acid are omitted from the cocktail (Table V). However, marked differences in attachment are observed on tissue culture plastic surfaces or on type I collagen-coated surfaces when either of these media supplements is omitted. (The overall efficiency of attachment in medium with all the supplements present was 48%, 57%, and 100% for cells plated on dishes coated with type I collagen, plastic, and type IV collagen, respectively, which confirms the selective attachment phenomenon in the serum-supplemented medium as presented in Table IV.)

Although it would be tempting to conclude that the decreased attachment on type I collagen or plastic surfaces when one of the growth factors was omitted from the serum-free medium cocktail was due to a diminished production of type IV collagen by the mammary cells, such a conclusion is not valid, since insulin does not differentially promote synthesis of this collagen species by mammary cells (Table II) [Salomon et al., 1981a]. It is possible that some other basement membrane component, such as laminin, heparan sulfate protoglycan, or fibronectin, is produced in rate-limiting amounts in the absence of insulin and consequently might reduce the cell attachment rate. Precedent for such a possibility has been established since Stephens et al. [1981] have shown that insulin and an insulin-like growth factor, MSA, promotes extracellular matrix glycosaminoglycan synthesis. More to the point, they have shown that the hormone effect was independent of the cell growth rate. Thus it seems plausible that even in the case of insulin, a major function of growth factors is to enhance the production of extracellular matrix components needed for cell attachment and flattening, the latter process believed to be essential for inducing the mitogenic process [Folkman and Moscona, 1978]. We are currently examining all of the factors listed in Table II to see whether they also coordinately stimulate production of heparan sulfate proteoglycan, laminin, and fibronectin as well as affecting type IV collagen synthesis. However, in light of the findings of Stephens et al. [1981], it will not be surprising to see some of the basal lamina components differentially affected by agents that stimulate mammary cell growth.

Stimulation of cell growth as well as cell attachment in serum-free medium is also dependent on the substratum provided to the mammary cells, as shown in Table VI. Cells were allowed to attach in medium in which a particular growth factor was omitted, and subsequent growth rates of the cells were determined in the continued absence of that factor. The most dramatic drop of cell proliferation was seen when EGF or dexamethasone was omitted from cell cultures grown on tissue culture plastic or type I collagen. Omission of either of these factors had little effect when the cells were grown on type IV collagen-coated dishes.

The above results show that in serum-free medium mammary cell growth is substantially better on type IV collagen than on plastic or on stromal collagen. In serum-supplemented medium, cell attachment is observed to be selective for basement membrane collagen but growth, following attachment, is similar regardless of the substratum type. This is not the case, however, if de novo collagen synthesis is blocked, for in this case growth on type IV collagen is significantly better than on type I collagen. Nandi's group [Yang et al., 1980] and Furmanski's group [Yang et al., 1981] have analyzed mammary cell growth both on and within rat tail collagen gels (primarily type I collagen and glycosaminoglycans) and have been successful in maintaining cell growth for a month or more. These results suggest that stromal elements may be important scaffolding upon which a completely assembled basement

TABLE VI. Effect of Serum-Free Medium Supplements on Mammary Cell Growth on Various Substrata

Factor omitted	% Decreased growth on:				
	P	I	IV	P/IV	I/IV
EGF	55	46	14	3.9	3.2
Insulin	38	31	32	1.2	1.0
Dexamethasone	58	46	13	4.4	3.5
Transferrin	24	35	15	1.6	2.3

Cells were plated either in complete medium with all the supplements present or the supplements were omitted individually. Twenty-four hours after plating, any unattached cells were removed and replaced with fresh medium with the same supplement factor omitted. The number of cells attached at 24 h and after 3 days subsequent growth was determined. The data are expressed as the percentage decreased growth rate of the cultures with a particular factor omitted when normalized against the control with all factors present on dishes with a particular substratum. The relative importance of a particular growth supplement on type I collagen or plastic surfaces is then expressed as a ratio. From the table it becomes apparent that EGF and dexamethasone are 3–4 times more potent growth stimulators for cells on type I collagen or plastic surfaces than on type IV collagen. Adapted from Salomon et al. [1981a]. P, plastic; I, type I collagen; IV, type IV collagen.

membrane can be deposited. This also may be inferred from reports from Bernfield's laboratory showing that glycosaminoglycan synthesis, processing, and turnover are facilitated in mouse mammary cells cultured on stromal collagen versus cultures on plastic [David and Bernfield, 1979]. We wish to emphasize that in relatively short-term cultures (up to 8 days and 3–4 cell doublings) we consistently see that purified type IV collagen is superior to purified type I collagen in sustaining normal rat mammary cell growth and viability.

Is the selective attachment of mammary cells on basement membrane collagen versus type I collagen a physiologically meaningful process, or a reflection of some surface charge density distribution different than that preferred by the mammary epithelium? It is not possible to unequivocally answer this question, but the cumulative evidence supports a selective, physiological recognition. The requirement of collagen IV production for growth and survival has been demonstrated, as mentioned earlier. Thus cis-hydroxyproline has been shown to selectively block collagen production and to ultimately produce mammary cell death both in vivo and in vitro [Wicha et al., 1979a, 1980]. Furthermore, the ability of this proline analog to kill mammary cells in culture is markedly reduced when the cells are cultured on type IV collagen in comparison to the effects on type I collagen [Wicha et al., 1979a].

The effects of other proline analogs on mammary cell killing in vivo and in vitro have tended to confirm those obtained with cis-hydroxyproline. For example, 4-thioproline, 3,4-dehydroproline, and L-azetidine-5-carboxylate have all been found to selectively block collagen synthesis by cultured ductal and alveolar cells and to inhibit mammary cell growth in proportion to their potency in blocking collagen production in vitro. This is presented in Table VII. These compounds are also very effective in blocking the growth of rat mammary adenocarcinomas, which are basement membrane-producing tumors, in intact animals (Taylor and Kidwell, in preparation). Their selectivity is exemplified by the fact that concentrations of the drugs that markedly arrest tumor growth have no detectable pathophysiological effects on the hosts.

SUMMARY

Herein we have reviewed our progress to date in evaluating in serum-free medium the effects of a variety of growth factors on basement membrane collagen synthesis. With only one exception, all agents that stimulate mammary cell growth also differentially stimulate synthesis of this basement membrane component. We also have shown that a number of factors that are growth-promoters for other cell types but not mammary cells do not stimulate

TABLE VII. Proline Analog Effects on Mammary Cell Growth and Collagen Synthesis

Analog	Relative potency in blocking collagen synthesis	I_D50 (μg/ml)
cis-4-Hydroxyproline	+++	30
L-Azetidine-5-carboxylic acid	++++	16
3,4-Dehydroproline	+	65
4-Thioproline	++++	25

Cells were plated in serum-free medium with all supplements listed in Table I. Twenty-four hours later the medium was changed and fresh medium with ^{3}H-lysine was added. In parallel experiments the ^{3}H-lysine was omitted and cell counts were performed after 3 days growth with varying concentrations of the proline analogs. The amount of ^{3}H-lysine incorporated into total cell protein versus collagenase-sensitive protein was estimated 24 h after addition of the proline analog (25 μg/ml) and the ^{3}H-lysine. I_D50: Concentration of analog required for 50% inhibition of growth. As is evident from the table, the more potent the analog is in blocking collagen labeling, the lower the concentration needed to block cell growth.

type IV collagen synthesis in mammary cells. Our presentation has also demonstrated that in serum-free medium mammary cells attach and proliferate better when provided a substratum of type IV collagen than stromal collagen or tissue culture plastic. The studies also have been partly extended to show that mammary cells are less dependent on a number of growth factors when cultured on a basement membrane collagen than on plastic-coated or type I collagen-coated surfaces. Taken together, these results lead to the conclusion that enhanced basement membrane production is one of the important responses of mammary cells to growth factors. It is probable that production of basement membranes is not only important, but essential, for the growth of the mammary epithelium.

REFERENCES

Bano M, Zweibel JA, Salomon D, Kidwell WR (1983): Detection and partial characterization of collagen synthesis stimulating activities in rat mammary adenocarcinomas. J Biol Chem 258:2729-2735.

Barrett AJ, Starkey PM (1973): The interaction of α_2-macroglobulin with proteinases. Biochem J 133:709-724.

Ben-David M (1968): Mechanism of induction of mammary gland differentiation by perphenazine. Endocrinology 83:1217-1223.

Bornstein P, Piez K (1966): The nature of the intramolecular cross-links in collagen. Biochemistry 5:3460-3473.

David G, Bernfield M (1979): Collagen reduces glycaminoglycan degradation by cultured mammary epithelial cells: Possible mechanism for basal lamina formation. Proc Natl Acad Sci USA 76:786-790.

Deutsch HF (1954): Fetuin, the mucoprotein of fetal calf serum. J Biol Chem 208:669-678.

Epstein EH (1974): [α1(111)]$_3$ human skin collagen. J Biol Chem 249:3225-3231.

Folkman J, Moscona A (1978): Role of cell shape in growth control. Nature 273:345-347.

Gospodarowicz D, Ill CR (1980): Do plasma and serum have different abilities to promote growth? Proc Natl Acad Sci USA 77:2726-2730.

Gospodarowicz D, Greenberg G, Birdwell CR (1978): Determination of cellular shape by the extracellular matrix and its correlation with growth. Cancer Res 38:4155-4177.

Hassell JR, Robey PG, Barrach H, Wilczek J, Rennard SI, Martin GR (1980): Isolation of a heparan sulfate containing proteoglycan from basement membrane. Proc Natl Acad Sci USA 77:4494-4498.

Kidwell WR, Wicha MS, Salomon DS, Liotta LA (1980a): Differential recognition of basement membrane collagen by normal and neoplastic mammary cells. In McGrath CM, Brennan CJ, Rich MA (eds): "Cell Biology of Breast Cancer." New York, Academic, pp 17-32.

Kidwell WR, Wicha MS, Salomon DS, Liotta LA (1980b): Hormonal controls of collagen substratum formation by cultured mammary cells. In Jiminez de Asua J, Levi-Montalcini R, Shields R, Iacobelli S (eds): "Control Mechanisms in Animal Cells." New York, Raven, pp 333-340.

Kidwell WR, Salomon DS, Liotta LA, Bano M (1982a): Effect of growth factors on mammary epithelial cell growth and basement membrane synthesis. In Sato G, Sirbasku D (eds): "Growth of Cells in Hormonally Defined Medium." Cold Spring Harbor, NY: Cold Spring Harbor Laboratory, pp 807-818.

Kidwell WR, Knazek RA, Vonderhaar BK, Losonczy I (1982b): Effects of unsaturated fatty acids on the development and proliferation of normal and neoplastic breast epithelium. In Arnott MS, van Eys J, Wang YM (eds): "Molecular Interrelations of Nutrition and Cancer." New York, Raven, pp 219-236.

Lewko WM, Liotta LA, Wicha MS, Vonderhaar BK, Kidwell WR (1981): Sensitivity of N-nitrosomethylurea-induced rat mammary tumors to cis-hydroxyproline, an inhibitor of collagen production. Cancer Res 41:2855-2862.

Liotta LA, Wicha MS, Rennard SI, Garbisa S, Kidwell WR (1980): Hormonal requirements for basement membrane collagen deposition by cultured mammary epithelium. Lab Invest 41:511-518.

Peterkofsky B (1972): The effect of ascorbic acid on collagen polypeptide synthesis and proline hydroxylation during the growth of cultured fibroblasts. Arch Biochem Biophys 152:318-328.

Rudland PS, Hallowes RC, Durbin H, Lewis D (1977): Mitogenic activity of pituitary hormones on cell cultures of normal and carcinogen-induced tumor epithelium from rat mammary glands. J Cell Biol 73:561-577.

Russo IH, Russo J (1978): Developmental stage of the rat mammary gland as a determinant of susceptibility to DMBA. J Natl Cancer Inst 61:1439-1459.

Salomon DS (1981): Correlation of receptors for growth factors on mouse embryonal carcinoma cells with growth in serum free, hormone supplemented medium. Exp Cell Res 128:311-327.

Salomon DS, Liotta LA, Kidwell WR (1981): Differential response to growth factor by rat mammary epithelium plated on different collagen substrata in serum free medium. Proc Natl Acad Sci USA 78:382-386.

Salomon DS, Bano M, Smith K, Kidwell WR (1982): Isolation and characterization of a growth factor (Embryonin) from bovine fetuin which resembles α_2-macroglobulin. J Biol Chem 257:14093-14101.

Smith BD, Martin GR, Miller EJ, Dorfmann A, Swarm R (1975): Nature of the collagen synthesized by a transplanted chondrosarcoma. Arch Biochem Biophys 166:181-186.

Spiro RG (1960): Studies on fetuin, a glycoprotein of fetal serum. J Biol Chem 235:2860-2869.

Stampfer M, Hallowes RC, Hackett AJ (1980): Growth of normal human mammary cells in culture. In Vitro 16:415-425.

Stephens RC, Nissley P, Kimura J, Rechler M, Caplan A, Hascall V (1981): Effects of insulin and MSA on proteoglycan biosynthesis in chondrocytes from the Swarm Chondrosarcoma. J Biol Chem 256:2045-2052.

Taylor-Papadimitriou J, Purkiss P, Fentiman IS (1979): Cholera toxin and analogues of cyclic AMP stimulate the growth of cultured mammary epithelial cells. J Cell Phys 102:317-321.

Timpl R, Martin GR, Bruckner P, Wich G, Wideman H (1978): Nature of the collagenous protein in a tumor basement membrane. Eur J Biol Chem 84:43-52.

Timpl R, Rhode H, Robey PG, Rennard SI, Foidart JM, Martin GR (1979): Laminin—A glycoprotein from basement membranes. J Biol Chem 254:9933-9937.

Uitto J, Prockop D (1977): Incorporation of proline analogs into procollagen. Arch Biochem Biophys 181:293-299.

Werb Z, Aggeler J (1978): Proteases induce secretion of collagenase and plasminogen activator by fibroblasts. Proc Natl Acad Sci USA 75:1839-1843.

Wicha MS, Liotta LA, Garbisa S, Kidwell WR (1979a): Basememt membrane collagen requirements for attachment and growth of mammary epithelium. Exp Cell Res 124:181-190.

Wicha MS, Liotta LA, Kidwell WR (1979b): Effects of free fatty acids on the growth of normal and neoplastic mammary epithelial cells. Cancer Res 39:426-435.

Wicha MS, Liotta LA, Vonderhaar BK, Kidwell WR (1980): Effects of inhibition of basement membrane collagen deposition on rat mammary gland development. Dev Biol 80:253-266.

Yang J, Richards J, Guzman R, Imagawa W, Nandi S (1980): Sustained growth in primary culture of normal mammary epithelial cells embedded in collagen gels. Proc Natl Acad Sci USA 77:2088-2092.

Yang NS, Kube D, Park C, Furmanski P (1981): Growth of human mammary cells on collagen gel surfaces. Cancer Res 41:4093-4100.

Methods for Serum-Free Culture of Cells of the Endocrine System,
pages 127–141

8
Isolation and Serum-Free Cultivation of Mammary Epithelial Cells Within a Collagen Gel Matrix

Walter Imagawa, Yasuhiro Tomooka, Jason Yang, Raphael Guzman, James Richards, and Satyabrata Nandi

Only a few years ago it was discovered that rodent and human mammary epithelial cells could be grown in primary cell culture if they were embedded within a collagen gel matrix [Yang et al., 1980]. The same cells plated on plastic would not undergo sustained (prolonged) growth [Richards et al., 1983] with the exception of human cells plated in the presence of conditioned medium [Stampfer et al., 1980]. Cell survival and sustained growth occurred in a variety of commercially available culture media such as Ham's F12, Dulbecco's modified Eagle's medium (DMEM), or Waymouth's medium but was dependent upon the presence of serum.

Although questions concerning the roles of mammogenic hormones and growth factors in the stimulation of the growth of mammary epithelial cells in vitro could now be asked, these questions could not be unequivocally answered using a culture system containing serum with its attendant unknown complexity [Yang et al., 1980]. Initial attempts to culture cells in serum-free Ham's F12 medium with supplements similar to those used successfully for serum-free culture of cell lines [Sato and Reid, 1978] were unsuccessful. More recently, we have succeeded in developing serum-free culture systems for mouse and human mammary epithelial cells [Imagawa et al., 1982; Yang et al., 1982].

The aims of this presentation are to describe the cell dissociation procedure that provides epithelial cells capable of growth under serum-free conditions,

Cancer Research Laboratory and Department of Zoology, University of California at Berkeley, Berkeley, California 94720

the collagen gel cell culture procedure, and, finally, the serum-free culture systems that have been used in the study of mammary gland biology. The discussion will be limited to the mouse mammary gland, although the procedures employed are generally applicable to human mammary tissue.

PREPARATION OF PRIMARY CULTURES OF MAMMARY EPITHELIAL CELLS
Isolation of Mammary Epithelial Cells

Collagenase dissociation. The mammary glands or mammary tumors are removed, weighed, and minced (under sterile conditions) with a razor blade until a "paste-like" consistency is achieved. The minced tissue is dissociated in a fluted Erlenmeyer flask in HEPES-buffered (10 mM) Medium 199 containing bovine serum albumin, fraction V at 1 mg/ml, and collagenase (Worthington III) at 1 g/liter. Approximately 1 g of tissue is used per 10 ml of dissociation medium. The final volume should be about one-third of the total volume of the chosen flask in order to obtain adequate agitation of the tissue pieces. The flask is shaken at 37°C in a gyratory water bath at 120-180 rpm. When a uniform suspension mostly devoid of large pieces of tissue and containing clean epithelial cell clumps is obtained (usually after 1-2 h), the dissociation is stopped and the suspension is filtered through 150 μm nitex. It should flow through the nitex easily. The cells are collected by gentle centrifugation and then subjected to a mild pronase treatment. The pronase (0.5-1 g/liter) digestion is done in a fluted flask containing 50 ml of HEPES-buffered Medium 199 and bovine serum albumin, fraction V (1 mg/ml). The flask is shaken very slowly for 30 min at 37°C. This step is included to break the large clumps of epithelial-stromal cells into smaller clumps composed of an estimated 10-100 cells. The cells are collected by gentle centrifugation, suspended in a small volume, and treated with a few drops of fresh DNase I (Sigma, 0.4 g/liter stock solution stored frozen in small aliquots). The suspension must consist of individual clumps of cells prior to the Percoll step.

The time of shaking, yield, and viability of the cells depends on the collagenase used. The expected yield (after the Percoll step described in the next section) from all 10 glands of a single 2-month-old virgin BALB/cCrgl mouse is (3-4) × 10^6 cells. The cell clumps should begin to spread within 24-48 h of culture. If yields are low, cell spreading is slow or nil, and contamination by stromal elements is prevalent, the collagenase preparation should be suspect. Different collagenase lots must be tested empirically (collagenase and protease activity are a poor index of performance) for their effectiveness.

The cell dissociation of human cells is similar to the procedure described here. Since these tissues contain a much larger stromal component, 1 gm/liter hyaluronidase is added to the collagenase digestion and the digestion time has to be extended [Yang et al., 1982].

Separation of stromal and epithelial cells. This step should be more properly called an enrichment step, since the complete separation of epithelial and stromal cells is usually not achieved. However, under serum-free conditions the growth of contaminating "fibroblast-like" cells is greatly reduced without the need for factors such as cholera toxin, which can inhibit fibroblast growth [Taylor-Papadimitriou et al., 1980]. Percoll (Pharmacia) gradient centrifugation is used to separate epithelial and stromal cells. The Percoll is adjusted to physiological salt and pH conditions by the addition of 1.2 ml of bicarbonate-free 10 × Waymouth's (powdered formula) medium and 16 ml of Medium 199 (Hanks' salts) to 10.8 ml of Percoll in a 30-ml screw-capped polycarbonate tube. The tube is spun at 20,000g in a fixed-angle rotor for 1 h prior to the loading of the cells. Approximately 20–30 million cells in no more than 2 ml are layered onto the preformed gradient and centrifuged at 800g (fixed-angle or swinging bucket rotor) for 15 min at room temperature. Usually three discrete regions or bands are seen: an upper band (lowest density) composed of stromal elements and cell debris, a lower band of higher density (1.05–1.07) than stromal cells composed of mostly epithelial cells, and a band of erythrocytes below the epithelial cells near the bottom of the tube. For mammary glands from virgin mice most of the cells loaded onto the gradient remain in the upper, stromal band. For glands from midpregnant mice, which contain a higher ratio of epithelial to stromal cells, the epithelial band is correspondingly larger. The epithelial cells are collected, washed, suspended in a small volume of HEPES-buffered Medium 199, and counted.

Collagen Gel Culture

Preparation of collagen. Rat tail (tails from young rats are preferred) collagen is obtained by breaking off small sections of intact, severed tails with pliers starting from the base of the tail. As each section is broken off the collagen tendons in that section remain behind, attached to the remainder of the tail. The tendons are cut with a razor blade, soaked in 70% ethanol for sterilization, dried, and weighed. This dried collagen can be stored at 0° for months.

The collagen is dissolved by adding 4 g to 1 liter of 0.017 M glacial acetic acid (made with sterile, double-distilled water) and stirring at 4°C for 48 h. The solubilized collagen is then centrifuged at 10,000g for 1 hour to remove undissolved material. The resulting collagen solution is usually too concentrated and can be diluted with cold acetic acid. The dilution factor is determined empirically by the gelation properties of a range of dilutions of the collagen solution.

Prior to determining the dilution factor for the collagen stock, the proper neutralizing solution for the gelation reaction (collagen fibers self-assemble, forming a hydrated gel when the pH is raised) must be determined. The desired neutralizing solution, composed of NaOH and 10 × Waymouth's medium (powdered formula MB 752/I), is one that will bring the pH of the collagen solution to 7.4 and the osmolarity to around 300 mosM. A series of neutralizing solutions (all solutions and collagen are kept on ice) composed of 1 ml of 0.34 N NaOH plus 2-1.5 ml, in 0.1-ml increments, of 10 × bicarbonate-free Waymouth's are prepared. (The NaOH and 10 × Waymouth's medium are stored at 4°C.) Each neutralizing mix is used to titrate a known volume of undiluted collagen stock to pH 7.4. The titration volume and NaOH:10 × Waymouth's ratio of the mix giving an osmolarity of about 300 mosM are noted. Usually a ratio of about 1.8 ml of 10 × Waymouth's to 1 ml of NaOH is used. About 1.5 ml of this mixture will neutralize 8 ml of collagen. The collagen dilution factor can now be determined with the proper neutralizing mix to produce gelation of different dilutions of the collagen stock. The desired dilution factor is the greatest dilution giving a firm gel within 5-10 min at room temperature without gelation when kept on ice. If the neutralized collagen gels too rapidly when kept on ice (cold retards gelation), there will be insufficient time to pipette the gel into numerous multiwells or culture dishes.

Embedding cells in collagen. All solutions including the diluted stock collagen, neutralizing mix, and final neutralized collagen are kept on ice. Just prior to use, the neutralizing mix is made by combining the NaOH and 10 × Waymouth's medium in the predetermined ratio (procedure described above).

Two neutralized collagen pools are needed. The first is used to place a bottom layer of collagen in the culture dish or multiwell. The bottom layer is needed to prevent cell attachment to the surface of the culture vessel. The appropriate volume of collagen (for a 1-cm well of a 24-well multiwell plate a 0.25-ml bottom layer is used) is titrated to pH 7.4 with the neutralizing mix by judging the color (rose pink) of the solution. The bottom layers are pipetted and allowed to gel by leaving the culture dishes undisturbed at room temperature. The second neutralized pool is prepared by again titrating the appropriate volume of collagen with neutralizing mix, followed by addition of the cells to achieve the desired cell density. The collagen, now containing cells, is pipetted on the top of the bottom layer. For a 24-well multiwell plate, a 0.5-ml top layer is used. When this top layer has solidified, medium is added and the culture dish is placed in a CO_2 incubator at 37°C.

Termination of cultures. At the end of the culture period, the gels from multiwells are transferred to 10-mm × 75-mm glass tubes with forceps and dissolved by the addition of 0.05 ml of 3.5 M acetic acid and incubation at 37°C. The cells are pelleted, extracted with approximately 1 ml of 70% ethanol, dried, and then assayed for DNA by a fluorometric assay [Hinegardner, 1971]. If the cells are to be passaged, they can be freed from the gels by collagenase treatment (0.1 ml of collagenase, 10 g/liter stock) followed by washing to remove residual collagenase.

SERUM-FREE CULTURE
Preparation of Media and Media Supplements

Preparation of media. All media are prepared with deionized, double-distilled water. The medium used for serum-free culture is a 1:1 mixture of Ham's F12 and Dulbecco's modified Eagle's medium, both from Gibco. The powdered media are dissolved in water, and sodium bicarbonate (culture grade) is added. The pH is adjusted to 7.4, the medium is filter-sterilized, and Amphotericin B (0.0025 g/liter) and Gentamycin sulfate (0.05 g/liter) are added. Prior to the development of serum-free culture conditions, these media along with Medium 199 and Waymouth's medium (powdered formula, Gibco) were tested for their growth-supporting capabilities, alone and in mixtures against a serum background. This particular mixture was found to be one of the most effective combinations for normal cells, superior to Ham's F12 or DMEM alone (unpublished observations). This mixture has also been found to be effective in the serum-free culture of a variety of cell types including epithelial cells [Barnes and Sato, 1980]. This medium can be used bicarbonate-buffered or HEPES-buffered (20 mM) with a reduction in the sodium bicarbonate concentration to 1.2 g/liter in a 5% carbon dioxide atmosphere. There seems to be no significant difference in the growth of the cells in bicarbonate- or HEPES-buffered media.

Preparation of media supplements. All medium supplements except epidermal growth factor (EGF, Collaborative Research) and selenous acid (Specpure) are from Sigma Chemical Company and are prepared with deionized, double-distilled water. Insulin (bovine) is dissolved in 0.01 N HCl and stored at 4° for several weeks; transferrin and EGF are dissolved in Puck's Saline A or medium and stored at 4° for months; bovine serum albumin, fraction V is dissolved in medium, the pH being adjusted to 7.4, and then is filter-sterilized before being added to the medium; cholera toxin is dissolved in water and stored at 4° for months; putrescine is dissolved in medium or Saline A and stored frozen; biotin and α-tocopherol succinate are dissolved in 100%

ethanol and stored at 0°; triiodothyronine is dissolved in 0.01 N NaOH and stored frozen; ascorbic acid is dissolved in water just prior to use and stored at 4° (in medium); selenous acid is dissolved in water and stored at 4°; linoleic acid is dissolved in an equimolar amount of 0.1 N NaOH in a nitrogen atmosphere, then incubated under nitrogen with essentially fatty acid-free bovine serum albumin (20 mg/ml) at 50° for 30 min. The linoleic acid-albumin complex is stored at 0°.

Growth in Serum-Free Medium

Dose-response studies. A serum-free medium composed of a 1:1 mixture of Ham's F12 and DMEM buffered with 20 mM HEPES and sodium bicarbonate (1.2 g/liter) and containing insulin (10 μg/ml), bovine serum albumin (fraction V, 5 mg/ml), cholera toxin (0.01 μg/ml), transferrin (10 μg/ml), and epidermal growth factor (0.1 μg/ml) was found to support the growth of normal and tumor mouse mammary epithelial cells [Imagawa et al., 1982]. Dose-response studies were done in which the concentration of each component of this medium was varied in turn while the others were maintained at the concentrations indicated above. Figure 1 shows the results of a typical experiment using cells from midpregnant BALB/cCrgl mice. Cells were seeded at an initial density of $(0.5-1) \times 10^5$ cells per well of a 24-well multiwell plate. At the end of 10-12 days, the cultures were terminated and DNA assays were performed. Figure 2 shows an epithelial colony growing in serum-free medium. There is no difference in colony morphology in serum-free or serum-containing medium. Similar results are obtained with cells from virgin BALB/cCrgl mice. The essential components are insulin, EGF (at an optimal concentration of 0.01 μg/ml), and bovine serum albumin V. Individual tumors from BALB/cfC3H mice varied in their growth requirements; although all require bovine serum albumin V and insulin, some can grow in the absence of EGF. The epithelial nature of the cells has been confirmed by the induction of casein synthesis in serum-free culture as well as the outgrowth of mammary glands in the parenchyma-free fat pads of syngeneic hosts after transplantation of cells cultured in serum-free medium (unpublished observations).

Nutritional requirements for growth. Although mouse mammary epithelial cells proliferate in medium containing only insulin, EGF, and bovine serum albumin fraction V (up to a 10-fold increase in cell number can occur in 10-12 days), occasionally some colonies are seen to degenerate. This degeneration occurs more often in cultures of cells from midpregnant animals and in cultures containing a high cell density (greater than 3×10^5 cells per 0.75 ml collagen). However, time course experiments show that cultures can

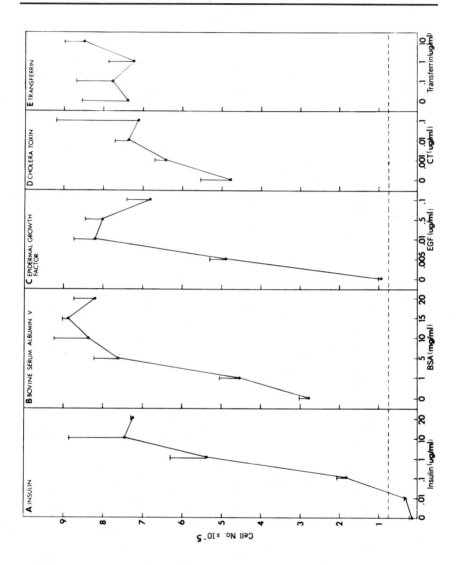

Fig. 1. Growth of cells from midpregnant mice cultured for 11 days in serum-free medium containing insulin (10 μg/ml), transferrin (10 μg/ml), EGF (0.1 μg/ml), cholera toxin (0.01 μg/ml), and BSA V (5 mg/ml). The concentration of each component was varied in turn as shown while the concentration of the other components was maintained at the above concentrations. ---, 0 time cell number. Data are expressed as means ± standard deviation for 3 gels.

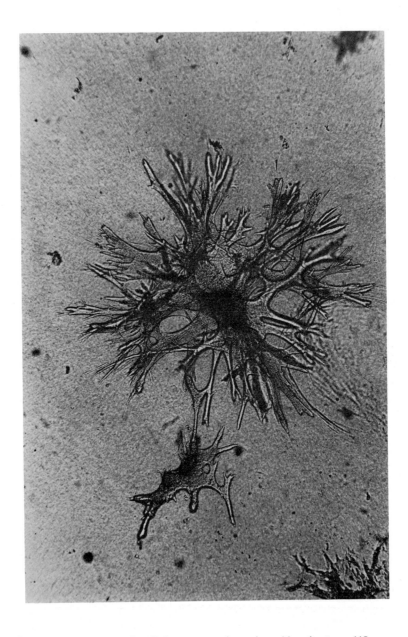

Fig. 2. An epithelial colony after 10 days in serum-free culture. Magnification ×118.

undergo sustained growth for at least 3 weeks without any growth decline [Imagawa et al., 1982]. The occasional degeneration may result from an omission of hormones or growth factors important for the maintenance of cell viability or the inclusion of factors that are toxic to a susceptible subset of cells. Alternatively, the basal medium composed of Ham's F12 and DMEM may be suboptimal for the primary culture of epithelial cells [Ham, 1982].

Of primary interest was the requirement for bovine serum albumin, which may contain a variety of contaminating factors such as hormones, vitamins, trace elements, and, most prominently, lipids. Bovine serum albumin V was delipidized by isopropyl ether:butanol extraction [Cham and Knowles, 1976] and/or dialyzed (M_r 3,000, Specpor) against deionized, double-distilled water. Figure 3 is a dramatic example showing how delipidation and dialysis, but not dialysis alone, of the albumin can reduce its ability to promote growth. Crystalline albumin does not support growth and may be toxic. Other supplements were added to serum-free medium containing insulin (10 μg/ml), EGF (0.01 μg/ml), transferrin (10 μg/ml), and either fatty acid-free (Sigma), delipidized/dialyzed, or untreated bovine serum albumin V and were tested for their effect upon the growth of cells from midpregnant mice. These supplements included vitamins such as ascorbic acid (1-50 μg/ml), α-tocopherol succinate (1-50 μg/ml), and biotin (0.1 -10 μg/ml), all of which had no effect upon growth regardless of the albumin preparation used. Other factors such as selenium, triiodothyronine, putrescine, and linoleic acid were tested as shown in Figures 4 and 5, and Tables I and II, respectively. Only putrescine (which is a component of Ham's F12) and linoleic acid stimulated growth. None of the supplements tested proved capable of eliminating the degeneration of some colonies described previously. These results do indicate that bovine serum albumin probably does not contribute low-molecular-weight substances but may provide lipid substrates to the cells that could reduce the metabolic demands upon the cells with a consequent enhancement of growth potential.

Applications and Perspectives

When investigators are faced with the problems of identifying those hormones and growth factors responsible for growth regulation in vitro, the composition of the serum-free medium to which these factors are added is a crucial variable. Hormonal effects can be antagonized or masked by a factor in the serum-free cocktail or, if growth in the basal cocktail is too rapid, more subtle growth stimulatory effects of added hormones or growth factors may be inapparent. Therefore, a variety of serum-free media should be used under conditions where growth is well below maximal.

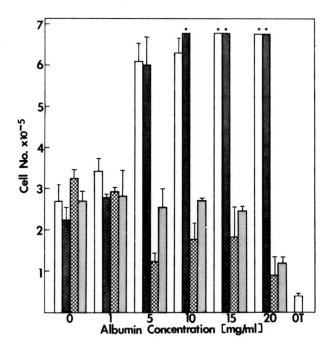

Fig. 3. Effect of different types of bovine serum albumin, fraction V (BSA V) upon the growth of cells from midpregnant mice cultured for 10 days in serum-free medium containing insulin (10 μg/ml), EGF (0.01 μg/ml), transferrin (10 μg/ml), and cholera toxin (0.01 μg/ml), Dialyzed BSA V, solid bars ■; untreated BSA V, open bars □; dialyzed/delipidized BSA V, gray bars ▨; crystalline BSA, hatched bars ▧. For each albumin type there was a separate no-added-albumin control. These controls are shown as growth at zero BSA. 0T, zero time cell number. *, minimum values. Data are expressed as mean ± standard deviation for three gels.

In order to find minimal serum-free conditions (that is, those in which cells survive, grow slowly, and remain growth-responsive) for testing the proliferative effect of mammogenic hormones, a series of media containing suboptimal concentrations of those factors required for growth were prepared. An optimal serum-free medium containing insulin (10 μg/ml), bovine serum albumin V (5 mg/ml), EGF (0.01 μg/ml), and transferrin (10 μg/ml) was prepared along with minimal media containing suboptimal concentrations of insulin (1 μg/ml), bovine serum albumin (1 mg/ml), or EGF (0.001 μg/ml). The minimal media contained one to all of these three factors at suboptimal concentrations. Transferrin was maintained at 10 μg/ml. Cells from midpregnant or virgin BALB/cCrgl mice were cultured for 6 days in minimal media and then switched to optimal medium for 6 more days. A parallel set of cultures was

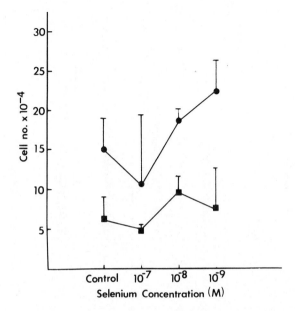

Fig. 4. Effect of selenium on the growth of cells from midpregnant BALB/cCrgl mice cultured in media containing insulin (10 μg/ml), EGF (0.01 μg/ml), transferrin (10 μg/ml), and untreated (5 mg/ml, circles) or delipidized/dialyzed bovine serum albumin, fraction V (5 mg/ml, squares). Data are expressed as mean ± standard deviation for three gels.

maintained in minimal medium for 12 days. Cultures were terminated at 6 and 12 days for DNA assay. Table III shows the results of one experiment done with cells from midpregnant mice. These results and other, similar results show that a 6-day exposure to suboptimal concentrations of one or two of the required components will not result in a general loss of cell viability and the cells will retain the capacity to grow when stimulated. Cell viability can decrease in complete minimal media (all components at suboptimal concentrations) or if the period in minimal media is extended beyond 10 days. These experiments demonstrate that suboptimization of the serum-free cocktail can be used to examine the proliferative capabilities of hormones and growth factors.

It is evident that the serum-free culture system for mouse mammary epithelial cells is highly manipulable. The essential supplements required for growth in Ham's F12/DMEM are few—insulin, serum albumin, and EGF—but growth can be enhanced by the addition of a variety of substances affecting different aspects of cellular metabolism. In fact, the "essential" factors may be, in turn,

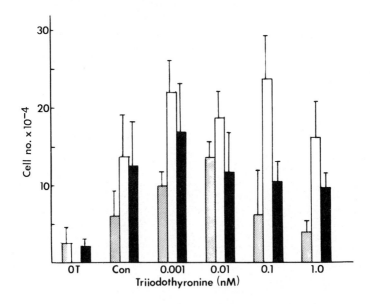

Fig. 5. Effect of triiodothyronine on the growth of cells from midpregnant BALB/cCrgl mice in media containing different bovine serum albumin, fraction V (BSA V) supplements. The medium contained insulin (10 μg/ml), EGF (0.01 μg/ml), transferrin (10 μg/ml), and BSA V as indicated. Diagonal slash bars ▨, 5 mg/ml dialyzed/delipidized; filled bars ■, 1 mg/ml essentially fatty acid-free; open bars □, untreated BSA V. 0T is starting cell number. Con is growth minus triiodothyronine. Mean ± standard deviation for three gels are shown.

manipulatable, for more recent work indicates that serum albumin may be replaceable by lipids and that EGF may not be required for growth under certain circumstances. Cell density, which changes during culture, may also play a modulatory role influencing growth requirements or hormonal responses. The basal medium itself is probably not an optimal medium for the growth of epithelial cells. It is well known that the composition of the medium can affect cellular requirements for growth factors and vice-versa [Ham, 1982; McKeehan, 1982]. Thus, the optimization of the culture medium may change not only the hormone and growth factor requirements for growth but cellular sensitivities to these factors as well.

Serum-free culture of mouse mammary epithelial cells is now routine. However, the serum-free culture system or systems in use must always be considered to be in a state of flux, for surely the systems will evolve as progress is made in defining the growth requirements and modulatory effects of both nutritional factors and hormones. The development of a completely defined serum-free medium is an attainable goal. For now, the serum-free culture of

TABLE I. Effect of Putrescine on Growth in Serum-Free Media Containing Different Albumin Preparations

Putrescine (μg/ml)	Untreated (5 mg/ml)	Delip/Dial (5 mg/ml)	Fatty acid-free	
			1 mg/ml	5 mg/ml
0	14.9 ± 3.2	6 ± 3.1	12.5 ± 5.6	14.5 ± 10.4
0.1	17.3 ± 4.6	8.8 ± 5.3	15.2 ± 5.2	17.6 ± 5.4
1	22.4 ± 6.5	8.3 ± 6.7	13.8 ± 2.2	18.8 ± 3.6
10	28.1 ± 17.3	17.3 ± 5.9	22.4 ± 2.6	34.6 ± 5.6
50	30.9 ± 3.9	15.2 ± 1.5	22.4 ± 6.8	32.4 ± 6.5

Mammary epithelial cells from midpregnant BALB/cCrgl mice were cultured in serum-free medium containing insulin (10 μg/ml), EGF (0.01 μg/ml), transferrin (10 μg/ml), and either untreated, delipidized and dialyzed, or fatty acid-free (Sigma) bovine serum albumin, fraction V. Putrescine was added (0.1-50 μg/ml) to the medium and the cultures were terminated after 10-12 days. The fatty acid-free albumin data are from the same experiment; the untreated, delipidized/dialyzed albumin data are a separate experiment. Initial cell number was (2-3) × 10^4 cells. Data are expressed as mean cell number × 10^{-4} ± standard deviation for three gels per experiment.

TABLE II. Effect of Linoleic Acid on Growth in the Presence of Fatty Acid-Free Albumin

Linoleic acid (μg/ml)	Albumin concentration	
	1 mg/ml	5 mg/ml
0	12.5 ± 5.6	14.9 ± 10.4
1	25.8 ± 7.4	15.2 ± 1.2
3	40.9 ± 7.5	24 ± 5.7
5	41.8 ± 6.2	36 ± 9.2
7	43.3 ± 6.3	32.8 ± 5.6
10	35.1 ± 6.5	47.8 ± 14
20	52.4 ± 7	37.9 ± 11.4

Mammary epithelial cells from midpregnant mice were cultured in serum-free medium containing insulin (10 μg/ml), EGF (0.01 μg/ml), transferrin (10 μg/ml), and fatty acid-free bovine serum albumin V (Sigma) at 1 or 5 mg/ml. Linoleate was added as a fatty acid-free bovine albumin V complex. Two separate experiments are shown. Initial cell number was (2-3) × 10^4 cells. Data are expressed as mean cell number × 10^{-4} ± standard deviation for three gels per experiment.

TABLE III. Growth in Minimal Media and Response to Medium Optimization

	Components			Days in culture		
	Insulin (μg/ml)	EGF (ng/ml)	BSA V (mg/ml)	6	12	6 Minimal + 6 Optimal
A	10	10	5	29 ± 6	76.4 ± 7.1	—
B	10	10	1	19.4 ± 4.6	39 ± 3.6	44.2 ± 1.6
C	10	1	5	17.3 ± 4.7	36 ± 0.4	46.8 ± 0
D	1	10	5	21 ± 1	44.7 ± 0	46.3 ± 2.5
E	10	1	1	11.2 ± 1.5	24.6 ± 3.6	33.9 ± 3.6
F	1	1	5	18.3 ± 1.6	24 ± 1	37.5 ± 8.3
G	1	10	1	20 ± 6.1	24 ± 2.1	34.4 ± 3.1
H	1	1	1	7.5 ± 0	13.7 ± 0	16.8 ± 0

Cells from midpregnant BALB/cCrgl mice were cultured in serum-free medium containing transferrin (10 μg/ml) and insulin, EGF, and bovine serum albumin, fraction V, at the indicated concentrations. Cells were cultured for 6 and 12 days in these media, then terminated for DNA assay. Parallel cultures for combinations B–H were changed to optimal medium (A) at 6 days and allowed to grow for 6 more days before DNA assay. The starting cell number was 4.3 ± 0.7 × 10^4. Data expressed as mean cell number × 10^{-4} ± standard deviation for 3 gels per combination.

mammary epithelial cells has permitted experimental approaches to questions concerning the interrelationships and direct effects of hormones and growth factors upon the growth of normal and tumor cells. In the future, serum-free culture may be of help in the discrimination of various types of normal cells as well as in the elucidation of differences between normal and transformed cells. Ultimately, the use of in vitro serum-free culture may lead to the understanding of in vivo phenomena that would otherwise remain resistant to experimental attack, mysteries within the complex world of the living organism.

ACKNOWLEDGMENTS

This investigation was supported by US Public Health Service grants numbers CA05388 and CA09041, awarded by the National Cancer Institute, DHHS and by the Committee of Research Funds from the University of California for the Department of Zoology, University of California, Berkeley.

REFERENCES

Barnes D, Sato G (1980): Methods for growth of cultured cells in serum-free medium. Anal Biochem 39:197-201.
Cham BE, Knowles BR (1976): A solvent system for delipidation of plasma or serum without protein precipitation. J Lipid Res 17:176-181.

Ham RG (1982): Importance of the basal nutrient medium in the design of hormonally defined media. In Sato GH, Pardee AB, Sirbasku D (eds): "Cold Spring Harbor Conferences on Cell Proliferation, Vol 9." Cold Spring Harbor, NY: Cold Spring Harbor Laboratory, pp 39-60.

Hinegardner RT (1971): An improved fluorometric assay for DNA. Anal Biochem 39:197-201.

Imagawa W, Tomooka Y, Nandi S (1982): Serum-free growth of normal and tumor mouse mammary epithelial cells in primary culture. Proc Natl Acad Sci USA 79:4074-4077.

McKeehan WL (1982): Growth-factor-nutrient interrelationships in control of normal and transformed cell proliferation. In Sato GH, Pardee AB, Sirbasku D (eds): "Cold Spring Harbor Conferences on Cell Proliferation, Vol 9." Cold Spring Harbor, NY: Cold Spring Harbor Laboratory, pp 65-74.

Richards J, Pasco D, Yang J, Guzman R, Nandi S (1983): Comparison of the growth of normal and neoplastic mouse mammary cells on plastic, on collagen, and in collagen gels. Exp Cell Res 146:1-14.

Sato G, Reid L (1978): Replacement of serum in cell culture by hormones. In Rickenberg HV (ed): "International Review of Biochemistry, Vol 20." Baltimore: University Park Press, pp 221-251.

Stampfer M, Hallowes RC, Hackett AJ (1980): Growth of normal human mammary cells in culture. In Vitro 16:415-425.

Taylor-Papadimitriou J, Purkis P, Fentiman IS (1980): Cholera toxin and analogues of cyclic AMP stimulate the growth of cultured human mammary epithelial cells. J Cell Physiol 102:317-321.

Yang J, Richards J, Guzman R, Imagawa W, Nandi S (1980): Sustained growth in primary culture of normal mammary epithelial cells embedded in collagen gels. Proc Natl Acad Sci USA 77:2088-2092.

Yang J, Larson I, Flynn D, Elias J, Nandi S (1982): Serum-free primary culture of human normal mammary epithelial cells in collagen gel matrix. Cell Biol Int Rep 6:969-975.

Methods for Serum-Free Culture of Cells of the Endocrine System,
pages 143–169
© 1984 Alan R. Liss, Inc., 150 Fifth Avenue, New York, NY 10011

9

Serum-Free Culture of the Isolated Whole Mammary Organ of the Mouse: A Model for the Study of Differentiation and Carcinogenesis

Mihir R. Banerjee and Michael Antoniou

CULTURE SYSTEMS OF MAMMARY TISSUE

Introduction

The growth and differentiation of the mammary gland is under the coordinated control of several peptide and steroid hormones [Banerjee, 1976; Forsyth and Hayden, 1977; Topper and Freeman, 1980]. Thus the mammary gland has proved to be an excellent model system for the study of hormone action [Banerjee et al., 1982; Houdebine, 1980; Rosen et al., 1980]. In addition, owing to the fact that breast tumors are the major cause of death from cancer among women in the western world today, the investigation of the mechanisms underlying both normal and neoplastic development of the mammary gland are an area of intense research.

Experiments performed over 20 years ago using hormone treatment of endocrinectomized animals [Lyons et al., 1958; Nandi, 1959] showed that estrogen, progesterone, prolactin, and growth hormone were required for the development of the mammary alveolar epithelial structures (mammogenesis). The principal hormones needed to induce the biosynthesis of milk (lactogenesis) were demonstrated to be prolactin and cortisol. However, it is apparent that the interpretation of results from such in vivo studies is made difficult by

Tumor Biology Laboratory, School of Biological Sciences, University of Nebraska, Lincoln, Nebraska 68588

systemic complexities. In order to avoid such problems, various culture models have been developed, each with its own advantages and disadvantages.

Epithelial cells obtained by the enzymatic dissociation of mammary tissue have been grown attached to the culture vessel [Ray et al., 1981a,b], on floating collagen membranes [Emerman et al., 1977], and embedded in collagen gels [Flynn et al., 1982; Pasco et al., 1982]. These systems offer the advantage of working with a relatively pure cell population. However, the cells in these culture models have been disrupted from their in vivo architectural organization, and serum needs to be included in the culture medium. That need makes it difficult to study the effect of specific hormones. The use of cultures consisting of intact alveoli may circumvent some of these problems [Carrington et al., 1981; Cline et al., 1982; Smith et al., 1982]. Explant organ culture of mammary gland from midpregnant or pseudopregnant animals has been extensively used [Forsyth, 1971]. In this culture system, fragments of mammary tissue are incubated in serum-free, chemically defined medium. Only studies of the hormonal regulation of milk production can be performed with mammary explants. The investigation of mammogenesis is not possible, since the explants are excised from tissue that has already undergone morphological development. A major drawback of the explant system is that tissue can be maintained in culture for at most 5 days. Thus the influence of hormones on the mammary gland in vivo will tend to "carry over" during the course of the experiments in vitro, which are generally conducted over a 2- to 3-day period. This is a very important consideration with regard to steroid hormones, which have been shown to persist at physiologically active levels for up to 2-3 days after mammary tissue has been placed in culture, in the absence of steroid hormones [Strobl and Lippman, 1979].

The problems inherent in the cell and explant systems are not present in the culture of the whole mammary gland from immature animals. The growth and differentiation of the whole mammary organ in vitro has been achieved for the rat [Dilley and Nandi, 1968] and the mouse [Ichinose and Nandi, 1966]. Through the use of different combinations of hormones in a serum-free chemically defined medium, the whole mammary organ can be induced to mimic the normal process of mammary development, namely mammogenesis, lactogenesis, and alveolar regression or involution [Wood et al., 1975; Terry et al., 1977]. The glands can be maintained in culture for at least a month and can be induced to undergo more than one cycle of morphological differentiation [Tonelli and Sorof, 1980]. Furthermore, as described in the section Transformation of the Mammary Cells in Organ Culture, the treatment of these murine mammary glands in culture with chemical carcinogens results in the neoplastic transformation of the epithelial cells associated with the appearance of nodules similar to that seen in the murine mammary gland in vivo [Banerjee et al., 1980]. The epithelial cells from these preneoplastic lesions can be serially transplanted into the mammary fat pad of virgin female mice indefinitely [Banerjee et al., 1980]. Thus the whole range of mammary development both normal and neoplastic can be studied within this culture system.

We describe here the method for culturing of the whole murine mammary gland and some of the results we have obtained by this system with regard to the mechanism of the hormonally induced expression of the milk protein genes and the process of chemical carcinogenesis.

Two-Step Method of Culture of the Whole Murine Mammary Organ

The culture of the whole mammary gland from mature virgin mice was first attempted by Prop [1961, 1966] with only limited success. Ichinose and Nandi [1964, 1966] were later able to obtain full development of the alveolar epithelial structures in the mammary organ from immature BALB/c female mice if the donor animals were first primed by daily injections of estrogen and progesterone. The culture method has since been further refined and extensively described [Wood et al., 1975; Lin et al., 1976; Banerjee et al., 1976]. A brief description is given below.

The mice used in our studies have been BALB/c virgin females 3–4 weeks old. Prior to dissection of the glands for culture, the mice receive nine daily subcutaneous injections of progesterone (1 mg) and 17β-estradiol (1 μg). The mammary gland from different strains of mice can be cultured successfully. However, the duration of the estrogen-progesterone priming has been found to be variable among different strains [Singh et al., 1970]. The mice are then sacrificed by cervical dislocation and the entire second thoracic mammary glands (including the primary duct and nipple) are excised and placed on Dacron rafts (Fig. 1A,B). The mammary gland attached to the raft is then placed in a plastic tissue culture dish containing serum-free Waymouth's medium (MB752/1) in the proportions of 1 ml of medium per gland. The raft floats on the medium with the mammary gland facing upwards (Fig. 1C). The culture medium is supplemented with the mammogenic hormone mixture insulin, prolactin, growth hormone (5 μg/ml of each), progesterone (1 μg/ml), and 17β-estradiol (1 ng/ml). The mammary glands are incubated in a humidified atmosphere of 95% oxygen and 5% carbon dioxide at 37°C. The medium is changed every alternate day. During the 6 days of this step I period of culture, the ductal parenchyma (Fig. 2A) proliferates to develop abundant alveolar epithelial structures, the site of milk biosynthesis (Fig. 2B). Step II incubation of the mammary glands in medium containing the lactogenic

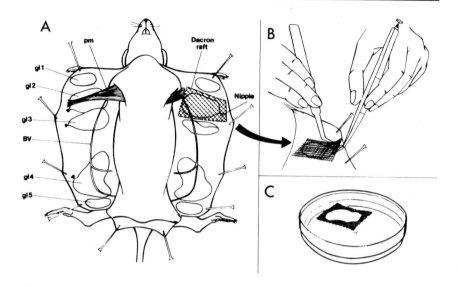

Fig. 1. The diagramatic illustration of the steps involved in the removal of, and explanation of, the murine second thoracic mammary gland in organ culture. A. Location of the second thoracic glands (gl 2). The pectoral muscle (pm) is shown on one side. B. Positioning of the Dacron raft and the dissection of the gland with a pair of forceps and a Dewcker scissors. C. Gland supported by the raft on the surface of the culture medium.

hormone combination of insulin, prolactin, and hydrocortisone (5 μg/ml of each) results in the appearance of a milk-like secretion (containing milk fat and proteins) within the lumen of the alveoli (Fig. 2C) [Wood et al., 1975; Terry et al., 1977]. Subsequent incubation of the glands for 10-12 days in the presence of only insulin (5 μg/ml) or insulin (5 μg/ml) and aldosterone (1 μg/ml) causes a regression of the alveolar structures leaving only the ductal parenchyma (Fig. 2D).

Thus, unlike the situation in vivo during pregnancy [Banerjee, 1976], the

Fig. 2. Growth and differentiation of the whole murine mammary gland in vitro. a. Second thoracic mammary gland from a 3- to 4-week-old female BALB/c mouse after nine daily injections of estrogen and progesterone. Only a ductal parenchyma is discernable. b. Gland after 6 days of culture in medium containing the mammogenic hormone mixture of insulin, prolactin, growth hormone, estrogen, and progesterone. Note the extensive development of alveolar epithelial structures. c. Histological section of a gland that was initially cultured as in panel b, and then incubated for a further 6 days in the presence of insulin, prolactin, and cortisol. The lumens of the alveoli are full of a milk-like secretion, containing proteins and fat droplets. d. Gland cultured as in b, followed by 12 days in medium containing insulin and aldosterone. The alveolar structures can be seen to have regressed, leaving only a ductal parenchyma.

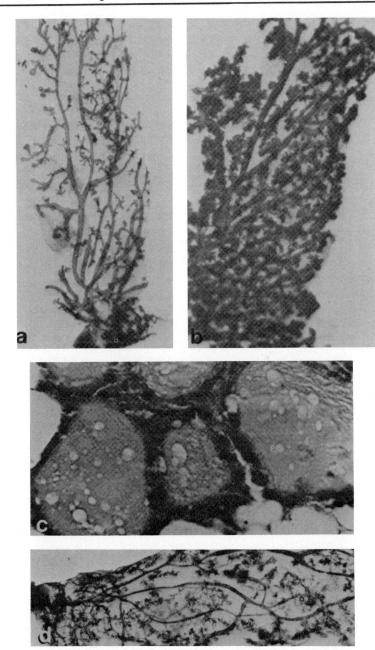

two-step culture of the whole murine mammary gland in a hormonally controlled environment exhibits the developmental stages of mammogenesis and lactogenesis in a sequential order. This in vitro system therefore provides an ideal model for the study of the influence of individual hormones on the expression of the milk protein genes.

Milk Protein Gene Expression During the Culture of the Whole Murine Mammary Organ

The expression of the genes for the major milk proteins (the caseins) during the culture of the whole murine mammary gland was initially measured by cell-free translation of RNA extracted from the glands [Terry et al., 1977]. A more accurate quantitation of the mRNAs for the caseins has been achieved through the use of a cDNA hybridization probe synthesized from an RNA fraction highly enriched for the casein mRNAs [Ganguly et al., 1979]. The results of the hybridization analysis between the casein cDNA and RNA extracted from the mammary glands at various points during the two-step period of culture are shown in Figure 3 [Mehta et al., 1980]. At the end of the step I incubation in the presence of the mammogenic hormone combination, a very low level of casein mRNAs are detectable. This is indicated by a high $eR_0t_{1/2}$ value ($524.8 \ \mathrm{mol \cdot sec \cdot liter^{-1}}$), which corresponds to 0.00067% of the total RNA or approximately 150 casein mRNA molecules per epithelial cell. Subsequent incubation of the glands in medium containing insulin, prolactin, and hydrocortisone results in a marked increase in the concentration of casein mRNAs. After 9 days of step II culture, casein mRNAs rise to account for 0.09% of the total RNA or about 37,500 mRNA molecules per mammary epithelial cell.

The accumulation of the mRNA for murine whey acid protein (WAP), the major milk whey protein [Zamierowski and Ebner, 1980; Piletz et al., 1981], shows a hormone dependence similar to that for the caseins (Antoniou, McDowell, and Banerjee, manuscript in preparation). WAP mRNA is virtually absent from the mammary glands after step I culture. This is indicated by only limited protection of the WAP cDNA hybridization probe even by an eR_0t value of $2{,}592 \ \mathrm{mol \cdot sec \cdot liter^{-1}}$ (Fig. 4A). However, after 3 days of incubation with the lactogenic hormone mixture of insulin, prolactin, and cortisol, the concentration of WAP mRNA increases to 0.005% of the total RNA (Fig. 4A). As in the case of the casein mRNAs [Banerjee et al., 1982], 3 days of step II culture in medium containing either insulin and prolactin or insulin and hydrocortisone alone does not promote an increase in the amount of WAP mRNA above the basal level already present in the glands at the end of the step I period of mammogenesis (Fig. 4B).

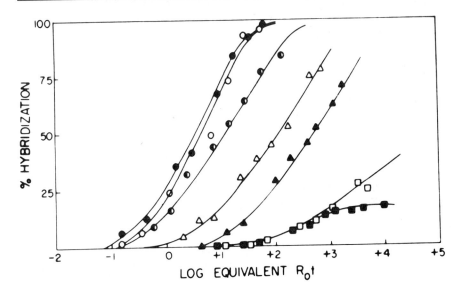

Fig. 3. Hybridization of casein cDNA to total RNA extracted from murine mammary glands at different stages of organ culture. Casein ^{3}H-cDNA (500 cpm per reaction) was hybridized under conditions of RNA excess for varying periods of time at 68°C. Total RNA was extracted from mammary glands at the following points of culture: ■—■, glands isolated from 3-week-old BALB/c virgin female mice; □—□, glands from BALB/c virgin female mice that had received nine daily subcutaneous injections of estrogen and progesterone; ▲—▲, glands grown for 6 days in mammogenic medium containing insulin (I), prolactin (Prl), estrogen (E), progesterone (P), and growth hormone (GH); △—△, glands cultured for 6 days with IPrlEPGH and 1 day with IPrl and cortisol (F); ◖—◖, 6 days IPrlEPGH + 3 days IPrlF; ○—○, 6 days IPrlEPGH + 6 days IPrlF; ●—●, 6 days IPrlEPGH + 9 days IPrlF. The casein cDNA hybridized to its template RNA with an $eR_0t_{1/2}$ value of 0.003 mol·sec·liter^{-1}

These results quite clearly demonstrate that accumulation of the milk protein mRNAs in the murine mammary organ in culture is dependent upon the presence of a glucocorticoid in medium containing prolactin.

Simultaneous occurrence of alveolar morphogenesis and expression of the casein genes can be induced in the mammary glands in culture by including hydrocortisone during the step I incubation [Ganguly et al., 1982b], or by culture in the presence of insulin, prolactin, and hydrocortisone (5 μg/ml of each), and aldosterone (1 μg/ml) [Ganguly et al., 1981]. In this respect the whole mammary organ in vitro mimics the pattern of milk protein gene expression during pregnancy in vivo [Banerjee, 1976]. Moreover, these observations further confirm that the presence of glucocorticoids are essential for the expression of the murine milk protein genes.

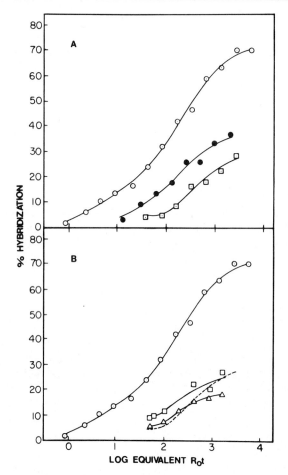

Fig. 4. The hormonally induced accumulation of whey acidic protein mRNA in the murine mammary gland in vitro. Whey acidic protein (WAP) mRNA was isolated from total poly(A)-containing RNA obtained from the mammary gland of lactating mice. The poly(A)-containing RNA was fractionated by preparative agarose gel electrophoresis in the presence of methylmercury hydroxide. An RNA fraction of approximately 700 nucleotides in length was assessed to consist largely of WAP mRNA by a combination of cell-free translation and immunoprecipitation. The ^{3}H-cDNA prepared from the WAP mRNA was then hybridized to total RNA extracted from mammary glands cultured in the presence of different hormone combinations. A. ▢ —▢ , 6 days with insulin, prolactin, 17β-estrodiol, progesterone, and growth hormone (I, Prl, E, P, GH); ●—● , 6 days with I, Prl, E, P, GH plus 1 day with insulin, prolactin, and hydrocortisone (I, Prl, F); ⊙ — ⊙ , 6 days with I, Prl, E, P, GH plus 3 days with I, Prl, F. B. □—□, 6 days with I, Prl, E, P, GH plus 3 days with I, Prl; △—△ , 6 days I, Prl, E, P, GH plus 3 days with I, F; ⊙ — ⊙ , 6 days with I, Prl, E, P, GH plus 3 days with I, Prl, F. The broken line in B indicates the position of the 6-day I, Prl, E, P, GH curve shown in A.

Earlier findings in which explants of mammary tissue from rats [Guyette et al., 1979] and rabbits [Devinoy et al., 1978] were used indicated that prolactin alone was sufficient to induce expression of the casein genes. Glucocorticoids were envisaged only to potentiate the effect of the polypeptide hormone. However, these conclusions were arrived at without taking into consideration the effect of residual steroid hormones present within the tissue [Bolander et al., 1979; Ganguly, 1980]. It is therefore quite conceivable that the stimulatory effect of prolactin on milk protein gene expression was evident only because of a synergistic action between the prolactin and the residual glucocorticoid in the explants.

Effect of Progesterone

The involvement of progesterone in the hormonal control of milk production has been known for many years. The drop in plasma progesterone during late pregnancy in the rat led Kuhn [1969] to postulate this event as the "trigger" for lactogenesis. It was subsequently demonstrated by hormone treatment of rabbits [Assairi et al., 1974; Houdebine and Gaye, 1975; Teyssot and Houdebine, 1981] and rats [Rosen et al., 1978] that exogenous progesterone inhibits milk protein gene expression. Similar results have been obtained with explant cultures of mammary tissue from rats in midpregnancy [Matusik and Rosen, 1978]. In all of these studies it was assumed that progesterone inhibits the expression of the casein genes by interfering with the action of prolactin. However, it has been shown that displacement of cortisol from its cytoplasmic receptors by progesterone inhibits the induction of murine mammary tumor virus (MTV) in murine mammary cells by the glucocorticoid [Shyamala and Dickson, 1976]. The possibility therefore exists that progesterone may be inhibiting the induction of milk protein gene expression by interfering with the action of glucocorticoids. We have tested this hypothesis in the culture of the whole murine mammary organ [Ganguly et al., 1982b].

Mammary glands were initially cultured for 6 days in the step I hormone mixture in order to induce morphogenesis of the alveolar structures. The glands were then transferred to the step II lactogenic medium, which in addition to the usual hormones contained varying amounts of progesterone. Increasing progesterone concentration resulted in greater degrees of inhibition of glucocorticoid binding to its specific cytoplasmic receptor. At a hydrocortisone-progesterone ratio of 1, a 60% inhibition of binding to its receptor was observed, with a corresponding decrease in the accumulation of casein mRNAs.

Recently, we have also shown that competition for the glucocorticoid receptor by progesterone reduces the binding of the glucocorticoid-receptor complex to the chromatin, which is accompanied by an inhibition of casein synthesis (Majumder, Antoniou, and Banerjee, unpublished results).

The necessity of nuclear binding of the glucocorticoid-receptor complex in order for the stimulation of milk protein gene expression to take place has also been demonstrated with pyridoxal-5'-phosphate [Majumder et al., 1983]. Pyridoxal-5'-phosphate inhibits the nuclear binding of the steroid-hormone receptor complex [Litwack, 1979]. The inclusion of 2 mM and 5 mM pyridoxal-5'-phosphate in the culture medium during 3 days of step II incubation of the mammary glands results in 52% and 92% inhibition, respectively, of ^{3}H-dexamethasone binding to the chromatin. A corresponding 10- and 20-fold decrease in casein mRNAs is observed. The effect of pyridoxal-5'-phosphate was found to be totally reversible after withdrawal of the vitamin B_6 analog from the medium.

Recombinant cDNA clones for the various murine milk protein mRNAs have recently been constructed in our own laboratory [Mehta et al., 1981; Antoniou, McDowell, Joshi, Mehta, and Banerjee, unpublished results] and elsewhere [Hennighausen and Sippel, 1982]. We are currently in the process of using these cDNA clones in conjunction with the whole mammary gland culture system to monitor the accumulation of individual milk protein mRNAs in response to different hormone combinations. In addition we are using the cDNA clones to determine more precisely the roles that each hormone plays during lactogenesis— that is, which hormone(s) act at the level of transcription and which are having an effect posttranscriptionally during the induction of milk protein gene expression. The latter study will be performed by assaying directly the transcripts generated in nuclei isolated from mammary glands subjected to different hormone treatments.

The experimental results presented here demonstrate that the whole mammary gland in culture retains all the characteristics of the organ in vivo. The precise nature in which the hormone environment can be controlled and the relative ease with which large amounts of tissue can be generated make the culture of the whole mammary organ an ideal system for studying mammogenesis and lactogenesis at a molecular biological level.

TRANSFORMATION OF THE MAMMARY CELLS IN ORGAN CULTURE
Background

The malignant diseases in human and in experimental animals are mostly of epithelial cell origin and the need for development of in vitro models for epithelial cell transformation has been emphasized [Heidelberger, 1970]. Although in recent years attempts to develop in vitro models for epithelial cell transformation have met with some success, the poor ability of the epithelial cells to maintain a state of differentiation and the absence of an in vitro marker of transformation have restricted reliable studies on the molecular and cell biology of the neoplastic process in the epithelial cell culture model. Moreover, the need for serum supplementation of the medium for most epithelial cell cultures contributes to additional complications. On the other hand, epithelial cells in pieces of tissue from various organs, including the mammary gland, exhibit the characteristics of differentiation in "organ culture," although cell proliferation in this culture model remains at the basal, steady-state condition. Studies [Lasnitzki, 1958, 1963; Heidelberger, 1973] have also shown that epithelial cells in pieces of mouse prostate tissue after exposure to the hydrocarbon carcinogen 3-methyl-cholanthrene (MCA) in culture show histopathological changes reminiscent of neoplastic tissue. Epithelial cells apparently transformed in organ culture, however, fail to produce tumor upon transplantation into syngeneic animals. This inability of the transformed cells to express as neoplasm in the animals may relate to the low levels of cell proliferation in organ culture. The low level of cell proliferation in the tissues may prevent "fixation" of the transformed cells and their subsequent expression.

Extensive studies have established [DeOme, 1966; Nandi and McGrath, 1973; Medina, 1974] that the multistep genesis of mammary tumors in mice is associated with the mitogenic action of the hormones; the transformation is marked by the initial appearance of precancerous hyperplastic alveolar nodules (HAN) in the mammary glands regardless of their virus, mouse mammary tumor virus (MTV), or chemical carcinogen etiology. After transplantation into the gland-free mammary fat pads of syngeneic virgin hosts, HANs initially produce serially transplantable hyperplastic alveolar outgrowths in syngeneic hosts, and mammary carcinomas subsequently appear in the HAN outgrowth tissue. Maintenance of the alveolar structures in the hyperplastic outgrowths through serial transplant generation in virgin hosts is indicative of irreversible escape of the epithelial cells from normal hormonal regulation. The lobuloalveolar structures in the HAN outgrowths also fail to show a normal response to the hormones regulating functional differentiation, as indicated by little or no expression of the milk-protein genes [Pauley and Socher,, 1980; Ganguly et al., 1982a]. Mitogenic hormone treatment of the animal stimulates macromolecular synthesis in the mammary epithelial cells of the virgin animals, and the hormone-mediated enhancement of DNA synthesis is conducive to neoplastic transformation of the mammary cells in mice [Banerjee and Rogers, 1971; Nandi, 1978].

As described in the introductory section, the discovery by Ichinose and Nandi [1966] that an isolated whole mammary organ obtained from immature female mice can develop pregnancy-like lobuloalveolar structures in a hormonally defined, serum-free medium made it feasible to promote the entire developmental cycle of the mammary gland in vitro. Studies in our laboratory have accomplished the sequential development of the lobuloalveolar structures, lactogenesis, and alveolar regression (involution) in the isolated whole mammary organ in serum-free medium, supplemented with the appropriate combinations of polypeptide and steroid hormones [Banerjee, 1976]. This remarkably faithful developmental process of the mammary parenchyma in vitro prompted the idea that the mammary gland during its development in vitro may also be susceptible to neoplastic transformation of the epithelial cells. Based on the observation described above, studies were undertaken to ascertain whether the mammary epithelial cells in the whole organ in culture respond to the transforming action of the carcinogenic hydrocarbons 7,12-dimethylbenz[a]anthracene (DMBA) and MCA. The results of these studies have been extensively described in a recent review [Banerjee, 1983] and a brief account is included in this chapter.

Preliminary Studies

In preliminary studies mammary tumor-prone, MTV-positive C3H female mice, foster nursed by MTV-negative C57Bl mice, were used. Foster nursing of C3H infants with C57Bl mothers prevents milk-borne transmission of MTV, and the mammary tumor incidence in the C3HfC57Bl mice remains very low. As usual after 9 days of hormonal priming of the immature female mice, the whole second thoracic mammary glands were incubated in Waymouth's synthetic medium containing the complete mitogenic hormone mixture insulin, prolactin, growth hormone, estrogen, progesterone, and aldosterone to stimulate lobuloalveolar morphogenesis [Banerjee et al., 1976]. During morphogenesis in vitro the glands were exposed to 1 μg/ml DMBA or 5 μg/ml MCA for a 24-h period between the 1st and 2nd day of culture. Each culture dish (Falcon plastic tissue culture dish, 60 $\times$ 15 cm) contained 1 ml of medium per gland and 3-4 glands were incubated in a dish. After the 24-h carcinogen treatment, the glands were incubated for another 8-9 days in carcinogen-free medium containing the same mitogenic hormone mixture to provide the promotive action. Additional incubation of the glands for 12-14 days in the medium containing only insulin caused complete regression of the alveolar structures in the control glands treated with DMSO used as solvent for the hydrocarbons. In the carcinogen-treated glands isolated areas of alveolar structures were retained in 26% of the regressed glands. Retention of the alveolar structures in the hormone-deficient medium indicates that the epithelial cells have escaped from the normal hormonal requirement for maintenance of the lobuloalveolar structures. Thus the characteristic escape of the alveoli in the glands in vitro from normal hormonal requirements resembles the similar loss of hormone responsiveness of the precancerous HAN seen in murine mammary glands in vivo after exposure of the animals to MTV or carcinogenic chemicals [DeOme, 1966; Nandi and McGrath, 1973; Medina, 1974].

In Vitro Model of Mammary Cell Transformation in Culture

Based on the observations of the preliminary studies described above, more detailed studies were performed with the mammary glands of BALB/c mice [Banerjee et al., 1980; Lin et al., 1976]. BALB/c female mice are MTV-free (unexpressed), and these animals are susceptible to exogenous MTV or chemical carcinogen-induced mammary carcinogenesis, sequentially producing HAN and mammary tumors in vivo [DeOme, 1966; Nandi and McGrath, 1973; Medina, 1974]. A concentration of 1 μg DMBA/ml of medium was used in the preliminary studies, because the same concentration of the hydrocarbon induces a high frequency of neoplastic transformation of fibroblasts in culture [Heidelberger, 1975]. However, in the organ culture model the mammary fat pad, by trapping the lipid-soluble hydrocarbons, may reduce the effective concentrations of the carcinogens, reaching the parenchymal cells. Thus a concentration of 2 μg (7.8 μM) DMBA per ml of medium was used. Studies in our laboratory showed that the minimal hormone combination of insulin, prolactin, and aldosterone is also highly mitogenic, stimulating full lobuloalveolar morphogenesis of the glands in vitro in absence of the ovarian steroids [Banerjee, 1976]. Moreover, glucocorticoids can enhance skin carcinogenesis apparently by augmenting metabolic activation of the hydrocarbon carcinogens [Briggs and Briggs, 1973]. Cortisol was included in the mammogenic hormone combination of insulin, prolactin, aldosterone, and cortisol.

As described in the introductory section, 3- to 4-week-old female mice were primed for 9 days by daily injections of estrogen and progesterone. The whole second thoracic mammary glands were excised and incubated in serum-free Waymouth's medium containing the hormones insulin, prolactin, aldosterone, and cortisol [Lin et al., 1976; Banerjee, 1983]. Measurement of ^{3}H-thymidine incorporation into the acid-insoluble material of the mammary glands showed that during the 6 days of the culture period, DNA synthesis rises in two waves, the first wave appearing between days 1 and 2, followed by a second wave between days 3 and 4. Scoring of the labeling index in autoradiographs of tissue sections further revealed that the increase is mostly due to DNA synthesis in the epithelial cells [Lin et al., 1976]. Hormone-induced DNA synthesis and accompanying cell proliferative activity are believed to promote the processes of neoplastic transformation [Nandi, 1978].

Thus the enhancement of DNA synthesis during morphogenesis of the glands in vitro is likely to be conducive to the transforming action of the carcinogenic chemicals.

Based on the rationale discussed above, the following experiments were done to determine the transforming action of DMBA in the whole mammary organ in culture. The glands were treated with DMBA for 24 h at different times during the 6 days of morphogenesis in medium containing the hormones insulin, prolactin, aldosterone, and cortisol [Banerjee et al., 1980; Lin et al., 1976; Banerjee, 1983]. Treatment of the glands with 7.8 μM DMBA between days 1 and 2 of culture caused a severe cytotoxic effect. The residual cells failed to complete the lobuloalveolar development during culture in the carcinogen-free medium containing the same mitogenic hormone mixture (Fig. 5). As indicated earlier, corresponding to the same period of carcinogen treatment between days 1 and 2, the glands also showed the first wave of DNA synthesis. It should be mentioned that priming of the young animals with estrogen and progesterone stimulates DNA synthesis in mammary glands in vivo [Banerjee, 1976], and the epithelial cells initiated into S phase in vivo are likely to be active in DNA synthesis during the period of carcinogen treatment and the cells actively synthesizing DNA are susceptible to cytotoxicity. The glands treated with DMBA between days 3 and 4 of culture also showed some cytotoxic effect, but a sufficient number of cells apparently remained viable, and the parenchyma completed a nearly normal lobuloalveolar development after subsequent incubation in the carcinogen-free medium containing the same mitogenic hormone mixture. The kinetics of DNA synthesis in the glands during the 6-day culture period showed that the 24-h period of carcinogen treatment between days 3 and 4 corresponds to a stage when the pool of proliferating epithelial cells are likely to be in transit from the G_1 to the S phase of the cell cycle entering the second wave of DNA synthesis [Lin et al., 1976]. The cell population in transit from the G to the S phase are less susceptible to cytotoxicity, and this conceivably allows maintenance of the critical cell density in the glands that favor subsequent morphogenesis. Corresponding to the reduced level of DNA synthesis in the glands during DMBA treatment between day 4-5 and day 5-6, the gland showed a decreased cytotoxic response and the parenchyma remained capable of full lobuloalveolar development. The observations described above indicate that after the initial 3 days of culture the cell density in the glands reaches a level that allows the parenchymal tissue to overcome the cytotoxic effect of 7.8 μM DMBA, and the residual cells remain capable of continued proliferation, completing nearly normal morphogenesis of the glands in vitro. Thus the mammary cells appear to be more susceptible to the transforming action of DMBA between day 3 and day 4 of culture.

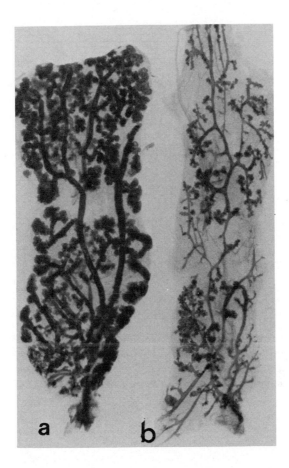

Fig. 5. Cytotoxic effect of 7.8 μM DMBA on the mammary glands in vitro. a. Control gland treated with DMSO showing full lobuloalveolar development. b. Gland treated with DMBA showing cytotoxic effect. From Lin et al. [1976], with permission.

After 24-h treatment with 7.8 μM DMBA between days 3 and 4, the glands were incubated for another 5-6 days in carcinogen-free fresh medium containing the same mitogenic hormone mixture to provide the promotive action. The glands were then incubated for an additional 12-14 days in medium with insulin and aldosterone to cause regression of the alveolar structures. Microscope examination of the stained whole-mount preparation of the glands showed that incubation in hormone-deficient medium containing insulin and aldosterone caused a complete regression of the alveolar structures, leaving a ductal parenchyma in the control glands treated with DMSO used as solvent for the hydrocarbon, and no nonregressed areas of alveolar structure were observed in these glands (0/30). In contrast, nodule-like alveolar lesions (NLAL) were present in 31/39 (79%) of the DMBA-treated glands, with an average of 8.4 lesions per gland [Lin et al., 1976] as illustrated in Figure 6. Maintenance of the lobuloalveolar structures in a hormone-deficient medium, which causes regression of the same structure under normal conditions, again indicates an escape of the epithelium in NLAL from normal hormonal requirements. Thus, DMBA-induced NLALs are considered to represent a trans-

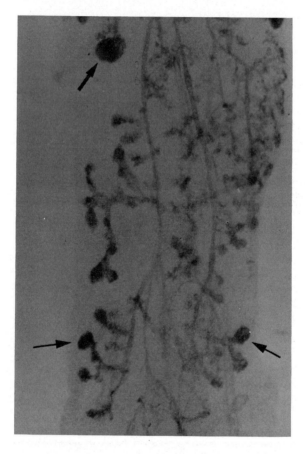

Fig. 6. Morphology of DMBA-induced NLAL (arrows) in the mammary glands in vitro. From Lin et al. [1976], with permission.

formed state of the mammary epithelial cells, and the glands showing NLAL are designated as transformed. The escape of the epithelium in NLAL from normal hormonal control also corresponds to similar characteristics of the precancerous HAN of mouse mammary glands in vivo [DeOme, 1966; Nandi and McGrath, 1973; Medina,, 1974; Pauley and Socher, 1980].

The gland treated with DMBA for a 24-h period between days 4–5 and 5–6 showed a progressively reduced level of transformation [Lin et al., 1976]. Thus the highest level of transformation is induced when most epithelial cells in the glands are likely to be in G_1 to S phase of the cell cycle during days 3 and 4 of culture. This suggests that DMBA transformation of the mammary epithelial cells in organ culture is cell cycle-related. This observation is consistent with the earlier finding that chemical carcinogen-induced in vitro transformation of the fibroblasts is also cell cycle-related [Heidelberger, 1975]. In addition to the importance of the cell cycle, combination of the mitogenic hormones also plays a role in enhancing the transformation process, apparently by providing the promotive action (Table I). The hormone combination insulin, prolactin, aldosterone, and cortisol was most conducive, showing a 79% transformation, whereas in the medium containing insulin, prolactin, and aldosterone the level of transformation was only 38%. No transformation was observed in medium containing insulin, prolactin, and cortisol, regardless of the time of treatment. It is also of interest that while the levels of the mitogenic action of the hormone mixtures insulin, prolactin, and aldosterone or insulin, prolactin, aldosterone, and cortisol were virtually identical, the frequency of transformation remained highest in the glands in the presence of glucocorticoid in the medium. This suggests that the glucocorticoid may act at a level other than stimulation of cell proliferation. Glucocorticoid has been reported to increase mouse skin carcinogenesis by enhancing the metabolic activation of hydrocarbons.

The results described above thus corroborate the findings of our preliminary studies in C3HfC57 mice showing that DMBA transformation of mammary

TABLE I. Influence of Different Hormone Mixtures on DMBA-Induced NLAL Incidence in the Mammary Gland In Vitro

Hormones[a]	24-h DMBA treatment at different times in culture				
	0–24 h	24–48 h	48–72 h	72–96 h	96–144 h
I, Prl, F	0	0	0	0	0
I, Prl, A	0	0	0	11/29 (38)[b]	9/26 (35)
I, Prl, A, F	0	7/21 (33)	12/21 (57)	31/39 (79)	14/21 (67)

[a]I, insulin; Prl, prolactin; A, aldosterone; F, cortisol.
[b]Figures in parentheses are percentages.

epithelial cells is inducible in the isolated whole mammary organ in vitro. Studies on the mammary glands of BALB/c mice further demonstrate that selection of the critical stage of cell cycle at the time of carcinogen treatment and an optimal mitogenic hormone environment in the medium can significantly enhance the frequency of transformation, rising to 79%. The hormones apparently play a role both at the initiation and the promotive stages of the transformation process. Parallel studies have shown that MCA also can induce a 40% incidence of NLAL in the glands under similar experimental conditions [Lin et al., 1976], and hydrocarbon carcinogens form a covalent adduct with mammary DNA in organ culture [Banerjee, 1983]. Thus the observations discussed above suggest the development of a new in vitro transformation model of the epithelial cells in an isolated whole mammary organ in hormonally defined serum-free medium, and suggest that NLAL in the glands constitutes an in vitro marker of transformation. An outline of this model is illustrated in Figure 7 [Banerjee et al., 1980].

In subsequent studies in our laboratory and others [Banerjee, 1983; Tonelli et al., 1979; Dickens and Sorof, 1980], NLAL-inducing ability of a variety of oncogenic chemicals, both direct-acting and those requiring metabolic activation, has been observed in the same organ culture transformation model, and the details of these studies have been recently reviewed [Banerjee, 1983].

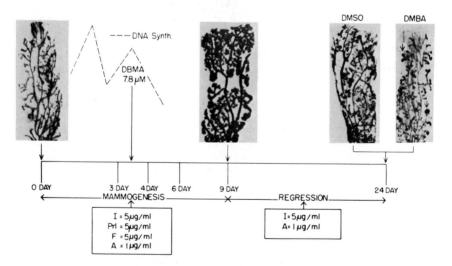

Fig. 7. Experimental model for chemical carcinogen transformation of the mammary epithelial cells in organ culture. For explanation of hormones see Table I.

Biochemical studies have further shown that the carcinogenic hydrocarbon binds to the DNA of the mammary glands in vitro, to form a DNA carcinogen adduct, suggesting metabolic activation of the procarcinogen to the ultimate carcinogenic derivatives in the mammary cells in organ culture [Banerjee, 1983].

Mammary Fat Pad Transplantation of the Transformed Cell In Vivo

Although NLAL provides an in vitro morphological marker of transformation, the escape of the epithelium from normal hormonal control alone does not consititute evidence of neoplastic changes of the epithelial cells in NLAL. The possible neoplastic potential of the cells transformed in vitro by DMBA was ascertained by transplantation of the cells into the animals, by the standard gland-free mammary fat pad transplantation procedure [Banerjee et al., 1980; Banerjee, 1983; DeOme et al., 1959]. As indicated earlier, in the mammary tumor system expression of the neoplastic cells is a multistep process, and the mammary fat pad transplantation procedure favors sequential expression of the tranformed cells, initially as hyperplastic lobuloalveolar structures with the subsequent appearance of mammary carcinomas [DeOme, 1966; Nandi and McGrath, 1973; Medina, 1974] in syngeneic virgin hosts. The same sequential appearance of hyperplastic outgrowth followed by the appearance of malignant tissue is maintained at each serial transplant generation. The gland-free mammary fat pad transplantation procedure developed by DeOme and his associates [1959] involves surgical removal of the rudimentary mammary parenchyma from the number 4 (inguinal) mammary glands of 3-week-old female mice. The remaining gland-free mammary fat pad then is used as the site of transplantation. This elegant procedure then permits transplantation of cells into the biologically preferred site of the mammary cells in the body. Normal mammary cells, either in pieces of tissue or in dissociated cell suspension after transplantation into the fat pad, rapidly proliferate and reconstitute a normal mammary tree filling the fat pad. The mammary tree derived from the normal mammary cells remains responsive to the endocrine environment of the host animals, whereas outgrowths of the transformed cells generally produce hyperplastic lobuloalveolar outgrowths that are nonresponsive to the host's hormonal environment.

Expression of Preneoplastic and Neoplastic Characteristics

Mammary cells in pieces of tissue from DMBA-treated glands (from NLAL areas of regressed glands) were transplanted into one gland-free mammary fat pad, and pieces of tissue from the control glands treated with DMSO were transplanted into the contralateral mammary fat pads of virgin syngeneic mice.

Host animals were given a supplemental hormone (prolactin) stimulation for the initial 6 weeks by a pituitary isograft into the renal capsule, and this mitogenic treatment apparently promoted enhanced expression of the transformed cells [Medina, 1978]. Ten weeks after removal of the grafted pituitary the fat pads were examined for the morphological characteristics of the outgrowth tissue produced by the implanted cells. In one series of these studies [Banerjee, 1983; Banerjee et al., 1980] 25 of 54 (46%) implants produced lobuloalveolar hyperplastic mammary cell outgrowths (MH-outgrowths) in the first generation, and mammary carcinomas subsequently appeared in 7 of the MH-outgrowths (Figs. 8 and 9). The remaining implants produced mostly ductal outgrowths and occasional outgrowths were composed of both ductal and lobuloalveolar structures. The implants from control glands consistently produced normal-like ductal outgrowth in the contralateral fat pad and no mammary tumor.

In another series of experiments [Banerjee, 1983; Banerjee et al., 1980] collagenase-dissociated epithelial cells from DMBA-treated glands were transplanted into the gland-free mammary fat pads of virgin mice, and the host animals were stimulated by pituitary isograft for 6 weeks. The mammary fat pads were then examined 10 weeks after removal of the pituitary. MH-outgrowths were present in 26 of 48 (54%) of these fat pads and mammary tumors subsequently appeared in 8 of the MH-outgrowths [Banerjee, 1983].

The results of the transplantation studies described above demonstrate that DMBA-transformed mammary epithelial cells in the isolated whole mammary organ in vitro are potentially neoplastic. Long-term studies [Banerjee, 1983; Iyer and Banerjee, 1981] have further shown that MH-outgrowth tissue is serially transplantable into virgin hosts without any supplemental hormone stimulation, indicating that escape of the epithelial cells in the MH-outgrowths from normal hormonal control is irreversible. Moreover, the pattern of sequential appearance of the MH-outgrowths and the mammary tumors at each transplant generation remained virtually identical to those of the preneoplastic HAN observed during murine mammary carcinogenesis in vivo. Assessment of 12 MH-outgrowth lines during serial transplantation into the gland-free mammary fat pad of syngeneic virgin hosts further showed that the characteristic growth potential and tumorigenicity of each outgrowth line are maintained through generations of transplantation.

The results described above thus present a demonstration that the mammary cells transformed after DMBA treatment in vitro are potentially neoplastic, and expression of the transformed cells exhibits a remarkable ability to mimic the complex developmental stages of murine mammary carcinogenesis in the animal. Thus the results described in this chapter present a new in vitro

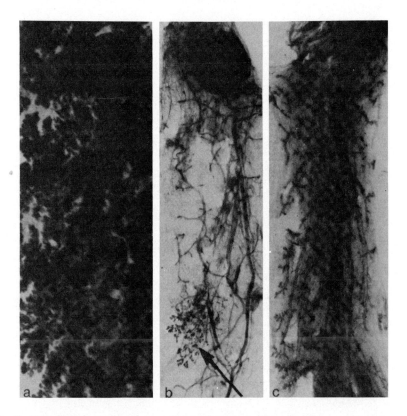

Fig. 8. Different morphological types of outgrowths derived from mammary cells transformed by DMBA in organ culture. a. Typical hyperplastic lobuloalveolar outgrowth. b. Mixed outgrowth containing lobuloalveolar stuctures in the ductal parenchyma. c. Ductal outgrowth derived from mammary cells treated wth DMSO, used as solvent for DMBA. From Telang et al. [1979], with permission.

model of epithelial cell neoplastic transformation in an isolated whole organ in a hormonally defined serum-free medium. This in vitro model also prescribes biological conditions of the mammary glands in the petri dish that are close to those present in the animal. Therefore this culture model provides conditions suitable for studies on the complex mechanisms of molecular and cell biology of mammary carcinogenesis in particular and epithelial cell neoplasia in general. The evidence presented in this chapter further demonstrates that the neoplastic process of the mammary epithelial cells is associated with the appearance of NLAL in the glands in vitro and that these appear to be analogous to the well-established precancerous HAN of murine mammary

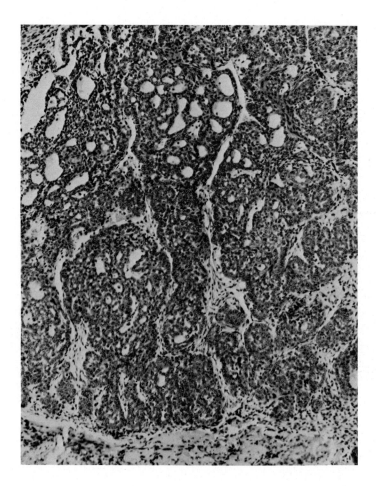

Fig. 9. Histology of a mammary carcinoma produced by a hyperplastic outgrowth derived from mammary cells transformed by DMBA in organ culture.

glands in the animals. Thus NLAL serves as a distinct in vitro transformation marker. At this time no other morphological or biochemical marker of epithelial cell transformation in vitro is known.

Chemoprevention of Mammary Cell Transformation in Organ Culture

Further studies in our laboratory and others using NLAL as in vitro marker of transformation have shown that retinoids can inhibit chemical carcinogen-induced transformation of the mammary cells in organ culture acting antipromotionally, and that estrogen plays an antagonistic role in the preventive action of the vitamin A analogs [Banerjee, 1983; Chatterjee and Banerjee, 1982a,b,c; Dickens et al., 1979]. Moreover, selenium and β-carotene also can cause a dose-dependent inhibition of DMBA transformation of the mammary cells in organ culture, acting both at the initiation and the promotional stages [Banerjee, 1983; Chatterjee and Banerjee, 1982c].

CONCLUDING COMMENTS

The neoplastic transformation model of the mammary cells in organ culture now makes it feasible to investigate the relationship between molecular events of chemical oncogenesis and chemopreventive agents in the same in vitro model. NLAL in the glands can be used as a morphological end point of transformation in vitro.

In conclusion, preceding discussions of the results presented in this chapter demonstrate that the culture model of the whole mammary organ of the mouse presents opportunities for reliable studies 1) on hormone-inducible selective gene expression leading to differentiation and 2) the molecular mechanisms of action of chemopreventive agents on chemically induced biochemical processes of neoplastic transformation of the epithelial cells in a major endocrine-dependent organ.

ACKNOWLEDGMENTS

The authors would like to thank Scott McDowell for technical assistance and Arvilla Kirchhoff for secretarial assistance. The work was supported by US Public Health Service grants CA11058 and CA25304 from the National Cancer Institute, National Institutes of Health.

REFERENCES

Assairi L, Delouis C, Gay P, Houdebine LM, Olliver-Bousquet M, Denamur R (1974): Inhibition by progesterone of the lactogenic effect or prolactin in the pseudopregnant rabbit. Biochem J 144:245-252.

Banerjee MR (1976): Responses of mammary cells to hormones. Int Rev Cytol 46:1-97.

Banerjee MR (1983): An in vitro model for neoplastic transformation of epithelial cells in an isolated whole mammary organ of the mouse. In Weber M, Sekely L (eds): "In Vitro Model for Cancer Research." Boca Raton, FL: CRC Press (in press).

Banerjee MR, Rogers FM (1971): Hormonal regulation of DNA polymerase activity and DNA synthesis in preneoplastic nodules of mouse mammary gland. J Endocrinol 49:39-49.

Banerjee MR, Wood BG, Lin FK, Crump LR (1976): Organ culture of the whole mammary gland of the mouse. In Sanford KK (ed): "Tissue Culture Association Manual." Rockville, MD: Tissue Culture Association, Vol 2, pp 457-462.

Banerjee MR, Ganguly N, Mehta NM, Iyer AP, Ganguly R (1980): Functional differentiation and neoplastic transformation in an isolated whole mammary organ in vitro. In McGrath C, Brennan M, Rich M (eds): "Cell Biology of Breast Cancer." New York: Academic, pp 485-516.

Banerjee MR, Mehta NM, Ganguly R, Majumder PK, Ganguly N, Joshi J (1982): Selective gene expression in an isolated whole mammary organ in vitro. In Sirbasku DA, Sato GH, Pardee AB (eds): "Growth of Cells in a Hormonally Defined Medium." Cold Spring Harbor, New York: Cold Spring Harbor Laboratory, pp 789-805.

Bolander FF Jr, Nicholas KR, Topper YJ (1979): Retention of glucocorticoid by isolated mammary tissue may complicate interpretation of results from in vitro experiments. Biochem Biophys Res Commun 91:247-252.

Briggs MH, Briggs M (1973): Induction by topical corticosteroids of skin enzymes metabolizing carcinogenic hydrocarbons. Br J Dermatol 88:75-81.

Carrington CA, Hosick HL, Forsyth IA, Dils RR (1981): Novel multialveolar epithelial structures from rabbit mammary gland that synthesize milk specific fatty acids in response to prolactin. In Vitro 17:363-368.

Chatterjee M, Banerjee MR (1982a): N-nitrosodiethylamine-induced nodule-like alveolar lesion and its prevention by a retinoid in BALB/c mouse mammary glands in the whole organ in culture. Carcinogenesis 3:801-804.

Chatterjee M, Banerjee MR (1982b): Influence of hormones on N-(4-hydroxyphenyl)retinamide inhibition of 7,12-dimethylbenz[a]anthracene transformation of mammary cells in organ culture. Cancer Lett 16:239-245.

Chatterjee M, Banerjee MR (1982c): Selenium mediated dose-dependent inhibition of 7,12-dimethylbenz[a]anthracene induced transformation of mammary cell in organ culture. Cancer Lett 17:187-195.

Cline PR, Zamora PO, Hosick HL (1982): Morphology and lactose synthesis in tissue culture of mammary alveoli isolated from lactating mice. In Vitro 18:694-702.

DeOme KB (1966): The mammary tumor system in mice. In Burdette J (ed): "Viruses Inducing Cancer." Salt Lake City: University of Utah Press, pp 127-137.

DeOme KB, Faulkin LT Jr, Bern HA, Blair PB (1959): Development of mammary tumors from hyperplastic alveolar nodule transplanted into gland-free mammary fat pad of female C3H mice. Cancer Res 19:515-520.

Devinoy E, Houdebine LM, Delouis C (1978): Role of prolactin and glucocorticoids in the expression of casein gene in rabbit mammary gland organ culture, quantification of mRNA. Biochim Biophys Acta 517:360-366.

Dickens MS, Sorof S (1980): Retinoid prevents transformation of cultured mammary glands but not by nonactivated procarcinogens. Nature 85:581-584.

Dickens MS, Custer RP, Sorof S (1979): Retinoid prevents mammary gland transformation by carcinogenic hydrocarbon in whole organ culture. Proc Natl Acad Sci USA 76:5891-5895.

Dilley WG, Nandi S (1968): Rat mammary gland differentiation in vitro in the absence of steroids. Science 161:59-60.

Emerman J, Enami J, Pitelka DR, Nandi S (1977): Hormonal effects on intracellular and secreted casein in cultures of mouse mammary epithelial cells on floating collagen membranes. Proc Natl Acad Sci USA 74:4466-4470.

Flynn D, Yang J, Nandi S (1982): Growth and differentiation of primary cultures of mouse mammary epithelium embedded in collagen gel. Differentiation 22:191-194.

Forsyth IA (1971): Organ culture techniques and the study of hormone effects on the mammary gland. J Dairy Res 38:419-444.

Forsyth IA, Hayden TJ (1977): Comparative endocrinology of mammary growth and lactation. Symp Zool Soc London 41:135-163.

Ganguly R, Mehta NM, Ganguly N, Banerjee MR (1979): Glucocorticoid modulation of casein gene transcription in mouse mammary gland. Proc Natl Acad Sci USA 76:6466-6470.

Ganguly R, Ganguly N, Mehta NM, Banerjee MR (1980): Absolute requirement of glucocorticoid for expression of the casein gene in presence of prolactin. Proc Natl Acad Sci USA 77:6003-6006.

Ganguly N, Ganguly R, Mehta NM, Crump LR, Banerjee MR (1981): Simultaneous occurrence of pregnancy-like lobuloalveolar morphogenesis and casein gene expression in a culture of the whole mammary gland. In Vitro 17:55-60.

Ganguly N, Ganguly R, Mehta NM, Banerjee MR (1982a): Growth and differentiation of hyperplastic outgrowths derived from mouse mammary epithelial cells transformed in organ culture. J Natl Cancer Inst 69:453-463.

Ganguly R, Majumder PK, Ganguly N, Banerjee MR (1982b): The mechanisms of progesterone-glucocorticoid interaction in regulation of casein gene expression. J Biol Chem 257:2182-2187.

Guyette WA, Matusik RJ, Rosen JM (1979): Prolactin mediated transcriptional and post-transcriptional control of casein gene expression. Cell 17:1013-1023.

Heidelberger C (1970): Chemical carcinogenesis, chemotherapy: Cancer's continuing core challenges. Cancer Res 30:1549-1569.

Heidelberger C (1973): Chemical carcinogenesis in culture. Adv Cancer Res 18:317-366.

Heidelberger C (1975): Chemical carcinogenesis. Annu Rev Biochem 44:79-121.

Hennighausen LG, Sippel A (1982): Characterization and cloning of the mRNAs specific for the lactating mouse mammary gland. Eur J Biochem 125:125-131.

Houdebine LM (1980): Role of prolactin, glucocorticoids and progesterone in the control of casein gene expression. In Dumont J, Nunez J (eds): "Hormones and Cell Regulation." Amsterdam: Elsevier/North-Holland, Vol 4, pp 175-196.

Houdebine L, Gaye P (1975): Regulation of casein synthesis in the rabbit mammary gland. Mol Cell Endocrinol 3:37-55.

Ichinose RR, Nandi S (1964): Lobuloalveolar differentiation in mouse mammary tissue in vitro. Science 145:496-497.

Ichinose RR, Nandi S (1966): Influence of hormones on lobuloalveolar differentiation of mouse mammary gland in vitro. J Endocrinol 35:331-340.

Iyer AP, Banerjee MR (1981): Sequential expression of preneoplastic and neoplastic characteristics of mouse mammary epithelial cells transformed in organ culture. J Natl Cancer Inst 66:893-905.

Kuhn NJ (1969): Progesterone withdrawal as the lactogenic trigger in the rat. J Endocrinol 44:39-54.

Lasnitzki I (1958): Br J Cancer 12:547.

Lasnitzki I (1963): Growth pattern of mouse prostate gland in organ culture and its response to sex hormones, vitamin A and 3-methylcholanthrene. Natl Cancer Inst Monogr 12:381.

Lin FK, Banerjee MR, Crump LR (1976): Cell cycle-related hormone carcinogen interaction during chemical carcinogen induction of nodule-like mammary lesions in organ culture. Cancer Res 36:1607-1614.

Litwack G (1979): Modulator and the glucocorticoid receptor. Trends Biochem Sci October, pp 217-220.

Lyons WR, Li CH, Cole RD, Johnson RE (1958): The hormonal control of mammary growth and lactation. Recent Prog Horm Res 14:219-248.

Majumder PK, Joshi JB, Banerjee MR (1983): Correlation between nuclear glucocorticoid receptor levels and casein gene expression in murine mammary gland in vitro. J Biol Chem 258:6793-6798.

Matusik RJ, Rosen JM (1978): Prolactin induction of casein mRNA in organ culture. J Biol Chem 253:2343-2347.

Medina D (1974): Mammary tumorigenesis in chemical carcinogen treated mice. I. Incidence in BALB/c and C57BL mice. J Natl Cancer Inst 53:213-221.

Medina D (1978): Preneoplasia in breast cancer. In McGuire WL (ed): "Breast Cancer." New York: Plenum, Vol 2, pp 47-102.

Mehta NM, Ganguly N, Ganguly R, Banerjee MR (1980): Hormonal moduation of the casein gene expression in a mammogenesis-lactogenesis two-step culture model of whole mammary gland of the mouse. J Biol Chem 55:4430-4434.

Mehta NM, El-Gewely MR, Joshi J, Helling RB, Banerjee MR (1981): Cloning of mouse β-casein gene sequences. Gene 15:285-288.

Nandi S (1959): Hormonal control of mammogenesis and lactogenesis in C3H/HeCrgl mouse. Univ Calif Publ Zool 65:1-129.

Nandi S (1978): Hormonal carcinogenesis: A novel hypothesis for the role of hormones. J Environ Pathol Toxicol 2:13-20.

Nandi S, McGrath CS (1973): Mammary neoplasia in mice. Adv Cancer Res 17:353-414.

Pasco D, Quan A, Smith S, Nandi S (1982): Effect of hormones and EGF on proliferation of rat mammary epithelium enriched for alveoli. Exp Cell Res 141:313-324.

Pauley RJ, Socher SH (1980): Hormonal influences on the expression of casein messenger RNA during mouse mammary tumorigenesis. Cancer Res 40:362-367.

Piletz JE, Hienlen M, Ganschow RE (1981): Biochemical characterization of a novel whey protein from murine milk. J Biol Chem 56:11509-11516.

Prop FJA (1961): Effects of hormones on mouse mammary glands in vitro: Analysis of factors that cause lobuloalveolar development. Pathol Biol 9:640-645.

Prop FJA (1966): Effect of donor age on hormone reactivity of mouse mammary gland organ cultures. Exp Cell Res 42:386-388.

Ray DB, Horst IA, Jensen RW, Kowal J (1981a): Normal mammary cells in long-term culture. I. Development of hormone dependent functional monolayer cultures and assay of alpha-lactalbumin production. Endocrinology 108:573-583.

Ray DB, Horst IA, Jensen RW, Mills NC, Kowal J (1981b): Normal mammary cells in long-term culture. II. Prolactin, corticosterone, insulin and triiodothyronine effects on alpha-lactalbumin production. Endocrinology 108:584-590.

Rosen JM, O'Neal DL, McHugh JE, Comstock JP (1978): Progesterone mediated inhibition of casein mRNA and polysomal casein synthesis in the rat mammary gland during pregnancy. Biochemistry 17:290-297.

Rosen JM, Matusik R, Richards DA, Gupta P, Rodgers JR (1980): Multihormonal regulation of casein gene expression at the transcriptional and posttranscriptional levels in the mammary gland. Recent Prog Horm Res 36:157-193.

Shyamala G, Dickson C (1976): Relationship between receptor and mammary tumor virus production after stimulation by glucocorticoid. Nature 262:107-112.

Singh DV, DeOme K, Bern HA (1970): Strain differences in response of the mouse mammary gland to hormones in vitro. J Natl Cancer Inst 45:657-675.

Smith JJ, Nickerson SC, Kennan TW (1982): Metabolic energy and cytoskeletal requirements for synthesis and secretion by acini from rat mammary gland. Int J Biochem 14:87-98.

Strobl JS, Lippman ME (1979): Prolonged retention of estradiol by human breast cancer cells in tissue culture. Cancer Res 39:3319-3327.

Terry PM, Banerjee MR, Lui RM (1977): Hormone-inducible casein messenger RNA in a serum-free organ culture of whole mammary gland. Proc Natl Acad Sci USA 74:2441-2445.

Teyssot B, Houdebine LM (1981): Role of progesterone and glucocorticoids in transcription of the β-casein and 28S ribosomal genes in the rabbit mammary glands. Eur J Biochem 114:597-608.

Tonelli QJ, Sorof S (1980): Epidermal growth factor requirement for development of cultured mammary glands. Nature 285:250-252.

Tonelli QJ, Custer RP, Sorof S (1979): Transformation of cultured mouse mammary glands by aromatic amines and amides and their derivatives. Cancer Res 39:1784-1792.

Topper YJ, Freeman CS (1980): Multiple hormone interactions in the developmental biology of the mammary gland. Physiol Rev 60:1049-1106.

Wood BG, Washburn LL, Mukherjee AS, Banerjee MR (1975): Hormonal regulation of lobuloalveolar growth, functional differentiation and regression of whole mammary gland in organ culture. J Endocrinol 65:1-6.

Zamierowski MM, Ebner KE (1980): A radioimmunoassay for mouse α-lactalbumin. J Immunol Methods 36:211-220.

Methods for Serum-Free Culture of Cells of the Endocrine System,
pages 171-182
© 1984 Alan R. Liss, Inc., 150 Fifth Avenue, New York, NY 10011

10
Growth of Human Mammary Epithelial Cells in Monolayer Culture

Martha Stampfer

The mammary gland represents an excellent source of human cells for culture, since abundant amounts of tissue are available from several commonly performed surgical procedures—reduction mammoplasties, biopsies, gynecomastias, and mastectomies. These various tissues can provide cells from individuals of all ages and breast pathologies. In particular, mammary gland epithelial cells in culture can be valuable substrates for studies on carcinogenesis, differentiation, and basic cellular and molecular mechanisms. In vivo, the breast glandular epithelial cells are the cell type responsible for expression of the differentiated functions associated with synthesis of milk products; this behavior is under specific hormonal control. The breast epithelial cells are also the source of the second most common cancer in this country.

Our laboratory has developed methods to utilize surgically removed tissue for growth of human mammary epithelial cells (HMEC) in monolayer culture [Stampfer et al., 1980; Smith et al., 1981; Stampfer, 1982]. Other laboratories have developed tissue culture methods using human mammary cells derived from lactation fluids [Taylor-Papadimitriou et al., 1980; Kirkland et al., 1979; Buehring, 1972] and surgically derived cells grow within collagen gels [Yang et al., 1981]. Our objectives in developing this system were 1) to obtain pure populations of epithelial cells, 2) to obtain sufficient number of cells from one individual to permit repetition of experiments from the same person, 3) to grow the cells in culture for enough population doublings and passages to allow numerous biologic and biochemical experiments, and 4) to be able to find culture conditions that would permit expression (and modula-

Division of Biology and Medicine, Lawrence Berkeley Laboratory, Berkeley, California 94720

tion) of normal, differentiated mammary epithelial functions. The following methods describe how we have accomplished the first three of these goals, and our present state of progress for the fourth objective.

TISSUE COLLECTION

Large quantities of human mammary tissues are readily available as discard material from several common surgical procedures: reduction mammoplasties, mastectomies, biopsies, and gynecomastias. These specimens can be stored (or shipped) at 4°C for up to 72 h without affecting subsequent viability, so that tissues can be utilized from nonlocal sources. If not used immediately, smaller specimens (e.g., tumors, biopsies) are stored in sterile medium containing 5% fetal calf serum (FCS) and antibiotics (100 U/ml penicillin, 100 μg/ml fungizone, 50 U/ml polymyxin B).

PROCESSING OF MAMMARY TISSUE

The glandular epithelial cells are separated from the stromal cells by a procedure involving dissection, enzymatic digestion, and filtration. In nontumor specimens, epithelial areas appear as white strands embedded in the stromal matrix of adipose tissue, connective tissue, and blood vessels. These areas are gently dissected out by use of a combination of scalpel, forcep, and scissor to scrape away the grossly fatty material and cut or lacerate the epithelial-appearing areas. Tumor tissue is processed by carefully mincing the whole specimen with scalpel and forcep. The minced epithelial-containing tissue is placed in a conical centrifuge tube (50 ml or 15 ml) with the tissue comprising no greater than a third of the volume of the tube. The tube is brought up to full volume, leaving only a small air space to allow for gentle mixing during rotation, using tissue digestion mixture (Ham's F-12, 10 μg/ml insulin, antibiotics) and a final concentration of 10% FCS, 200 U/ml crude collagenase (Sigma type I), and 100 U/ml hyaluronidase (Sigma). The tubes are placed on a tube rotator and incubated overnight at 37°C. The next day, the tubes are centrifuged at 600g for 5 min, the pelleted material is resuspended in fresh tissue digestion mixture, FCS, and enzymes, and the tubes are reincubated with rotation at 37°C. Most tissues require an additional round of centrifugation and resuspension overnight in fresh tissue digestion/ enzyme mixture. The incubation is completed when microscopic examination shows clumps of cells (organoids) with ductal, alveolar, or ductular-alveolar structures (Fig. 1) free from attached stroma. For tumor tissues, the cellular clumps may not display this normal glandular morphology, and only unstructured clumps of epithelial cells may be visible.

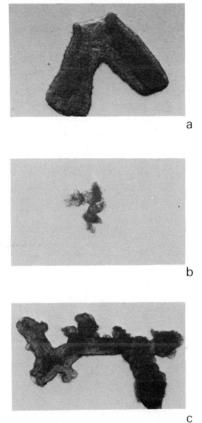

a

b

c

Fig. 1. Organoids derived from enzymatic digestion of reduction mammoplasty tissue. Ductal (a), alveolar (b), ductular-alveolar-like (c) structures. ×34. From Stampfer et al. [1980], with permission.

When digestion is completed, the material is centrifuged and resuspended in a small volume of medium. It is then placed on a sterile polyester filter of 150-μm pore size (Pecap Monofilament polyester screen, Tetko, Inc., Monterey Park, CA), consisting of a 3″ × 3″ piece of filter screen held rigid between two metal plates containing a 2″ diameter center opening. After collection of a filtrate by gravity, the material remaining of the filter is collected by inverting the filter and washing the collected material into a 50-ml centrifuge tube. The material remaining in the filtrate is placed on a 51-μm filter, and the collection process is repeated to harvest the smaller epithelial clumps. For some tumor tissues, which contain only small clumps, only one filtration through a 95-μm or 51-μm filter is performed. The material collected on the different-sized filters, and the filtrate, are each centrifuged and the pellets are resuspended in cell preservative medium (Dulbecco's modified Eagle's medium [DME], 15% FCS, 10% dimethylsulfoxide [DMSO]), with a 10:1 volume of medium to volume of the packed cell pellet. Aliquots containing about 0.1 ml each of pelleted cells are slowly frozen to $-70°C$ and then transferred to storage in liquid nitrogen. Depending upon the amount of tissue obtained and utilized, and the epithelial content of that tissue, one can typically generate approximately 10-150 ampules per reduction mammoplasty, 4-40 per nontumor mastectomy tissue, 2-15 per biopsy and gynecomastia tissue, and 0-20 per tumor tissue. These organoids have been stored frozen in liquid nitrogen for 6 years with no apparent reduction in viability. The pools of larger organoids (150 μm) contain nearly pure populations of epithelial cells. The smaller organoid pools (95 μm, 51 μm) may additionally contain some incompletely digested blood vessel elements. The filtrate contains a mixed population of small epithelial and vascular cell clumps, plus single epithelial and stromal cells.

CELL CULTURE MEDIUM

We have used two different kinds of medium to achieve prolonged reproducible and rapid growth of the HMEC (see Tables I and 2). These two media produce different patterns of cell growth, and perhaps different states of functional differentiation of the HMEC.

Our originally developed medium, designated MM, contains several hormones and growth factors, FCS, and conditioned medium (CM) from three human cell lines. The rapid cell growth observed with MM is dependent upon the CM from the human fetal intestine cell line fHs74Int and/or the bladder line Hs767B1 developed by Owens et al. [1976]. Other human fetal intestine lines tested were also effective. Unfortunately, the nature of the growth factor in the CM has not been determined. CM from the putative myoepithelial cell line Hs578Bst [Hackett et al., 1977] is not required for rapid growth, but it is included since initial experiments indicated that it increased HMEC attachment to the plastic substrate. All three cell lines are available from the American Type Culture Collection, Rockville, MD. To prepare CM, cells are grown in T-75 flasks and fed with a basal medium (Table I). The supernatant is collected from subconfluent to confluent cultures every 48-72 h. The CM may be stored frozen and sterilized by filtration before use. The fHs74Int and Hs767B1 cell lines are maintained with 1:3 splits every 2-3 weeks; the Hs578Bst is split 1:2 every 3-4 weeks. The proliferative capacity of these lines appears to decline around passages 22-26 and they are then discarded.

TABLE I. Contents of Cell Culture Media

Basal medium [7.5% CO_2 atmosphere] (for fibroblasts; cell lines used to produce conditioned media)	
Ham's F12	47.5%
Dulbecco's modified Eagle's Medium	47.5%
Fetal calf serum	5.0%
Insulin	5 $\mu g/ml$
MM [7.5% CO_2 atmosphere]	
Ham's F12	30%
Dulbecco's modified Eagle's medium	30%
Fetal calf serum	0.5%
Conditioned media	
fHs74Int and/or Hs767B1	30%
Hs578Bst	9.5%
Insulin	10 $\mu g/ml$
Hydrocortisone	0.1 $\mu g/ml$
Epidermal growth factor	5 ng/ml
Triiodothyronine	10^{-8} M
Estradiol	10^{-9} M
Cholera toxin	1 ng/ml
Penicillin	100 U/ml
Streptomycin	100 $\mu g/ml$
MCDB170 [2% CO_2 atmosphere]	
Basal MCDB170	100%
Insulin	5 $\mu g/ml$
Hydrocortisone	0.5 $\mu g/ml$
Epidermal growth factor	5 ng/ml
Ethanolamine	10^{-4} M
Phosphoethanolamine	10^{-4} M
Transferrin	10 $\mu g/ml$
Bovine pituitary extract	70 $\mu g/ml$

More recently, a serum-free medium, designated MCDB170, has been developed in Dr. Richard Ham's laboratory. This medium currently contains only one undefined element, bovine pituitary extract (BPE). The exact content of this medium is reported elsewhere [Hammond et al., 1983].

INITIATION OF CELL GROWTH

Cultures are initiated by quickly thawing frozen organoids and seeding them into T-25 flasks. One ampule containing approximately 0.1 ml of pelleted organoids in a 1-ml volume of cell preservative medium is generally seeded into six T-25 flasks. To ensure an even distribution and rapid attachment, the organoids are carefully dripped onto the surface of the flask with a

TABLE II. Comparison of Cell Growth in MM vs. MCDB170

	MM	MCDB170
Cell passages with active growth	2-4	10-20
Density of seeding	$(3-5) \times 10^3$ cells per cm^2	$(3-5) \times 10^3$ cells per cm^2
Density at subculture	$(3-5) \times 10^4$ cells per cm^2	$(3-5) \times 10^4$ cells per cm^2
Maximal doubling times	18-24 h	36-72 h
Colony-forming efficiency	2-40% with feeder layer cells	5-30%
Keratin	Present	Present
Cell-associated fibronectin pattern	Powdery, punctate	Powdery, punctate
Milk fat globule antigen	Positive mainly on larger, squamous-appearing cells	Rare positive
Pattern of glucose metabolites	Large amounts of glycogen, lactic acid, some specific amino acids, and hexose phosphates	Little glycogen, hexose phosphates, and amino acids, less lactic acid, more TCA cycle intermediates
Morphology of cells that no longer divide	Large, squamous, vacuolated, smooth-edged	Elongated large, flat, striated, irregular edges (2-4 passage); large, vacuolated, smooth edged (10-20 passage)

1-ml pipette. Then 2 ml of medium is added. By 24 h, most organoids should appear firmly attached to the flask, and an additional 2 ml of medium is added. Cultures are routinely fed three times a week.

Cell migration from the organoids is visible by 24-48 h after seeding (Fig. 2). In MM, mitotic activity is visible by 48 h, and there is subsequent rapid growth to near confluence within 5-8 days after seeding. Cell growth in MCDB170 is slower, 10-14 days being required to achieve confluence.

Occasionally, some fibroblastic cell growth can be observed in primary cultures, particularly with tumor specimens or material collected on a filter smaller than 150 μm. These fibroblasts can usually preferentially be removed by performing a differential trypsinization [Owens et al., 1974]. The cultures are exposed to STV (saline, 0.05% trypsin, 0.02% versene) at room temperature for a short period of time (~1-2 min), and the detached cells are removed. At these time periods, most of the fibroblasts are removed because they are less adherent, whereas the epithelial cells remain attached to the substrate.

SUBCULTURE OF HMEC

To subculture, the cell monolayer is washed once with STV, a small volume of STV is added to just cover the cells, and the flask is left at room temperature

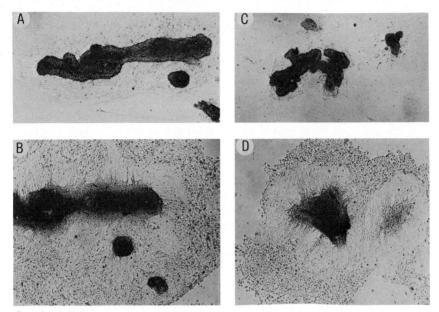

Fig. 2. Outgrowth of mammary epithelial cells from specimen H184 organoids. A. Culture in MM 2 days after seeding. B. The same culture in MM 4 days after seeding. C. Culture in MCDB170 2 days after seeding. D. Culture in MCDB170 5 days after seeding. ×38.

until the desired number of cells have detached. Cells grown in MM are removed with 2-4 ml of MM, counted in a hemocytometer, and plated directly into new dishes. Detached cells from cultures grown in the serum-free MCDB170 are washed off with 5 ml of buffer, counted, brought up to 10 ml in buffer, and pelleted at 600g for 5 min to remove the cells from the trypsin. The pelleted cells are resuspended in fresh medium and replated. For primary cultures, we generally do not subculture all of the cells at once, but perform a partial trypsinization, by which approximately half of the cells are removed to second passage. The cells remaining in the primary flask display rapid re-growth to near confluence and need to be subcultures again within 48 h (in MM) or 96 h (in MCDB170). Also for MCDB170, the cells remaining in the flask need an additional wash with buffer before refeeding to remove any residual trypsin. This partial trypsinization procedure can be performed 3-6 times with subsequent active growth in the second-passage cells, thus gener-ating larger cell numbers spaced over time. Secondary-passage cells in mass culture are seeded at a density of $(3-5) \times 10^3$ per cm^2. Clonal growth, with efficiencies of 5-30%, is supported by MCDB170. To achieve clonal growth (with efficiencies of 2-40% in second passage) in MM, the single epithelial cells need to be seeded onto dishes containing 10^3 cells per cm^2 of UV-inactivated fibroblasts [Smith et al., 1981].

To maintain active growth upon subculture, it is essential that the primary culture not be permitted to remain at confluence. Cells at confluence, especially those grown in MM, will start to grow in multilayers and form domes and ridge-like structures [Stampfer et al., 1980]. Once this occurs, subsequent growth capacity and colony-forming ability is diminished. We have observed that the presence of cholera toxin in primary cultures in MM produces cell growth in multilayers well before outgrowth to confluence, and we therefore omit cholera toxin in primary cultures of nontumor specimens. Additionally, cells grown in MM need to have the pH carefully monitored, since they produce large quantities of acid products, particularly lactic acid; as cultures near confluence, they may become overly acidic. Normally the cells are maintained at a pH range of 6.9-7.3, corresponding to an orange-red color with phenol red as a pH indicator. If the culture medium becomes yellow-orange, the flasks should be removed from a 7.5% CO_2 atmosphere to a lower CO_2 concentration ($\sim 2\%$).

PROPAGATION OF HMEC

In MM, most cells from premenopausal nontumor tissue show a similar growth pattern, although interindividual differences may exist [Stampfer et al., 1982] (we have examined about 40 such specimens). Secondary and tertiary cultures grow rapidly (doubling times of 18-48 h) to visual confluence in 5-6 days and need to be subcultured at that time (cell density $\sim 5 \times 10^4$ per cm^2), before multilayering occurs. By fourth passage, most specimens show a decreased growth rate, and by fifth passage, there is little net increase in cell numbers, although areas of mitotic activity are sometimes still visible. As the cell's proliferative capacity decreases at higher passage, the cell population can be observed to contain an increased percentage of large, squamous-looking cells, which do not undergo further cell divisions (Fig. 3).

Variability in growth patterns is observed when postmenopausal or tumor tissues are examined. In general, cells from postmenopausal tissues display active growth for fewer subcultures (1-2), whereas growth of cells from tumor tissues may range from activity equal to that of normal cells to poor growth even at secondary passage. Occasional tumor specimens have also not shown any growth in primary culture, but in most of these cases the tumor specimen obtained was extremely small, and little if any epithelial tissue was present after enzymatic digestion.

Thus far we have examined much fewer specimens (a total of eleven) in MCDB170 and cannot yet be sure what variability will exist in growth patterns

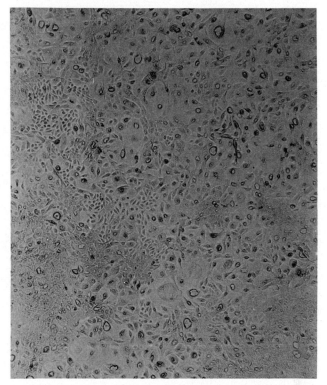

Fig. 3.   Confluent fourth-passage culture of specimen H184 mammary epithelial cells grown in MM. Note the heterogeneity in cell morphology, with areas of small refractile growing cells, tightly packed areas of small nongrowing cells, and large squamous vacuolated cells. ×32.

between individuals and tissue types. In the light microscope, proliferating cell populations appear morphologically similar to cells grown in MM (Fig. 4A,B); however, growth rates are slower (doubling times of 36–72 h).

The most striking difference between the cells grown in MCDB170 vs. MM is that more population doublings occur in the serum-free medium; however, only a small subpopulation of the cells is capable of this more extended growth. Depending upon the individual, at passage 2–4 two morphologically distinct cell populations appear (Fig. 4C). One type maintains the same morphology and growth rate as that initially observed, but the second type appears larger and flatter, with less-defined cell borders and little proliferative capacity. Results thus far indicate that the percentage of growing cells present at passages 2–4 can be increased by addition of agents which increase intracellular levels of cAMP. For some individuals, such agents are required to maintain any growing cell population. Observation of single-cell colony growth

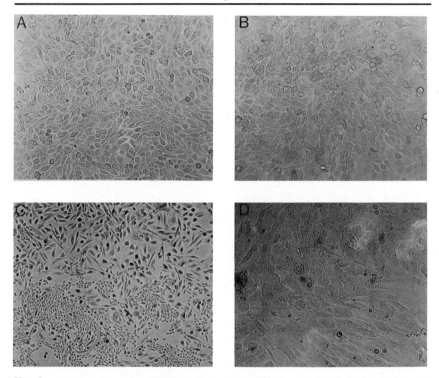

Fig. 4. Cells from specimen H161 grown in MCDB170. A. Confluent primary culture. B. Confluent ninth-passage culture. ×152. Note the similar epithelial cobblestone morphology in early- and late-passage cells, with mitoses continuing in confluent populations. C. Third-passage culture. ×38. Note the two distinctly different cell morphologies. The smaller refractile cells appear similar to those in A and B. The larger, elongated cells do not maintain mitotic activity. D. Sixteenth-passage cells. ×152. Note the heterogenity in cell size compared to cells in A and B. Cells become larger and more elongated with some vacuolization, but maintain a cobblestone appearance and some mitotic activity.

at passages 2–3 shows that growing populations of the smaller, more refractile cells can become colonies of nongrowing larger cells, with various intermediate morphologies occurring during the course of this change-over. The smaller, growing cell population reestablishes itself as the only cell type within 1–2 passages, and thereafter only rare flattened cells are visible. Active cell growth is maintained for about 45 population doublings, or 10–20 passages. After that point, increased heterogeneity in cell size and much decreased mitotic activity is observed (Fig. 4D).

Single-cell populations grown in MM or MCDB170 can be stored frozen at any passage level. Cells grown in MM are preserved in 6% DMSO, 44% FCS, 50% DME. Cells grown in MCDB170 are preserved in 10% glycerol,

15% FCS, 75% basal MCDB170; when thawed, these cells are pelleted at 600g for 5 min to remove them from the serum.

CHARACTERIZATION OF CELL POPULATIONS

The mammary epithelial nature of the cells grown in these media can be established by several criteria (see Table II). Morphologically, the cells in MM and MCDB170 have a typical epithelial polygonal, cobblestone appearance in the light microscope, and they contain epithelial characteristics (microvilli, perinuclear bundles of tonofilaments, desmosomal junctions) in the electron microscope [Stampfer et al., 1980]. As visualized by the technique of indirect immunofluorescence, cells grown in MM, as well as early- and late-passage cells grown in MCDB170, contain epithelial specific keratin. These cell populations all also have the same powdery punctate epithelial pattern of cell-associated fibronectin [Stampfer et al., 1981]. However, cells grown in MM differ from those in MCDB170 in their expression of the human mammary epithelial-specific milk fat globule antigen [Taylor-Papadimitriou et al., 1981], in that few cells (< 5%) grown in MCDB170 are positive for this antigen, whereas cells grown in MM contain 5-30% bright positive cells, depending upon the individual specimen and passage level. All specimens thus far tested are negative for factor VIII, a marker of endothelial cells. These immunofluorescence assays are simple, quick methods to determine the epithelial purity of the cell populations. Preliminary experiments examining the pattern of glucose metabolites produced by the HMEC suggest that this method [Emerman et al., 1981] can be used to identify these cells as mammary epithelial. It is also possible that the patterns of glucose metabolites may be useful as an assay for the state of functional differentiation in the HMEC. Preliminary results show that the pattern observed appears dependent upon the growth medium used (see Table II).

ACKNOWLEDGMENTS

The author gratefully acknowledges the excellent technical assistance of Annie Pang and Kristy Mathews. This work was supported by the U.S. Public Health Service grants CA24844 and CA30228 from the National Cancer Institute.

REFERENCES

Buehring GC (1972): Culture of human mammary epithelial cells: Keeping abreast with a new method. J Natl Cancer Inst 49:1433-1434.

Emerman JT, Bartley JC, Bissell MJ (1981): Glucose metabolite patterns as markers of functional differentiation in freshly isolated and cultured mouse mammary epithelial cells. Exp Cell Res 134:241-250.

Hackett AJ, Smith HS, Springer EL, Owens RB, Nelson-Rees WA, Riggs JL, Gardner MB (1977): Two syngeneic cell lines from human breast tissue: The aneuploid mammary epithelial (Hs578T) and the diploid myoepithelial (Hs578Bst) cell lines. J Natl Cancer Inst 58:1795-1806.

Hammond SL, Ham RG, Stampfer MR (1983): Defined medium for normal human mammary epithelial cells. In Vitro 19:252. (Also submitted to Proc Natl Acad Sci).

Kirkland WL, Yang N, Jorgensen T, Longley C, Furmanski P (1979): Growth of normal and malignant human mammary epithelial cells in culture. J Natl Cancer Inst 63:29-41.

Owens RB, Smith HS, Hackett AJ (1974): Epithelial cell cultures from normal glandular tissue of mice. J Natl Cancer Inst 53:261-269.

Owens RB, Smith HS, Nelson-Rees WA, Springer EL (1976): Epithelial cell cultures from normal and cancerous human tissues. J Natl Cancer Inst 56:843-849.

Smith HS, Lan S, Ceriani RL, Hackett AJ, Stampfer M (1981): Clonal proliferation of cultured nonmalignant and malignant human breast epithelia. Cancer Res 41:4637-4643.

Stampfer MR (1982): Cholera toxin stimulation of human mammary epithelial cells in culture. In Vitro 18:531-537.

Stampfer MR, Hallowes R, Hackett AJ (1980): Growth of normal human mammary cells in culture. In Vitro 16:415-425.

Stampfer MR, Vlodavsky I, Smith HS, Ford R, Becker FF, Riggs J (1981): Fibronectin production by human mammary cells. J Natl Cancer Inst 67:253-261.

Stampfer MR, Hackett AJ, Hancock MC, Leung J, Edgington T, Smith HS (1982): Growth of human mammary epithelium in culture and expression of tumor specific properties. Cold Spring Harbor Conf Cell Prolif 9:819-830.

Taylor-Papadimitriou J, Purkis P, Fentiman IS (1980): Cholera toxin and analogues of cyclic AMP stimulate the growth of cultured human mammary epithelial cells. J Cell Physiol 101:317-321.

Taylor-Papadimitriou J, Peterson JA, Arklie J, Burchell J, Ceriani RL, Bodmer WF (1981): Monoclonal antibodies to epithelium specific component of the human milk fat globule membrane: Production and reaction with cells in culture. Int J Cancer 28:17-21.

Yang J, Elias JJ, Petrakis NL, Wellings SR, Nandi S (1981): Effects of hormones and growth factors on human mammary epithelial cells in collagen gel culture. Cancer Res 41:1021-1027.

Methods for Serum-Free Culture of Cells of the Endocrine System,
pages 183–200
© 1984 Alan R. Liss, Inc., 150 Fifth Avenue, New York, NY 10011

11
Definition of Hormones and Growth Factors Required for Optimal Proliferation and Expression of Phenotypic Responses in Human Breast Cancer Cells

Marc E. Lippman

It is the purpose of this review to fulfill three principal objectives. First, we will provide a review of individual hormonal factors known to influence the growth of human breast cancer either in vivo or in vitro. In this section we will also consider some of the difficulties encountered when attempting to extrapolate from in vitro models to regulation of growth of human breast cancer in vivo. Second, we will provide information on the specific growth requirements of a single human breast cancer cell line (ZR-75-1) that has been adapted by us to growth in serum-free medium. Finally, we will conclude with some illustrative examples of the sorts of experiments that can be accomplished under these conditions with respect to hormonal regulation of growth and specific gene products.

It is obviously the goal of in vitro cell culture studies to understand the regulation of normal or neoplastic cells in vivo. Clearly, development of defined media in which a group of specific factors can be shown to be required either for growth or regulation of specific gene products is a potential means of achieving this goal. However, the demonstration that a specific factor is or is not regulatory in vitro may not necessarily provide useful information concerning regulation of growth in vivo. In order to illustrate this point, it is

Medical Breast Cancer Section, Medicine Branch, National Cancer Institute, National Institutes of Health, Bethesda, MD 20205

worthwhile to examine some problems associated with in vitro cell culture systems particularly as they pertain to human breast cancer.

First, virtually all breast cell lines have been established from malignant effusions. As such, they represent a subset of the original tumor population that had the ability to metastasize and grow in a specific environment completely unlike that of the primary tumor. Not only may this represent clonal evolution in vivo, but, by the time the tumor sample is collected for culture, a number of therapies, such as irradiation, cytotoxic drugs, and hormonal manipulations, may have produced even greater restriction of the cell population and limited substantially the responses to many growth factors of the surviving cell population.

Second, conditions selected for initiation of culture may immediately lead to selection of cells capable of growth in the absence of factors omitted from the original medium. In addition, culture conditions almost invariably select against slower-growing populations of cells. Since differentiation frequently is related inversely to growth rate, many populations of cells that may express those hormonal responses of greatest interest may be overgrown by hormone-independent cell populations before experiments can be undertaken.

Third, in an effort to provide some assurance of a homogeneous population of cells, cloning may result in selection of a population of cells possessing a limited repertoire of the total responses of a given tumor. Conceivably, multiple sublines of a given heterogeneous tumor contribute to a given phenotypic group response.

Fourth, viral or mycoplasma contamination of cultures can occur, leading to substantial alterations in expression of some phenotypic effects.

Fifth, cells grown in tissue culture are denied many factors that may be critical to the expression of a given response. Adherence to a basement membrane or substratum, a polarized orientation, additional supporting cell types, or growth factors may all be absolutely essential to the expression of any given response. For example, androgen-provoked regressions of mammary tissue are due to effects on surrounding fibroblasts and not a response of the mammary cells themselves. Observation of an androgen effect in vitro would require the presence of both mammary and stromal elements [Dürnberger et al., 1978]. Estrogen-induced hormones, such as putative estromedins (discussed elsewhere in this volume), represent a similar phenomenon.

Sixth, it is possible to misinterpret lack of responsiveness of a cell line because it is assumed incorrectly that the hormone is a mitogen or an inducer of a given product. For example, the MCF-7 cells will grow optimally in insulin and charcoal-treated calf serum in the absence of estradiol. If one adds estrogen to this system, no further stimulation of growth is observed and the cells might therefore be considered hormone-independent. On the other hand, progesterone receptor is completely inducible under these same conditions. As another example, vasopressin stimulates fatty acid synthesis, phospholipid turnover, and accumulation of protein within cells without having any mitogenic effect in a cell line derived from a rat breast cancer induced by 7,12-dimethylbenz[a]-anthracene (DMBA) [Monaco et al., 1978]. Thus, failure to observe responses to a given hormone may be dependent on the phenomenon measured.

Finally, and most pernicious of all, a cell line may be thought to be unresponsive to a given factor because it is incorrectly assumed that this factor has been removed from the medium. Sera contain high concentrations of many growth factors, including steroids [Esber et al., 1973]. We have shown that under certain conditions, up to 2 weeks may be required to remove physiologic concentrations of estradiol from cells in culture [Strobl and Lippman, 1979; Strobl et al., 1980]. Cells are capable of concentrating estrogens tenfold over the ambient medium concentration via a process not requiring receptor. Thus, any attempt to demonstrate responsiveness to this hormone that does not adequately control for this phenomenon would artifactually fail to demonstrate hormone responsiveness.

All of the above caveats make firm conclusions concerning the absence of a given hormonal response particularly difficult to interpret. On the other hand, positive experiments are substantially less ambiguous; however, even in this setting, it is possible for mistakes to occur. For example, it is well known that most DMBA-induced rat mammary tumors are prolactin-dependent. Initial studies with a tissue culture cell line derived from one of these tumors suggested that it was prolactin-dependent; but careful, subsequent studies revealed that the response was due to contaminating vasopressin in the prolactin preparations [Monaco et al., 1980]. Similarly, we reported that the MCF-7 human breast cancer cell line contained androgen receptor and responded to androgen administration [Lippman et al., 1976a]. Subsequently, it has been suggested that the response to nonphysiologic concentrations of androgen was due to interaction of the androgen with the estrogen receptor and response system of these cells [Zava and McGuire, 1978]. Even more recently it has been demonstrated that these cells do respond to androgens but not by alterations in growth rate [MacIndoe and Etre, 1980].

Despite these many difficulties, there are many advantages to the cell culture approach to the study of hormonal interactions with human breast cancer. First, by using cells derived from a human neoplasm, many of the difficulties associated with species differences are eliminated. This may be a great advantage with such hormones as prolactin. Second, the use of a single, cloned cell type allows great confidence to be placed in what the primary responding cell type is, assuming an effect is seen. Thus, an unequivocal demonstration of an estrogen effect on a cloned cell type rules out the need for an intermediary effector system. Third, it recently has become possible to do many experiments in defined medium systems. In such situations, one can be certain that the hormonal effect studied is not mediated by some additional unknown factor in serum, etc. Fourth, cell culture systems are particularly advantageous for the study of drug and hormone metabolism as tissue redistribution, plasma binding, and nontarget tissue sites of metabolism and excretion can be eliminated. Finally, and most importantly, it is possible to develop drug- and hormone-resistant variant sublines derived from wild-type parental cell lines. With appropriate biochemical and genetic complementation techniques, it is possible to gain new insights into the mechanisms of hormonal dependency. Such an approach recently has been employed by selecting antiestrogen-independent human breast cancer cell variants and it will briefly be described later.

With all of these considerations in mind, it is possible to enumerate those hormones now known to influence either growth or differentiated functions of human breast cancer cells. In addition, there is a shorter list of hormones for which specific receptors have been demonstrated but for which no response has as yet been shown.

HORMONES KNOWN TO AFFECT GROWTH
OF HUMAN BREAST CANCER
Estrogens

For nearly a century, it has been known that removal of the ovaries would lead to objective improvement in some patients with metastatic breast cancer. Later, it was, of course, appreciated that many breast cancers in both humans and experimental animals were estrogen-dependent. Nonetheless, it is only within the past 5 years that an estrogen-responsive cell system has been described. Following the initial description of the MCF-7 human breast cancer cell line [Soule et al., 1973], Brooks et al. [1973] demonstrated that these cells contained estrogen receptor (ER). Shortly thereafter, we showed that these cells showed a variety of growth responses to physiologically relevant concentrations of estrogen as well as inhibition [Lippman et al., 1976a, 1977a]. A variety of specific products also have been shown to be under estrogenic control in these cells, including thymidine kinase (TK) [Bronzert et al., 1981], progesterone receptor [Horwitz and McGuire, 1978], lactic dehydrogenase (LDH) isoenzymes [Burke et al., 1978], a secreted protein of unknown function [Westley and Rochefort, 1980], plasminogen activator [Butler et al., 1979], and a cytoplasmic protein of 26 kdaltons [Edwards et al., 1980]. In addition, we have characterized a second human breast cancer cell line (ZR-75-1) that also has ER [Engel et al., 1978]. In defined medium, this cell line can be shown to be dependent on estrogen for its growth [Allegra and Lippman, 1978], as well as having an estrogen-inducible secreted protein [Westley and Rochefort, 1980]. Several other groups have reported that estrogens can alter growth rate of human breast cancer cell lines [Weichsel-baum et al., 1978; E.R. Jensen et al., personal communication], whereas others have failed to demonstrate growth responses to estrogen [Barnes and Sato, 1979; Shafie, 1980].

The presence of antiestrogen inhibition, which is reversible by estrogen, and the presence of many functions that are estrogen-inducible is, however, seemingly unequivocal. In many cases, the failure to demonstrate estrogenic effects seems clearly attributable to failure either to adequately remove endogenous hormone or failure to remove insulin from the medium, because insulin can serve as an alternative growth factor. In fact, when such efforts are made, it is possible to obtain estrogenic effects where previously they had been unobtainable [C. McGrath et al., personal communication; Vignon et al., 1982; Adams et al., 1982]. More recently, work by numerous other groups with the above cell lines as well as other breast cancer cell lines (T47D and CAMA-1) have all shown direct regulation of growth by estrogens.

Recently, we have used a variety of novel probes for measuring DNA synthesis rate and pyrimidine biosynthesis [Aitken and Lippman, 1980]. These techniques reveal that some of the previous failure to obtain estrogenic responses is due to massive inhibition of the de novo pathway of pyrimidine biosynthesis by estrogen starvation, which can be partially overcome by thymidine adminstration. Under such circumstances in which the intracellular pool of de novo synthesized thymidine is low, thymidine administration alone can function as a growth factor. When true DNA synthesis rates are measured or quantification of the de novo pathway is accomplished, dramatic stimulation of DNA synthesis by estrogen is apparent. In addition, a variety of enzymes involved in DNA synthesis, including carbamyl phosphate synthetase, aspartate transcarbamylase, dihydroorotase, thymidylate synthetase, and dihydrofolate reductase (DHFR), are all induced.

By cloning hormone-responsive human breast cancer cells in soft agar in the presence of lethal concentrations of antiestrogens, we have been able to develop hormone-independent variants of MCF-7 cells with a variety of interesting phenotypes [Nawata et al., 1981a,b]. These include one variant that retains estrogen responsiveness with a complete loss of antiestrogenic response. In this cell line, activation of receptor in vivo is different from wild-type MCF-7 cells. In another variant that retains minimal antiestrogenic inhibition but has lost responsiveness to estrogens, including progesterone receptor inducibility, the receptor has an abnormal chromatographic profile on DNA cellulose, eluting at a higher salt concentration. Thus, in both of these variants, the defect appears to be expressed at the level of receptor but at some site removed from the initial binding of ligand (estrogen or antiestrogen), which is entirely normal. We believe that such variants can add substantial insight into the mechanisms by which estrogens stimulate growth in human breast cancers.

Glucocorticoids

It has long been appreciated that a small minority of patients with metastatic breast cancer will have beneficial although brief responses to exogenously administered glucocorticoids. Although several mechanisms may account for this effect, including modulation of the immune system or effects on supporting stroma, it is clear that direct inhibitory effects also are possible. In tissue culture, glucocorticoid hormones exert a variety of inhibitory effects on breast cell growth [Lippman et al., 1976d] as well as antagonizing the trophic effects of insulin [Osborne et al., 1979]. These effects are mediated by glucocorticoid receptors found in these cells. Cell lines that lack high-affinity glucocorticoid receptors fail to respond to glucocorticoids. Although such receptors are found in about half of human breast cancer biopsies [Allegra et al., 1979], they do not appear to have significant associations with biological responses to classical endocrine therapies.

Androgens

It has been observed empirically that some human breast cancers will improve with androgen therapy, although the basis for this response is unknown [Stoll, 1972]. In addition, about one-third of human breast cancers contain androgen receptors. Androgen dependence has been shown in at least one rodent breast cancer cell line [Smith and King, 1972]. Several human breast cancer cell lines contain androgen receptor that is readily distinguished from ER [Lippman et al., 1976b; Engel et al., 1978]. We initially demonstrated that androgens could increase thymidine incorporation and protein synthesis in MCF-7 cells, but concentrations required were supraphysiologic and vastly in excess of those required to saturate androgen receptors [Lippman et al., 1976a]. We also demonstrated that these cells could rapidly metabolize dihydrotestosterone (DHT) to androstanediols and more polar conjugates. We suggested that, because of this metabolism, nonphysiologic concentrations of androgen were required. Subsequently, it was shown that

these high concentrations of androgen were capable of occupying and trans-
locating the ER as well as antagonizing the inhibitory effects of antiestrogens
[Zava and McGuire, 1978]. MacIndoe and Etre [1980] have recently shown
that androgen can profoundly regulate estrogen effects on progesterone receptor. These experiments are performed under circumstances that strongly
suggest direct action via androgen receptor.

Iodothyronines

Although some epidemiologic evidence has suggested that derangements
in thyroid function are associated with an altered rate of breast cancer incidence, an unequivocal association of therapeutic benefit for thyroid hormone
replacement has not been demonstrated. Nonetheless, MCF-7 human breast
cancer cells contain classical high-affinity nuclear receptors for thyroid hormone and have a growth response to physiologic concentrations of thyroid
hormones [Burke and McGuire, 1978]. The ZR-75-1 cell line has an absolute
dependence on physiologic concentrations of triiodothyronine (T_3) when
grown in defined medium [Allegra and Lippman, 1978]. Working also in
defined medium, Barnes and Sato [1979] have been able to demonstrate the
thyroid hormone dependence of MCF-7 cells. Thus, human breast cancer cell
lines appear to be an exciting system for the study of thyroid hormone
interaction with human breast cancer.

Insulin

Insulin is a critical hormone in the normal differentiation of the mammary
gland and is required for normal lactogenesis in rodents. Major derangements
in glucose homeostasis induced by surgical or chemical interference with
pancreatic function are associated with altered tumor growth rates in several
murine systems. An important regulatory role for insulin in human breast
cancer has not been established. With this in mind, it was reasonable to study
the effects of insulin on human breast cancer cell lines grown in tissue culture.
In 1976, we reported that physiologic concentrations of insulin strongly stimulated the growth of both human [Osborne et al., 1976] and rodent mammary
cancer cell lines [Monaco et al., 1978]. In human cell lines, high-affinity,
specific receptors for insulin readily are demonstrable, and binding and biologic effects are well correlated [Osborne et al., 1978]. Mitogenic effects of
insulin can be seen in defined medium for both the MCF-7 cell line [Barnes
and Sato, 1979] and the ZR-75-1 cell line [Allegra and Lippman, 1978].
Insulin also induces increases in fatty acid synthesis by increasing the activity
of acetyl coenzyme A carboxylase [Monaco et al., 1980] as well as increasing
the enzyme thymidine kinase [Lippman et al., 1976e; Bronzert et al., 1981].

Retinoids

Vitamin A derivatives are required for normal epithelial differentiation and long have been known to have an antipromotional effect in a variety of carcinogenesis assays. The appearance of DMBA-induced breast cancers can be substantially decreased by the administration of vitamin A derivatives to rats [Moon et al., 1976]. In addition, specific binding activities for vitamin A derivatives have been demonstrated in some human breast tumor cytosols [Ong et al., 1975]. For these reasons, we decided to study the effects of retinoids on human breast cancer cell lines in tissue culture. We found that several lines of human breast cancer contained separable binding activities for retinol and retinoic acid [Lacroix and Lippman, 1980]. Vitamin A derivatives induced several effects on cell growth, depending on the cell lines studied. These included a slower growth rate but identical confluent density, slower rate but a lower confluent density, and cell death following a period of increasing growth inhibition. These effects were reversible by removal of retinoids. Although no direct evidence has been obtained proving that these binding activities serve as true receptors for retinoids, there is good agreement between relative binding affinity and biologic effectiveness. Clinical trials are under way at several institutions examining any activity of 13-cis-retinoic acid as an antineoplastic agent in breast cancer. Thus far, initial therapy trials at the National Cancer Institute have not been encouraging [Cassidy and Lippman, 1982].

Epidermal Growth Factor

Epidermal growth factor is a peptide first purified from the rodent submaxillary gland. It was later shown to have growth-promoting activity for several fibroblast and epithelial cell lines in culture. Its identification as a true hormone in humans has not been accomplished. Nonetheless, this peptide has been shown to function as a mitogen for MCF-7 human breast cancer cells in serum [Osborne et al., 1980] and in defined medium as well [Barnes and Sato, 1979]. Other cell lines such as MDA-MB-231 were not stimulated by equivalent concentrations of hormone. Interestingly, an effect of epidermal growth factor could not be demonstrated in the presence of optimal concentrations of either serum or insulin. Whether epidermal growth factor is an important hormone in regulation of breast cancer cell growth factor for mammary cancer cells will require further investigation.

Vitamin D

A substantial body of data has suggested that, in many respects, the mechanism of action of vitamin D is highly analogous to that of the steroid hormones. Cytoplasmic receptor proteins have been described whose binding specificities closely parallel the known biologic potencies of vitamin D analogs. Recently, vitamin D receptors have been described in human breast cancer tumor samples and the MCF-7 human breast cancer cell line [Eisman et al., 1980]. These receptors are highly similar in both physical characteristics and binding properties to those described in intestinal mucosa. Human breast cancer has a remarkable propensity to metastasize to bone and to induce hypercalcemia. Whether some direct responsiveness of tumor cells to vitamin D is involved is conjectural but appealing as a hypothesis based on these binding studies.

Progestins

Data derived from normal endometrial tissue have suggested that progesterone receptor activity is regulated by estrogens. Similar information has accumulated concerning human breast cancer. Both MCF-7 and ZR-75-1 human breast cancer cell lines contain progesterone receptor [Lippman et al., 1976d; Engel et al., 1978], and in both cases this receptor has been shown to be regulated by estrogens [Horwitz and McGuire, 1978]. However, in no breast cancer cell line has a direct action of progestins been identified.

Prolactin

The exact role of prolactin (if any) in human breast cancer is equivocal. No really substantial evidence has ever been presented proving prolactin dependence of human breast cancer. For example, the response rate to drugs such as ergoline derivatives and L-dopa are nil in patients with metastatic disease. Many of the patients who benefit from hypophysectomy can be shown to have higher plasma prolactin levels following therapy. For these reasons, it would be of great interest to define specific responses of human breast cancer cells to prolactin. Reports have appeared suggesting that prolactin may increase ER concentrations or growth rate [Shafie and Brooks, 1977] in MCF-7 human breast cancer cells. Neither has been confirmed. Recently, specific prolactin receptors have been described in the MCF-7 cell line [Shiu, 1979]. These receptors have the usual binding affinity and specificities of other prolactin receptors and undergo internalization following occupancy by hormone [Shiu, 1980]. This important observation also awaits confirmation.

SPECIFIC GROWTH REQUIREMENTS OF ZR-75-1 HUMAN BREAST CANCER CELLS IN SERUM-FREE MEDIUM

In this section we will consider some of the properties of ZR-75-1 cells and the definition of conditions which are able to maintain their growth and define serum-free medium.

ZR-75-1 cultures were derived from a malignant ascitic effusion in a 63-year-old white female who had undergone modified radical mastectomy 34 months previously for infiltrating duct carcinoma of the right breast. She was receiving postmenopausal estrogen therapy with conjugated equine estrogens (Premarin) at the time of primary diagnosis. Among the chemotherapeutic agents subsequently employed without apparent benefit were Tamoxifen (ICI 46474, an antiestrogen) and fluoxymesterone (Halotestin). The effusion from which ZR-75-1 cells were derived was obtained 3 months after the beginning of antiestrogen therapy.

Establishment and characterization of the cell line has been previously described (for detailed methodology, see Engel et al. [1978]). Briefly, the salient features are as follows:

1. The morphology of the cells in culture is clearly epithelial and is similar to that seen in biopsy material and in preparations of exfoliated cells from the original patient.

2. They exhibit ultrastructural features characteristic of breast carcinoma cells, such as desmosomes, tonofibrils, and intracytoplasmic ductlike vacuoles [Buehring and Hackett, 1975].

3. They possess human chromosomes (modal number 74–75) with markers different from those of HeLa cells by trypsin-Giemsa banding techniques and a distinct allozyme phenotype, which further serve to assure their non-HeLa origin and distinctness from other breast cell lines.

4. They possess specific receptors for glucocorticoids, estrogens, androgens, progestins, insulin, retinoids, and prolactin.

The line has been maintained in serial culture for 5.5 years through approximately 275 passages.

The cell line was initially established and maintained in RPMI 1640 medium supplemented with 25 mM N-2-hydroxyethyl-piperanzine-N'-2-ethanesulfonic acid buffer, 100 units/ml penicillin, 100 g/ml streptomycin, 75 g/ml neomycin, and fetal calf serum (FCS). Later, any of several tissue culture media (Ham's F10, improved minimal essential medium [IMEM], or minimal essential medium [MEM]) supplemented as above proved equally satisfactory.

IMEM [Richter et al., 1972] supplemented with L-glutamine (0.6 g/liter), pencillin (62 mg/liter), and streptomycin (135 mg/liter) was the basic culture medium to which hormones and growth factors were added. Transferrin (Sigma) was added at a final concentration of 1 μg/ml. T_3 (Sigma) 10^{-5} M stock solution was prepared in 0.1 N NaOH and added to medium to yield a final concentration of 10^{-8} M. Insulin U-100 (Eli Lilly and Co.) was added at a concentration of 5×10^{-7} M. 17β-estradiol and dexamethasone (DEX)(Sigma) in benzene-ethanol were evaporated to dryness, dissolved in ethanol, and stored at $-20°C$ until use. Final concentration of ethanol is 0.1%, and this concentration has no effect on the growth of the cells. IMEM supplemented with estradiol, T_3, insulin, DEX, and transferrin at the above concentrations is referred to as IMEM-HS. Tamoxifen (ICI 46474) was similarly prepared. Fibroblast growth factor (FGF)(Collaborative Research) at a concentration of 0.025 $\mu g/ml$ was added to the tissue culture flasks when the cells were subcultured in addition to nucleosides (10^{-8} M cytidine, uridine, thymidine, and adenine [Sigma]) and nonessential amino acids. Other factors tested for growth-promoting activity include epidermal growth factor (EGF) (Collaborative Research), 5-dihydrotestosterone (Steraloids Inc.), vasopressin (Calbiochem), oxytocin (Sigma), and human placental lactogen (Sigma). Effects of ZR-75-1-conditioned medium will also be considered. ZR-75-1 cells grow in this medium at a rate equivalent to optimal supplementation with fetal calf serum. Cells can be passaged by either scraping with a rubber policeman or with EDTA. Plating efficiency is approximately 1.2% in IMEM-HS but can be increased to 3.4% by additional supplementation with cytidine, uridine, thymidine, and adenosine (all at 10^{-8} M), with nonessential amino acids, and with fibroblast growth factor (0.025 $\mu g/ml$). Conditioned medium derived from ZR-75-1 cells, human placental lactogen, epidermal growth factor, androgens, vasopressin, or oxytocin had no further effect on either growth or plating efficiency at any concentrations we employed. It is worth mentioning that in data not presented in this report conditioned medium was found to have profound growth-promoting activity on MCF-7 cells. Cells have been maintained under these conditions for at least 6 months through 13 passages without obvious morphologic change or alterations in hormonal responsiveness.

Control cells in IMEM alone remain viable for a variable period of time up to about 7 days. Conditions prior to the initiation of the experiment (density, charcoal-treated calf serum vs fetal calf serum, etc.) strongly influence this period of preserved viability. Omission of transferrin from the medium results in cell death after about 4–5 days in culture. As low a concentration as 0.25 $\mu g/ml$ can stimulate cell number over control cells. About 2.5 $\mu g/ml$ is optimal. If either triiodothyronine (T_3), estradiol, or insulin is omitted from the medium, the cells grow slowly for 4–7 days and then enter a prolonged period (lasting up to at least 3 weeks) during which there is no net increase in cell number. T_3 stimulates growth at 10^{-10} M but 10^{-8} M provides greatest stimulation. Insulin is active at 10^{-11} M and maximal at 10^{-10} M. We use 10^{-7} M insulin since these higher concentrations are no less stimulatory and since the ZR-75-1 cells can metabolize insulin so rapidly [Osborne et al., 1978]. If estradiol is removed from IMEM-HS, the cells double approximately once and then there is no net growth.

It is important to note that while there is no net change in cell number in cells deprived of estradiol, this does not appear to be due simply to cessation of growth for the following reasons: First, estradiol-free cells continue to incorporate thymidine though at a lower rate than do hormone-treated cells; second, if the cells are prelabeled with thymidine, there is a loss of radioactivity into the medium in estrogen-deprived cells but not in estrogen-treated cells (estrogen-treated cells, 1% loss; estrogen-deprived cells, 60% loss); third, there is an obvious decrease in cell adhesiveness in estrogen-deprived cells, and detached cells are easily seen in the medium. Thus, it is likely that the ZR-75-1 cells are capable of low growth in estrogen-free medium, an effect masked by continued cell loss from the dish and replenishment. If estradiol is removed from cells in IMEM-HS, they double about once and then enter the prolonged phase of no net growth previously described. As shown, the continued presence of estradiol in IMEM-HS induces exponential growth of ZR-75-1 cells until density-induced inhibition of cell proliferation is achieved. These effects are paralleled by effects on mitotic index (Table I).

This experiment strongly suggests that estradiol is an immediate mitogen of at least some estrogen-dependent human breast cancer cells. Of course, it is possible that estrogen induces increases in the activity of a diffusable mitogen for breast cancer cells. This appears unlikely for two reasons: 1) Conditioned medium obtained from ZR-75-1 cells grown in IMEM-HS will not stimulate other ZR-75-1 cells nor support the growth of MCF-7 serum-free growth; 2)

TABLE I. Effect of Estradiol on the Mitotic Index of MCF-7 Cells

Expt. No.	Control cells			Estradiol-treated cells		
	MI[a] (%)	Cells counted	Fields counted	MI (%)	Cells counted	Fields counted
1[b]	1.28	2196	8	1.94	2988	8
2[c]						
24 h	3.43	611	4	4.74	674	8
48 h	4.89	429	11	8.45	331	10
72 h	4.48	735	10	15.34	1199	7
96 h	8.96	736	18	5.07	1044	7

[a]MI, mitotic index = cells in mitosis/total cells.
[b]In experiment 1, control cells were grown in serum-free medium and estradiol-treated cells in serum-free medium + 2 nM estradiol for 72 h. Colchicine was added 4 h before harvesting the cells.
[c]In experiment 2, control cells were grown in medium supplemented with 1% charcoal-treated calf serum and estradiol-treated cells in medium supplemented with 1% charcoal-treated calf serum + 2 nM estradiol. Different flasks of cells were harvested at 24, 48, 72, and 96 h after colchicine addition at 20, 44, 68, and 92 h.

conditioned medium plus IMEM-HS without estradiol will not replace estradiol as a stimulator of ZR-75-1 cells.

While not directly part of the work on ZR-75-1, we have recently reexamined the effects of conditioned medium on another human breast cancer cell line, MCF-7. Data presented by Vignon and colleagues [1982] have strongly suggested that MCF-7 cells may provide a factor that is under estrogenic control and that stimulates growth rate. In an independent set of as yet unpublished observations, we have noted that conditioned media obtained from MCF-7 cells is capable of markedly enhancing proliferative rate and estrogen stimulatory effects seen following cell growth inhibition by amino acid deprivation, and capable of strongly down-regulating estrogen receptor. These effects are enhanced by the simultaneous addition of estradiol to the medium.

REGULATION OF GROWTH AND PROGESTERONE RECEPTOR IN ZR-75-1 CELLS IN DEFINED MEDIUM

As previously described, addition of estradiol is required for continued growth of ZR-75-1 cells in defined medium. If experiments are performed with cells previously growing in serum-containing medium (and thus exposed to physiologic concentrations of circulating estrogens), great care must be taken to assure that endogenous estradiol is removed from the cells. For example, in an experiment previously described [Strobl and Lippman, 1979], cells were exposed to tritiated estradiol for 3 h and for the next 14 days medium was exchanged daily for fresh hormone and serum-free medium. Nearly 12 days were required for 100-fold reduction in intracellular hormone concentration. Thus, during this time period demonstration of an effective exogenous estradiol would be unlikely, although antiestrogen activity might be expected. We explored the quantitative effects of estrogens and antiestrogens in greater detail. Following a prolonged period of daily medium exchange for ZR-75-1 cells into IMEM-HS without estradiol, nearly 11 days of medium exchange into IMEM-HS minus estradiol are required to induce a complete cessation of net cell growth. Under these conditions, we find that as little as 10^{-11} M estradiol stimulates cell division. This stimulation is about half as effective as 10^{-10} M and 10^{-9} M estradiol, which is optimally active; 10^{-8} M estradiol is about equal to 10^{-11} M estradiol, and 10^{-7} M estradiol is substantially less stimulatory. Whether or not these suboptimal effects of higher concentrations of estradiol are simply nonspecifically toxic or specific regulatory mechanisms analogous to the inhibitory effects of high concentrations of estrogen on human breast cancer cell growth is unknown at the present time.

Using a similar strategy to rid the cells of endogenous estradiol, we find that addition of the antiestrogen Tamoxifen (ICI 46474) at a concentration of

10^{-6} M results in the rapid appearance of cell detachment and death. This effect of Tamoxifen is not likely to be due to competition with estradiol remaining within the cells, because of the prolonged daily medium changes that we have previously shown effectively rid the cells of endogenous estradiol. While it is possible that the cells may be able to synthesize biologically active estrogens from small molecules, this seems unlikely for several reasons. While all cells capable of growth in defined medium must be able to synthesize cholesterol, at least six separate enzymatic biotransformations would have to occur to reach estradiol from cholesterol, and most of these enzymes have not been found outside the gonads and adrenals. Second, if estradiol was synthesized slowly by these cells in culture, one would expect that after a few days in IMEM-HS without exogenous estradiol, concentrations would approach those required for growth stimulation. We have not observed this phenomenon. Third, radioimmunoassay of supernatant medium following prolonged maintenance in IMEM-HS without exogenous estradiol fails to reveal significant concentrations of estradiol. On the other hand, the effects of Tamoxifen are not explainable on the basis of nonspecific toxicity. We have previously shown [Lippman et al., 1976a,b] that antiestrogen effects are seen only in estrogen receptor-containing cells and are preventable by simultaneous addition of estradiol, and finally that, once initiated, they are reversible by subsequent addition of estradiol. Thus, the inhibitory effects of tamoxifen in the absence of estradiol is somewhat puzzling. Several possible explanations suggest themselves. First, one may imagine some intrinsic activity of the estrogen receptor in the absence of hormone. This activity is stimulated by hormone and inhibited by antihormone. Alternatively, it is possible that human breast cancer cells produce some gene product required for growth. In the absence of hormone receptor complexes, DNA segments required for growth are transcribed at some constitutive rate consistent with cell survival. The addition of an agonist hormone results in substantial activation by hormone receptor complexes, leading to enhanced cell growth. Antiestrogen bound to estrogen receptor complexes may translocate to the nucleus and further suppress transcription of the segments of the genome being transcribed at a low rate in the absence of estradiol. A third and important potential explanation may lie in the antiestrogen binding sites [Sutherland and Foo, 1980] recently described in these cells. Conceivably, at least some of the effects of antiestrogen are mediated directly through a class of sites that have no affinity for estradiol.

We next turn to a consideration of progesterone receptor regulation in ZR-75-1 cells in defined medium. Approximately one-third of patients with metastatic breast cancer respond to endocrine therapy. Knowledge of a tumor's estrogen receptor status greatly enhances the clinician's ability to predict which patients will respond to a hormonal therapy. Patients with estrogen receptor-positive tumors have an objective response rate of approximately 60%, whereas those with estrogen receptor-negative tumors respond less than 10% of the time [McGuire, 1977]. Unfortunately, 40% of patients with estrogen receptor-positive tumors do not respond to endocrine manipulation. Estrogen receptor is therefore necessary but not sufficient to label a tumor as hormone-dependent, and progesterone receptor synthesis is known to be controlled by estrogen in the uterus. Horwitz et al. have postulated that progesterone receptor might serve as a marker of estrogen action and hormone dependence in human breast cancer. Furthermore, Horwitz et al. [1975] have demonstrated that progesterone receptor activity is regulated by estrogens in the MCF-7 human breast cancer cell line.

We therefore studied the regulation of progesterone receptor in the ZR-75-1 human breast cancer cell system. The average progesterone receptor concentration in cells growing optimally in hormone-supplemented medium IMEM-HS is 150 ± 26 fmoles/10^6 cells (10 experiments; mean $\pm$ SEM). The average K_D was 6.4×10^{-10}. For comparison, cells growing in IMEM supplemented with 5% fetal calf serum (normal growth conditions) have an average progesterone receptor concentration of 140 ± 31 fmoles/10^6 cells (mean $\pm$ SEM). The average of K_D was 7×10^{-10} M. This appears to be the induced level of synthesis in this cell line. It is worth noting that fetal calf serum thus appears to contain optimal concentrations of estrogen for progesterone receptor induction.

Over an 8-day period in IMEM-HS, the concentration of progesterone receptor in these cells does not vary. Removal of insulin leads to no significant change in progesterone receptor concentration. However, removal of estradiol leads to a dramatic fall in progesterone receptor, and by day 5 progesterone receptor activity is undetectable. Readdition of estradiol to these cells on day 5 results in reappearance of progesterone receptor activity.

The effect of hormones on progesterone receptor concentration can be separated from general effects leading to cell growth. For example, removal of insulin from IMEM-HS leads to a cessation of growth, whereas addition of insulin leads to exponential growth. Regardless of the growth rate of the cells, progesterone receptor activity is maintained as long as the medium contains estrogen.

Estradiol concentrations of 10^{-8} M and 10^{-10} M are most effective in stimulating progesterone receptor. No inductive effect is seen at either 10^{-6} M or 10^{-12} M estradiol. Interestingly, no concentration of Tamoxifen tested (10^{-6} M, 10^{-7} M, or 10^{-8} M) shows any ability to increase progesterone receptor activity.

CONCLUDING REMARKS

Clearly, the material presented serves more as a progress report than a finished story. Optimal cloning, long-term growth, and a complete demonstration of a full panoply of hormonally inducible effects under totally defined conditions remain goals rather than achievements. Nonetheless, given the progress thus far with both breast cancer cell lines and other cell culture systems, this eventual goal appears attainable.

REFERENCES

Adams DJ, Edwards DP, Ciocca DR, Hajj H, McGuire WL (1982): Monoclonal antibodies against an estrogen-regulated protein in human breast cancer. Endocrine Society Abst 715.

Aitken SC, Lippman ME (1977): A simple computer program for quantification and Scatchard analysis of steroid receptor proteins. J Steroid Biochem 8:77.

Aitken SC, Lippman ME (1980): Hormonal regulation of net DNA synthesis in human breast cancer cells in tissue culture. In Jimenez de Asua L et al (eds): "Control Mechanisms in Animal Cells." New York: Raven, p 133.

Allegra JC, Lippman ME (1978): Growth of a human breast cancer cell line in serum-free hormone-supplemented medium. Cancer Res 38:3823.

Allegra JC, Lippman ME, Thompson EB, Simon R, Barlock A, Green L, Huff K, Do HMT, Aitken S, Warren R (1979): Relationship between the progesterone, androgen and glucocorticoid receptor and response rate to endocrine therapy in metastatic breast cancer. Cancer Res 39:1973.

Barnes D, Sato G (1979): Growth of a human mammary tumor cell line in a serum free medium. Nature 281:388.

Bronzert DA, Monaco ME, Pinkus L, Aitken S, Lippman ME (1981): Purification and properties of estrogen responsive to thymidine kinase from human breast cancer. Cancer Res 41:604.

Brooks SC, Locke ER, Soule HD (1973): Estrogen receptor in a human cell line (MCF-7) from breast carcinoma. J Biol Chem 248:6251-6253.

Buehring GC, Hackett AJ (1975): Human breast tumor cell lines: Identify evaluation by ultrastructure. J Natl Cancer Inst 53:621.

Burke RE, McGuire WL (1978): Nuclear thyroid receptor in a human breast cancer cell line. Cancer Res 38:3769.

Burke RE, Harris SC, McGuire WL (1978): Lactate dehydrogenase in estrogen responsive human breast cancer cells. Cancer Res 38:2773.

Butler WB, Kirkland WL, Jorgenson TI (1979): Induction of plasminogen activation by estrogen in a human breast cancer cell line (MCF-7). Biochem Biophys Res Commun 90:1328.

Cassidy J, Lippman ME (1982): Phase II trial of 13-cis-retinoic acid in metastatic breast cancer. Eur J Cancer (in press).

Dürnberger H, Heuberger B, Schwartz P, Wasner G, Kratochwil K (1978): Mesenchyme-mediated effect of testosterone on embryonic mammary epithelium. Cancer Res 38:4066-4070.

Edwards DP, Adams DJ, Squage N, McGuire WL (1980): Estrogen induced synthesis of specific proteins in human breast cancer cells. Biochem Biophys Res Commun 93:804.

Eisman JA, Martin TJ, MacIntyre I, Framptin RJ, Moseley JM, Whitehead R (1980): 1,25-Dihydroxy vitramin D_3 receptor in a cultured human breast cancer cell line (MCF-7 cells). Biochem Biophys Res Commun 93:9.

Engel LW, Young NA, Tralka TS, Lippman ME, O'Brien S, Joyce MJ (1978): Breast carcinoma cells in continuous culture: Establishment and characterization of three new cell lines. Cancer Res 38:3352.

Esber H, Payne I, Bogden A (1973): Variability of hormone concentrations and ratios in commercial sera used for tissue culture. J Natl Cancer Inst 50:559.

Horwitz KB, McGuire WL (1978): Estrogen control of progesterone receptor in human breast cancer. J Biol Chem 253:2223.

Horwitz KB, McGuire WL, Pearson OH, Segaloff A (1975): Predicting response to endocrine therapy in human breast cancer: A hypothesis. Science 189:726.

Lacroix A, Lippman ME (1980): Binding of retinoids to human breast cancer cell lines and their effects on cell growth. J Clin Invest 65:586.

Lippman ME, Bolan G, Huff K (1976a): The effects of androgens and antiandrogens on hormone-responsive human breast cancer in long-term tissue culture. Cancer Res 36:4610.

Lippman ME, Bolan G, Huff K (1976b): The effects of estrogens and antiestrogens on hormone-responsive human breast cancer in long-term tissue culture. Cancer Res 36:4595.

Lippman ME, Bolan G, Huff K (1976c): Interactions of antiestrogens with human breast cancer in long term tissue culture. Cancer Treat Rep 60:1421.

Lippman ME, Bolan G, Huff K (1976d): The effects of glucocorticoids and progesterone on hormone-responsive human breast cancer in long-term tissue culture. Cancer Res 36:4602.

Lippman ME, Bolan G, Monaco ME, Pinkus L, Engel L (1976e): Model systems for the study of estrogen action in tissue culture. J Steroid Biochem 7:1045.

Lippman ME, Huff K, Bolan G, Neifeld JP (1977a): Interactions of R5020 with progesterone and glucocorticoid receptors in human breast cancer and peripheral blood lymphocytes in vitro. In McGuire WL et al (eds): "Progesterone Receptors in Normal and Neoplastic Tissues." New York: Raven, p 193.

Lippman ME, Monaco ME, Bolan G (1977b): Effects of estrone, estradiol and estriol on hormone-responsive human breast cancer in long term tissue culture. Cancer Res 37:1901.

MacIndoe JH, Etre LA (1980): Androgens inhibit estrogen action in MCF-7 human breast cancer cells. Life Science 27:1643-1648.

McGuire WL (1977): Physiological principles underlying endocrine therapy of breast cancer. In McGuire WL (ed): "Breast Cancer Advances in Research and Treatment." New York: Plenum, Vol 1, p 217.

Monaco ME, Lippman ME, Knazek R, Kidwell WR (1978): Vasopressin stimulation of acetate incorporation into lipids in a dimethylbenz(a)-anthracene-induced rat mammary tumor cell line. Cancer Res 38:4101.

Monaco ME, Strobl J, Allegra JC, Lippman ME (1979): Interactions of steroid hormones with human breast cancer in vitro. In Thompson EB, Lippman ME (eds): "Steroid Receptors and the Management of Cancer." Cleveland: CRC Press, Vol 2, p 32.

Monaco ME, Kidwell WR, Kohn PH, Strobl JS, Lippman ME (1980): Neurohypophysial hormones and cancer. In Iacobelli S et al (eds): "Hormones and Cancer." New York: Raven, p 165.

Moon RC, Grubbs CJ, Sporn MB (1976): Inhibition of 7,12-dimethyl benz(a)anthracene-induced mammary carcinogenesis by retinyl acetate. Cancer Res 36:2626.

Nawata H, Bronzert D, Lippman ME (1981a): Isolation and characterization of a tamoxifen-resistant cell line derived from MCF-7 human breast cancer cells. J Biol Chem 256:5016.

Nawata H, Chong M, Bronzert D, Lippman ME (1981b): Estradiol independent growth of a subline of MCF-7 human breast cancer cell in culture. J Biol Chem 256:6895.

Ong DE, Page DL, Chytil F (1975): Retnoic acid binding protein: Occurrence in human tumors. Science 190:60.

Osborne CK, Bolan G, Monaco ME, Lippman ME (1976): Hormone responsive human breast cancer in long term tissue culture: Effects of insulin. Proc Natl Acad Sci USA 73:4536.

Osborne CK, Monaco ME, Lippman ME, Kahn CR (1978): Correlation among insulin binding, degradation, and biological activity in human breast cancer cells in long-term tissue culture. Cancer Res 38:94.

Osborne CK, Monaco ME, Kahn CR, Lippman ME (1979): Direct inhibition of growth and antagonism of insulin action by glucocorticoids in human breast cancer cells in culture. Cancer Res 39:2422.

Osborne CK, Hamilton B, Titus G, Livingston RB (1980): Epidermal growth factor stimulation of human breast cancer cells in culture. Cancer Res 40:2361.

Richter A, Sanford KK, Evans VJ (1972): Influence of oxygen and culture media on plating efficiency of some mammalian tissue cells. J Natl Cancer Inst 49:1705.

Shafie SM (1980): Estrogen and the growth of breast cancer: New evidence suggests indirect action. Science 209:701.

Shafie S, Brooks SC (1977): Effect of prolactin on growth and the estrogen receptor level of human breast cancer cells (MCF-7). Cancer Res 37:792.

Shiu RPC (1979): Prolactin receptors in human breast cancer cells in long term tissue culture. Cancer Res 39:4381.

Shiu RPC (1980): Processing of prolactin by human breast cancer cells in long term tissue culture. J Biol Chem 255:4278.

Smith JA, King RJB (1972): Effects of steroids on growth of an androgen dependent mouse mammary carcinoma in cell culture. Exp Cell Res 73:351.

Soule HD, Vazquez J, Long A, Albert S, Brennan M (1973): A human cell line from a pleural effusion derived from a breast carcinoma. J Natl Cancer Inst 51:1409.

Stoll BA (1972): "Endocrine Therapy in Malignant Disease." London: Saunders.

Strobl JS, Lippman ME (1979): Prolonged retention of estradiol by human breast cancer cells in tissue culture. Cancer Res 39:3319.

Strobl JS, Monaco ME, Lippman ME (1980): The role of intracellular equilibria and the effect of antiestrogens on estrogen-receptor dissociation kinetics from perfused cultures of human breast cancer cells. Endocrinology 107:450.

Sutherland RL, Foo MS (1980): Synthetic oestrogen antagonists in chick oviduct: Antagonist activity and interactions with high-affinity cytoplasmic binding sites. In Sutherland RL, Jordan VC (eds): "Non-Steroidal Antioestrogens." New York: Academic, pp 195–213.

Vignon F, Chalbos D, Derocq D, Rochefort H (1982): Stimulation by estrogens of the proliferation of T47D and MCF-7 human breast cancer cells: possible mediation by released proteins. Endocrine Soc Abstr 719.

Weichselbaum RR, Hellman S, Piro AJ, Nove JJ, Little JB (1978): Proliferation kinetics of a human breast cancer cell line in vitro following treatment with 17B-estradiol and 1-α-D-arabinofuranosylcytosine. Cancer Res 38:2329.

Westley B, Rochefort H (1980): A secreted glycoprotein induced by estrogen in human breast cancer cell lines. Cell 20:253.

Zava DT, McGuire WL (1978): Human breast cancer androgen action mediated by estrogen receptor. Science 199:787–788.

Methods for Serum-Free Culture of Cells of the Endocrine System,
pages 201–216

12
Serum-Free Cell Culture of MCF7 Human Mammary Carcinoma

David W. Barnes

The MCF7 human mammary carcinoma cell line, established in culture from a metastatic pleural effusion [Soule et al., 1973], retains many of the properties one might expect of differentiated mammary epithelium in vitro and has been used by many laboratories as a model for the study of a number of aspects of normal and neoplastic mammary cell biology [Lippman et al., 1977; Engel and Young, 1978; McGuire and Horwitz, 1979; Lippman, this volume]. MCF7 cells in vitro express specific receptors for estrogen, androgen, glucocorticoid, progesterone, insulin, epidermal growth factor (EGF), prolactin, and triiodothyronine [Brooks et al., 1973; Horwitz et al., 1975; Lippman and Bolan, 1975; Lippman et al., 1975; Horwitz and McGuire, 1978; Osborne et al., 1976, 1980; Shiu, 1979; Burke and McGuire, 1978; Barnes and Sato, 1979, 1980c; Lippman et al., 1976]. The cells in high-density cultures form hemicysts or domes, characteristic of transporting epithelium, and can also form duct-like structures under appropriate culture conditions [Soule et al., 1973; Lippman et al., 1977; Russo et al., 1976b]. The cells synthesize α-lactalbumin and express antigens that are immunologically related to antigens of human milk fat globules [Rose and McGrath, 1975; Ceriani et al., 1977; Engel and Young, 1978]. MCF7 in culture is reported to shed a virus-like particle with antigenic similarity to murine mammary tumor virus, and the cells contain nucleic acid sequences similar to those found in murine mammary tumor virus RNA [McGrath et al., 1974; Soule et al., 1976; Das and Mink, 1979]. MCF7 cells when injected into athymic mice will form tumors that are both pituitary- and ovary-dependent [Russo et al., 1976a; Shafie, 1980].

Department of Biological Sciences, University of Pittsburgh, Pittsburgh, Pennsylvania 15260

In this chapter are described methods for the long-term growth of the MCF7 cell line in serum-free medium [Barnes and Sato, 1979, 1980c; Barnes et al, 1981]. This medium provides technical advantages in the execution of experiments designed to examine a number of interesting questions regarding the cell biology of normal and neoplastic human mammary epithelium [Barnes and Sato, 1980a, 1980b; Barnes, 1984a,b]. It should prove useful, for example, in the examination of products secreted into the medium, allowing isolation of these products in the absence of the large amount of exogenous protein present in conventional culture medium that employs serum as a growth-stimulatory supplement. Serum-free cell culture also should allow the study in a precise way of nutritional requirements of these cells, as well as allowing examination of hormone responses in the absence of effects of hormonal serum components. Serum-free cell culture, in addition to more conventional techniques [Lippman, this volume], also can be used to select for cells within the population that express altered responses to the various factors affecting the growth of this line.

MATERIALS

Bovine insulin, human transferrin, prostaglandin F_2-α, 4-(2-hydroxyethyl)-1-piperazineethanesulfonic acid (HEPES), soybean trypsin inhibitor, antibiotics, and steroid hormones can be obtained from Sigma Chemical Company, St. Louis. Powdered formulations of Ham's F12 and Dulbecco-modified Eagle's medium (DME) can be obtained from Grand Island Biological Company, Grand Island, NY. Fetal calf serum was obtained from Reheis, Irvine, CA. Many other serum sources are acceptable. Epidermal growth factor (EGF) and human plasma fibronectin (cold-insoluble globulin or CIg) may be obtained from Meloy Laboratories, Springfield, VA, Bethesda Research Laboratories, Gaithersburg, MD, or Collaborative Research, Inc., Waltham, MA. Sodium selenite can be obtained from Fisher Chemical Company, Pittsburgh, or from Difco. Water for culture medium is freshly prepared, either by triple distillation in glass containers [Barnes and Sato, 1980a] or by passage through a Milli-Q water purification system (Millipore). MCF7 cells used in these studies were obtained from Dr. William McGuire, University of Texas, San Antonio, TX, and Dr. Marvin Rich, Michigan Cancer Foundation, Detroit.

PREPARATION OF CULTURE MEDIUM AND SUPPLEMENTS

The basal nutrient formulation to which are added supplements stimulatory of MCF7 cell growth is one-to-one mixture of DME and Ham's F12 [Mather and Sato, 1979] supplemented with 1.2 g/liter sodium bicarbonate, 15 mM HEPES, pH 7.4, 10^{-8} M sodium selenite, 200 IU/ml penicillin, 200 μg/ml streptomycin, and 25 μg/ml ampicillin (F12:DME). HEPES, selenite, and the antibiotics are maintained as 100-fold-concentrated stock solutions in highly purified water. For the preparation of 2 liters of F12:DME, powdered medium in 1 liter, preweighed packets (one F12 packet and one DME packet) is added to approximately 500 ml highly purified water and stirred until dissolved. To this is added 20 ml of concentrated HEPES stock, followed by concentrated stock solutions of the antibiotics and sodium selenite. The solution is then brought to nearly 2,000 ml with additional highly purified water, sodium bicarbonate is added, and the final adjustment to 2,000 ml is made.

The medium is immediately membrane-filtered for sterilization by passage through plastic disposable 0.2-μ filter units and stored frozen in 200-ml aliquots in sterile, disposable 75-cm^2 surface area (T75) tissue culture flasks. In general, storage of basal nutrient medium for long periods of time, even in the frozen form, is not recommended. In practice, our laboratory makes medium in 2-liter batches as needed, and the medium is usually used within 2 weeks. While this approach is time-consuming, it minimizes the chances of inadvertant use of F12:DME in which some decomposition of components has occurred during storage. Such problems are of little concern when the basal nutrient medium is supplemented with serum, but they may have serious consequences for serum-free cell culture [Ham, 1984].

Growth-stimulating supplements are prepared and maintained as sterile, concentrated stock solutions. Insulin is stored at 4°C at 1 mg/ml in 0.05 M HCl. Transferrin is stored frozen in 1-ml aliquots at 1 to 5 mg/ml in phosphate-buffered saline (PBS). Both of these solutions can be membrane-filtered for sterilization after the commercially available powders are dissolved. EGF and fibronectin may be obtained commercially as sterile lyophilized powders that can be reconstituted with sterile solutions, or as frozen sterile solutions. Optional concentrations of these factors from commercial sources may vary from batch to batch (e.g., 10-100 ng/ml for EGF, 2-15 μg/ml for fibronectin). Alternatively, these components can be isolated from primary sources, as discussed elsewhere [Yamada and Akiyama, 1984; Rubin and Bradshaw, 1984; Savage and Harper, 1984; Carpenter and Cohen, 1979; Hynes and Yamada, 1982]. Concentrated stocks of these factors can be maintained at 0.5-1.0 mg/ml (fibronectin) and 50-100 μg/ml (EGF). Care must be taken to prevent frequent freezing and thawing of fibronectin solutions in order to avoid aggregation, and it is best to store fibronectin in small aliquots of frozen stocks. General approaches to the use of fibronectin and similar factors in serum-free cell culture are described elsewhere [Barnes, 1984c]. Prostaglandin is prepared as a concentrated (0.25 mg/ml) stock in 95% ethanol and stored at $-20°$.

Serum spreading factor is prepared as described elsewhere [Barnes and Silnutzer, 1983; Silnutzer and Barnes, 1984]. This material is obtained in the final purification step in 0.1 M NaCl with 50 mM sodium phosphate buffer, pH 7.0. Because considerable losses are encountered upon sterilization of serum spreading factor by membrane filtration, and because this protein exhibits a strong affinity for the plastic tissue culture substratum and is effective as a substratum coat, serum spreading factor is presented to cells in the following manner. For use of serum spreading factor in 35-mm-diameter plates, the purified protein in unfiltered, concentrated solution (0.1–0.5 mg/ml) is diluted directly into 1 ml of F12:DME in the culture dish and this solution is incubated 1 h at 37°C in 95% air–5% CO_2. This solution is removed by aspiration; then 0.5 ml of 70% ethanol is added to the plate under sterile conditions and immediately removed, and the plate is washed five times with PBS under sterile conditions. In these circumstances, biologically active serum spreading factor adheres to the surface of the culture dish and is not inactivated by the sterilizing ethanol solution.

TRYPSINIZATION AND PLATING OF MCF7 IN SERUM-FREE MEDIUM

Passage of MCF7 cells is accomplished first by incubation of culture dishes with 0.1% crude trypsin in PBS with 1.0 mM ethylenediaminetetraacetate (EDTA) at 37° until the cells are detached. The cell suspension is then diluted into F12:DME containing 0.1% soybean trypsin inhibitor, and the cells are centrifuged from suspension at low speed and resuspended in fresh F12:DME. For serum-free plating in 35-mm-diameter dishes, cells are diluted in F12:DME to give the final cell density desired and added in 1-ml aliquots to dishes containing 1 ml of F12:DME previously equilibrated for 30 min in a 37° incubator in 5% CO_2–95% air atmosphere. Dishes that are to receive substratum modifications, such as exposure to serum spreading factor, also should have undergone pretreatment with such factors prior to preequilibration and cell seeding. Other growth-stimulating supplements are then added directly to the cells immediately after plating. Supplements are added as small volumes (e.g., 20 μl per plate) of sterile, concentrated stocks. Prostaglandin F_2-α is diluted into F12:DME from stocks containing 95% ethanol to provide an intermediate concentration from which the final dilution is made directly into the plates. Fresh intermediate dilutions of prostaglandin F_2-α are made in F12:DME from stock each time this factor is added to cells.

Care should be taken to prevent exposure of the cells to extremes of pH and temperature during the passaging process. Trypsinization, centrifugation, and resuspension should be accomplished as quickly and efficiently as possible so that cells spend as little time exposed to these conditions as can be reasonably achieved. Liberties that may be taken in the passage of these and other cell types when serum-containing media are used may result in greatly reduced cell survival upon passage when the cells are cultured under serum-free conditions. It may be helpful to change the medium the day after passaging the cells under serum-free conditions, in order to reduce the level in the medium of hydrolase activity released from cells damaged in the passaging procedure. Effects of hydrolytic enzyme activities on cell viability may not be of consequence in serum-containing media because these activities may be inhibited by serum factors, but the presence of these enzymes may represent a problem when passaging cells under serum-free conditions. Long-term growth of MCF7 in serum-free medium is best achieved in dishes rather than flasks. The reason for this is unclear, and this phenomenon is not generally observed for other cell types.

GROWTH CHARACTERISTICS OF MCF7 CELLS IN VITRO

MCF7 cells do not require high concentrations of fetal calf serum as a growth-stimulating supplement (Fig. 1); less than 5% is adequate to support optimal cell growth in several different basal nutrient media formulations. These cells in 5% or 10% fetal calf serum will grow exponentially with a doubling time of about 36 h. In F12:DME supplemented with insulin (0.25 μg/ml), transferrin (25 μg/ml), EGF (100 ng/ml), fibronectin (7.5 μg/ml), and prostaglandin F_2-α (25 ng/ml), MCF7 cells will grow continuously with a generation time equal to that of these cells in serum-supplemented media (Fig. 2) [Barnes and Sato, 1979, 1980c]. MCF7 cells can be passaged in this serum-free medium and will continue to proliferate for months in the absence of serum with no significant reduction in growth rate. In most experiments cell number in serum-supplemented medium at any point in the growth curve is higher than that of cells in the serum-free medium. This reflects a higher initial plating efficiency in serum-supplemented medium compared with serum-free medium, but it does not represent a significantly lower doubling time in the serum-free medium.

The choice of basal nutrient medium is critical for the growth of MCF7 cells in the absence of serum under the conditions described. These cells will not proliferate in DME supplemented with insulin, transferrin, prostaglandin F_2-α, EGF, and fibronectin; growth is seen, however, in F12 or F12:DME supplemented with the above components (Table I) [Barnes and Sato, 1980c]. At low cell densities, on the order of 5×10^3 cells per 35-mm-diameter culture

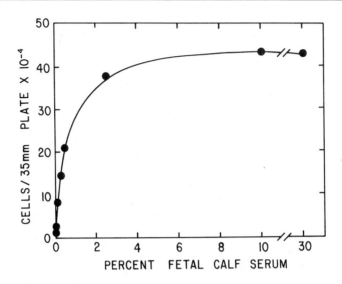

Fig. 1. Fetal calf serum concentration dependence of growth of MCF7 cells. Cells were plated at 2×10^4 per 35-mm-diameter dish in F12:DME with the indicated concentration of fetal calf serum. Number of cells per dish was determined 7 days after plating. For counting, cells were treated with trypsin-EDTA, sheared through a 22-gauge hypodermic needle to produce a single cell suspension, and counted in a Coulter particle counter.

dish, F12 supplemented with the five factors is as good as the F12:DME mixture as a basal nutrient medium supporting serum-free growth of MCF7; at higher cell densities, F12:DME is a somewhat better basal nutrient medium. Little difference between F12, DME, and F12:DME is observed when MCF7 cell growth is examined in the presence of 10% fetal calf serum (Table I).

With the exception of insulin, none of the medium supplements used for the serum-free growth of MCF7 are capable of significantly stimulating the proliferation of these cells when added alone in the absence of serum (Table II) [Barnes and Sato, 1980c]. However, the combination of the supplements is effective at stimulating growth, and effects of each factor can be demonstrated in the presence of the others (Figs. 3–7). No effect on cell growth can be demonstrated for serum spreading factor in the presence of insulin, EGF, transferrin, prostaglandin F_2-α, and fibronectin, but marked effects of this factor on MCF7 cell morphology in serum-free medium are observed (Fig. 8) [Barnes and Sato, 1979; Barnes et al., 1983; Silnutzer and Barnes, 1984].

A large number of other hormones, growth factors, and preparations at various states of purity have been tested for growth-promoting activity on MCF7 in F12:DME. Among those exhibiting growth-promoting activity are

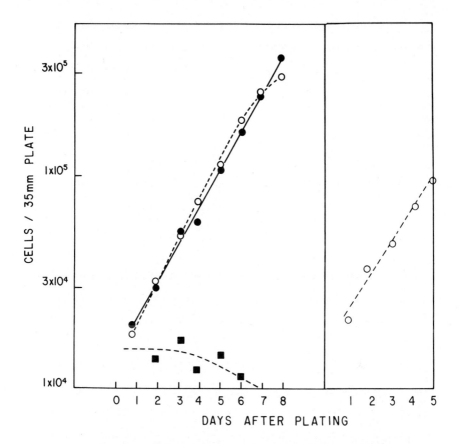

Fig. 2. Growth of MCF7 cells in serum-free medium. Left panel: Stock cultures grown in F12:DME supplemented with 10% fetal calf serum were detached from flasks with 0.1% trypsin-1.0 mM EDTA in PBS, treated with 0.1% soybean trypsin inhibitor in F12:DME, and plated at 3×10^4 cells per 35-mm-diameter dish in 2 ml medium supplemented with insulin (250 ng/ml), transferrin (25 µg/ml), EGF (100 ng/ml), prostaglandin F_2-α (100 ng/ml), and fibronectin (7.5 µg/ml) (○). Control plates contained F12:DME with 10% fetal calf serum (●) or F12:DME with no stimulatory supplements (■). Right panel: Cells grown with weekly passage (3 months) in serum-free medium containing the five supplements given above were plated in serum-free medium containing the five supplements as described, and number of cells was determined daily. From Barnes and Sato [1979], with permission.

TABLE I. Serum-Free Growth of MCF7 Cells in F12, DME, and F12:DME

Basal nutrient medium	Supplements	Cells per 35-mm-diameter plate
F12:DME	None	8.0×10^4
F12	Five factors	3.8×10^5
F12	Fetal calf serum (10%)	4.9×10^5
DME	Five factors	6.0×10^4
DME	Fetal calf serum (10%)	5.1×10^5
F12:DME	Five factors	4.7×10^5
F12:DME	Fetal calf serum (10%)	5.2×10^5

Cells grown in F12:DME containing 10% fetal calf serum were removed from flasks and replated at 5×10^4 cells per 35-mm-diameter plate in F12, DME, or F12:DME containing no supplements, 10% fetal calf serum, or the following five factors: insulin (250 ng/ml), transferrin (25 μg/ml), EGF (25 ng/ml), prostaglandin F_2-α (25 ng/ml), and fibronectin (7.5 μg/ml). Cells were counted 6 days after plating.

TABLE II. Effect of Estradiol on Growth of MCF7 Cells in Serum-Free Medium

	Cells per 35-mm-diameter plate	
Supplements	Without estradiol	With estradiol
None	4.22×10^4	4.83×10^4
EGF	4.62×10^4	5.00×10^4
Prostaglandin F_2-α	4.1×10^4	5.04×10^4
Insulin	12.2×10^4	13.6×10^4
Insulin, transferrin, EGF, prostaglandin F_2-α, fibronectin, serum spreading factor	20.2×10^4	20.0×10^4

Cells grown in F12:DME containing 10% fetal calf serum were removed from flasks and replated at 5×10^4 cells per 35-mm-diameter plate in F12:DME with the indicated supplements and with or without estradiol (10^{-9} M). Concentrations of the supplements were: insulin, 250 ng/ml; transferrin, 25 μg/ml; EGF, 25 ng/ml; prostaglandin F_2-α, 25 ng/ml; fibronectin, 7.5 μg/ml; serum spreading factor, 2μg/ml. Data shown are the average of five experiments. Cells are counted 6 days after plating.

partially purified preparations of ovine and bovine prolactin and partially purified urokinase (D. Barnes, unpublished observations). Prolactin is effective only at supraphysiologic concentrations, and the effect of crude prolactin preparations may be the result of contamination with other growth-promoting components found in the pituitary. A growth-promoting activity for normal human mammary epithelial cells also has been identified in pituitary extracts

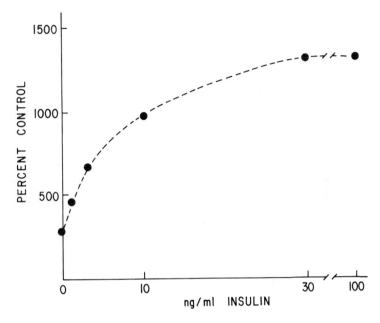

Fig. 3. Stimulation of MCF7 cell proliferation in serum-free medium by insulin. Cells were plated as described in Figure 2, except that the concentration of insulin varied as indicated. Number of cells was determined 7 days after plating. Number of cells per dish in unsupplemented F12:DME at the time of the experimental determination represents a control value of 100%.

[Stampfer, this volume]. Several growth-promoting factors have been identified in urine, and the effect of preparations of partially purified urokinase may be due to the presence of such factors. Partially purified preparations of pregnant mare serum gonadotropin also are growth-stimulating when used at microgram per milliliter concentrations (D. Barnes, unpublished observations). These commercially available preparations are rather crude, and mitogenic effects observed on MCF7 may be the result of contaminating serum growth factors. Effects of extracellular matrix material on MCF7 cells in serum-free medium also have been reported [Gospodarowicz et al., 1982; Mai and Chung, 1984], and MCF7 cells themselves synthesize an extracellular matrix [Mai and Chung, 1984], although the components or biologic effects of this matrix have not yet been examined in detail.

Although MCF7 cells express specific receptors for triiodothyronine and four classes of steroid hormones and are capable of exhibiting biologic responses to these factors under some conditions [Soule et al., 1973; Lippman et al., 1975, 1976, 1977; Lippman, this volume; Brooks et al., 1973; Horwitz

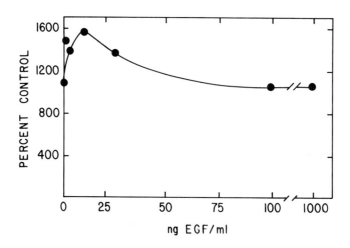

Fig. 4. Stimulation of MCF7 cell proliferation in serum-free medium by EGF. Cells were plated as described in Figure 2, except that the concentration of EGF varied as indicated. Number of cells was determined 9 days after plating; 100% control is number of cells in unsupplemented F12:DME.

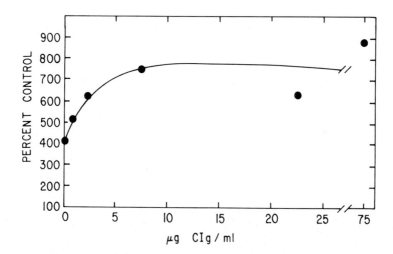

Fig. 5. Stimulation of MCF7 cell proliferation in serum-free medium by human plasma fibronectin or cold-insoluble globulin (CIg). Cells were plated as described in Figure 2, except that the concentration of fibronectin varied as indicated. Number of cells was determined 5 days after plating; 100% control is number of cells in unsupplemented F12:DME.

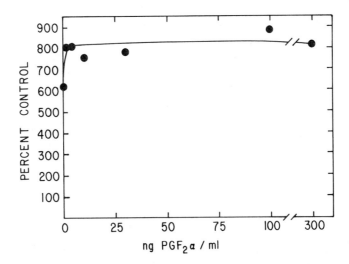

Fig. 6. Stimulation of MCF7 cell proliferation in serum-free medium by prostaglandin F_2-α. Cells were plated as described in Figure 2, except that the concentration of prostaglandin F_2-α varied as indicated. Number of cells was determined 5 days after plating; 100% control is number of cells in unsupplemented F12:DME.

et al., 1975; Lippman and Bolan, 1975; Horwitz and McGuire, 1978; Burke and McGuire, 1978], no marked growth-promoting effects of these factors are observed in the serum-free medium described. No consistent effect of physiologic concentrations of androgens or progesterone on MCF7 proliferation in serum-free medium is seen, and dexamethasone and hydrocortisone are strongly growth-inhibiting in serum-containing or serum-free medium [Lippman et al., 1976]. We have observed morphologic effects of triiodothyronine on MCF7 in the serum-free medium described, but we have not seen effects of this hormone on proliferation [Barnes and Sato, 1979]. Growth-promoting effects of estradiol in serum-containing or serum-free medium are quite small in our hands and are observed only in serum-free medium under conditions in which growth is otherwise suboptimal (Fig. 9, Table II) [Barnes and Sato, 1979, 1980c].

The difficulty in demonstrating large or consistent estrogen effects on MCF7 may stem from a number of factors. These cells may be stimulated by unoccupied nuclear estrogen receptors, independently of the presence of estrogen [Zava et al., 1979; Zava and McGuire, 1977]. Alternatively or additionally, the long-term retention of estradiol by these cells may make it difficult to reach a background in culture in which cells are not stimulated by

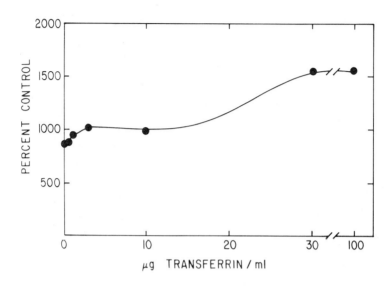

Fig. 7. Stimulation of MCF7 cell proliferation in serum-free medium by transferrin. Cells were plated as described in Figure 2, except that the concentration of transferrin varied as indicated. Number of cells was determined 7 days after plating; 100% control is number of cells in unsupplemented F12:DME.

residual intracellular estrogen [Strobl and Lippman, 1979]. Quantitative differences in estrogen effects also may exist among different sublines of MCF7. Sublines obtained from different laboratories have been found to differ in the levels of nuclear or cytoplasmic estrogen receptor and in at least one biochemical marker of estrogen effects [Edwards et al., 1980; Westley and Rochefort, 1980]. Another explanation for possible differences in the size of observed effects is that estrogen effects have been observed to be synergistic with other hormones, such as prolactin [Leung et al., 1978]. Despite numerous explanations enlisted to explain the difficulties in demonstrating more than marginal estrogen effects on MCF7 cells, a paradox remains between the moderately estrogen-responsive MCF7 cells in culture and the almost totally estrogen-dependent tumor arising from injection of these cells into athymic mice [Russo et al., 1976a; Shafie, 1980]. One idea advanced to explain this dichotomy suggests that estrogen in vivo acts to increase production of a second hormone-like factor, or estromedin, that acts as the major mitogen, much as growth hormone in vivo stimulates production of somatomedin [Sirbasku, 1978]. Studies of MCF7 proliferation in serum-free medium, in which the

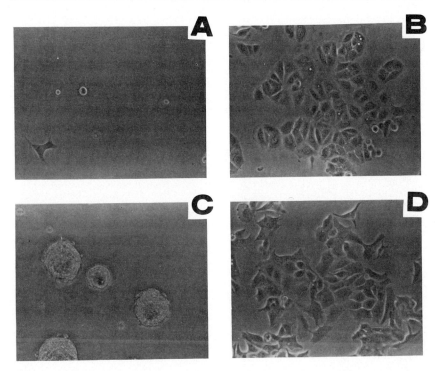

Fig. 8. Effect of serum spreading factor on attachment and spreading of MCF7 cells in serum-free medium. Cells were incubated for three days in F12:DME with no stimulatory supplements (A); F12:DME supplemented with 10% fetal calf serum (B); F12:DME supplemented with five factors as indicated in Figure 2 (C); F12:DME supplemented with five factors as indicated in Figure 2 plus serum spreading factor (2.5 μg/ml) (D). From Barnes and Sato [1979], with permission.

extracellular environment of the cells can be controlled in an absolute and precise manner, may help to answer questions of this type, which are of clear relevance to the physiology of the whole animal.

ACKNOWLEDGMENTS

This work was supported by American Cancer Society grant BC-368 and National Institutes of Health grant CA-35214. The author thanks G.H. Sato, R. Ham, M. Stampfer, D. Sirbasku, and J. Silnutzer for helpful discussions and suggestions.

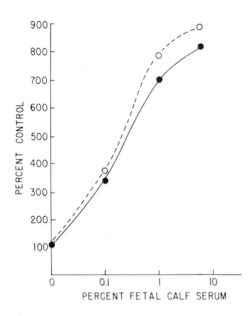

Fig. 9. Growth of MCF7 cells in serum-containing medium in the presence (○) and absence (●) of estradiol. Cells were plated at 5×10^4 per 35-mm-diameter dish in F12:DME with the indicated concentration of fetal calf serum, with or without added estradiol (10^{-9} M). Number of cells per dish was determined 5 days after plating; 100% control is number of cells in unsupplemented F12:DME.

REFERENCES

Barnes DW (1984a): Hormonally-defined serum-free media for epithelial cells in culture. In Taub M (ed): "Tissue Culture in the Study of Epithelial Transport." New York: Plenum (in press).

Barnes D (1984b): Nutritional and hormonal requirements of mammalian cells in culture. World Rev Nutr Diet (in press).

Barnes D (1984c): Attachment factors in cell culture. In Mather J (ed): "The Use of Serum-Free and Hormone-Supplemented Media." New York: Plenum, pp 195–237.

Barnes D, Sato G (1979): Growth of a human mammary tumor cell line in a serum-free medium. Nature 281:388–389.

Barnes D, Sato G (1980a): Methods for growth of cultured cells in serum-free medium. Anal Biochem 102:255–270.

Barnes DW, Sato GH (1980b): Serum-free cell culture: A unifying approach. Cell 22:649–655.

Barnes D, Sato G (1980c): Factors that stimulate proliferation of breast cancer cells in vitro in serum-free medium. In McGrath C, Brennan M, Rich M (eds): "Cell Biology of Breast Cancer." New York: Academic, pp 277–287.

Barnes D, Silnutzer J (1983): Isolation of human serum spreading factor. J Biol Chem 258:12548–12552.

Barnes DW, van der Bosch J, Masui H, Miyzaki K, Sato G (1981): The culture of human tumor cells. Methods Enzymol 79:368-391.

Barnes DW, Silnutzer J, See C, Shaffer M (1983): Characterization of human serum spreading factor with monoclonal antibody. Proc Natl Acad Sci USA 80:1362-1366.

Brooks S, Locke ER, Soule HD (1973): Estrogen receptor in a human cell line (MCF-7) from breast carcinoma. J Biol Chem 248:6251-6253.

Burke RE, McGuire WL (1978): Nuclear thyroid receptors in a human breast cancer cell line. Cancer Res 38:3769-3773.

Carpenter G, Cohen S (1979): Epidermal growth factor. Annu Rev Biochem 48:193-216.

Ceriani RL, Thompson K, Peterson JA, Abrahams S (1977): Surface differentiation antigens of human mammary epithelial cells carried on the human milk fat globule. Proc Natl Acad Sci USA 74:582-586.

Das MR, Mink MM (1979): Sequence homology of nucleic acids from human breast cancer cells and complementary DNAs from murine mammary tumor and Mason-Pfizer monkey virus. Cancer Res 39:5106-5113.

Edwards DP, Adams DJ, Savage N, McGuire WL (1980): Estrogen induced synthesis of specific proteins in human breast cancer cells. Biochem Biophys Res Commun 93:804-812.

Engel W, Young NA (1978): Human breast carcinoma cells in continuous culture: A review. Cancer Res 38:4327-4339.

Gospodarowicz D, Lui GM, Gonzales K (1982): High-density lipoprotein and the proliferation of human tumor cells maintained on extracellular matrix-coated dishes and exposed to defined medium. Cancer Res 42:3704-3713.

Ham R (1984): Formulation of basal nutrient media. In Barnes DW, Sirbasku DA, Sato GH (eds): "Cell Culture Methods for Molecular and Cell Biology." New York: Alan R. Liss, Vol 1, pp 3-21.

Horwitz KB, McGuire WL (1978): Estrogen control of progesterone receptor in human breast cancer. J Biol Chem 253:2223-2228.

Horwitz KB, Costlow ME, McGuire WL (1975): MCF-7: A human breast cancer cell line with estrogen, androgen, progesterone and glucocorticoid receptors. Steroids 26:785-795.

Hynes RO, Yamada KM (1982): Fibronectins: Multifunctional modular glycoproteins. J Cell Biol 95:369-378.

Leung BS, Qureshi S, Leung J (1978): Effect of prolactin and estrogen on human breast cancer cells in long-term tissue culture. Proceedings of the 60th Meeting of the Endocrine Society, p 130.

Lippman ME, Bolan G (1975): Oestrogen-responsive human breast cancer in long-term tissue culture. Nature 256:592-593.

Lippman ME, Bolan G, Huff K (1975): Human breast cancer responsive to androgen in long-term tissue culture. Nature 258:339-341.

Lippman M, Bolan G, Huff K (1976): The effects of glucocorticoids and progesterone on hormone-responsive human breast cancer in long-term culture. Cancer Res 36:4602-4609.

Lippman ME, Osborne CK, Knazek R, Young N (1977): In vitro model systems for the study of hormone-dependent human breast cancer. N Engl J Med 296:154-159.

Mai S, Chung AE (1984): Cell attachment and spreading on extracellular matrix coated beads. In Barnes DW, Sirbasku DA, Sato GH (eds): "Cell Culture Methods for Molecular and Cell Biology." New York: Alan R. Liss, Vol 1, pp 321-337.

Mather JP, Sato GH (1979): The use of hormone-supplemented serum-free media in primary cultures. Exp Cell Res 124:215-221.

McGrath CM, Grant PM, Soule HD, Glancy T, Rich MA (1974): Replication of oncornavirus-like particle in human breast carcinoma cell line, MCF-7. Nature 252:247-250.

McGuire WL, Horwitz KB (1979): Action of estrogen and antiestrogen in human breast cancer cell. In Ross S, Sato G (eds): "Hormones and Cell Culture." Cold Spring Harbor, New York: Cold Spring Harbor Laboratory, pp 937-947.

Osborne CK, Bolan G, Monaco ME, Lippman ME (1976): Hormone responsive human breast cancer in long-term tissue culture: Effect of insulin. Proc Natl Acad Sci USA 73:4536-4540.

Osborne CK, Hamilton B, Titus G, Livingston RB (1980): Epidermal growth factor stimulation of human breast cancer cells in culture. Cancer Res 40:2361-2366.

Rose HN, McGrath CM (1975): Alpha lactalbumin production in human mammary carcinoma. Science 190:673-675.

Rubin JS, Bradshaw RA (1984): Preparation of guinea pig prostate epidermal growth factor. In Barnes DW, Sirbasku DA, Sato GH (eds): "Cell Culture Methods for Molecular and Cell Biology." New York: Alan R. Liss, Vol 1, pp 139-145.

Russo J, Brennan MJ, Rich MA (1976a): Induction of tumor growth by inoculation of a human breast cancer cell (MCF-7) into ovary or pituitary grafted nude mice. Proc Am Assoc Cancer Res 17:116.

Russo J, Soule HD, McGrath C, Rich MA (1976b): Reexpression of the original tumor pattern by a human breast carcinoma cell line (MCF-7) in sponge culture. J Natl Cancer Inst 56:279-282.

Savage CR, Harper RA (1984): Purification of human epidermal growth factor from urine. In Barnes DW, Sirbasku DA, Sato GH (eds): "Cell Culture Methods for Molecular and Cell Biology." New York: Alan R. Liss, Vol 1, pp 147-158.

Shafie S (1980): Estrogen and the growth of breast cancer: New evidence suggests indirect action. Science 209:701-702.

Shiu RPC (1979): Prolactin receptors in human breast cancer cells in long-term tissue culture. Cancer Res 39:4381-4386.

Silnutzer J, Barnes DW (1984): Human serum spreading factor (SF): Assay, preparation and use in serum-free cell culture. In Barnes DW, Sirbasku DA, Sato GH (eds): "Cell Culture Methods for Molecular and Cell Biology." New York: Alan R. Liss, Vol 1, pp 245-268.

Sirbasku DA (1978): Estrogen induction of growth factors specific for hormone-responsive mammary, pituitary, and kidney tumor cells. Proc Natl Acad Sci USA 75:3786-3790.

Soule HD, Vazquez J, Long A, Albert S, Brennan M (1973): A human cell line from a pleural effusion derived from a breast carcinoma. J Natl Cancer Inst 51:1409-1416.

Soule HD, McGrath CM, Long A, Rich MA (1976): Hormonal stimulation of a virus-related antigen in a human breast carcinoma cell line, MCF-7. Proc Am Assoc Cancer Res 17:167.

Strobl JS, Lippman ME (1979): Prolonged retention of estradiol by human breast cancer cells in tissue culture. Cancer Res 39:3319-3327.

Westley B, Rochefort H (1980): A secreted glycoprotein induced by estrogen in human breast cancer cell lines. Cell 20:353-362.

Yamada K, Akiyama S (1984): Preparation of cellular fibronectin. In Barnes DW, Sirbasku DA, Sato GH (eds): "Cell Culture Methods for Molecular and Cell Biology." New York: Alan R. Liss, Vol 1, pp 215-230.

Zava DT, McGuire WL (1977): Estrogen receptor-unoccupied sites in nuclei in a breast tumor cell line. J Biol Chem 252:3703-3708.

Zava DT, Chamness GC, Horowitz KB, McGuire WL (1979): Human breast cancer: Biologically active estrogen receptors in the absence of estrogen? Science 196:663-664.

Methods for Serum-Free Culture of Cells of the Endocrine System, pages 217–241

13
General Methods for Isolation of Acetic Acid- and Heat-Stable Polypeptide Growth Factors for Mammary and Pituitary Tumor Cells

Tatsuhiko Ikeda, David Danielpour, Peter R. Galle, and David A. Sirbasku

The development of serum-free culture methods has allowed the identification of many biologic responses by cells in culture that were previously difficult to demonstrate in serum-containing medium. For example, in experiments measuring cell growth or differentiated function responses to steroid hormones, the problem of removing the endogenous pools of these hormones from any animal serum has not been resolved satisfactorily. The usual procedures of dextran-coated charcoal extraction at 56°C [Kirkland et al., 1976] did not remove these hormones completely, and in addition removed other hormones (i.e., thyroid hormones and insulin) and nutrients that might have resulted in identification or suppression of cellular responses not related to the in vivo effects of steroid hormones. Similarly, use of steroid hormone-deficient serum obtained from castrated animals presented potential problems since endocrine ablation changed the concentrations of many serum hormones and nutrients. Use of serum-free culture methods has at least in part overcome these problems. Examples of the study of the roles of steroid hormones in mammary tumor cell growth in serum-free medium have been presented elsewhere [Barnes and Sato, 1979]. In addition, Ambesi-Impiombato et al. [1982] have presented remarkable new data showing that the mitogenic and differentiation effects of the polypeptide hormone thyrotropin-stimulating hor-

Faculty of Nutrition, Kobe-Gakuin University, Igawadani-cho Arise, Nishi-ku, Kobe, Japan 673 (T.I.) and Department of Biochemistry and Molecular Biology, University of Texas Medical School, Houston, Texas 77225 (D.D., P.R.G., D.A.S.)

mone (TSH) on primary cultures of thyroid cells were readily demonstrable under serum-free hormonally defined conditions but not when these same cells were cultured in serum-containing medium. From data just cited as well as those presented in these volumes, it is apparent that the use of serum-free culture methods will allow study in vitro of a broad range of cellular physiology previously only accessible by in vivo methods.

In this report, we describe the general methods of isolation of a new family of mitogenic factors for the human T47D and MCF-7 mammary tumor cell lines [Soule et al., 1973], for the MTW9/PL rat mammary tumor cells [Sirbasku, 1978a], and for the GH3/C14 rat pituitary tumor cells [Sorrentino et al., 1976a,b]. The point most pertinent to these volumes was that these activities were identified only under serum-free conditions; when attempts were made to measure the mitogenic effects of these new activities on appropriate target cells maintained in serum-containing medium, the mitogenic activity was completely suppressed [Ikeda and Sirbasku, 1984]. In the following sections, we describe the methods for assaying these polypeptide growth factors and procedures for the isolation of each.

MATERIALS AND METHODS
Cell Lines Used

The MTW9/PL cells used in this study were shown previously to form estrogen-responsive tumors [Sirbasku, 1978a], thyroid hormone-responsive tumors [Sirbasku, 1978a], and pituitary hormone- or pituitary-origin growth factor-responsive tumors [Sirbasku et al., 1982] in W/Fu rats. These cells possess estrogen-specific receptors [Leland et al., 1982], and under serum-free culture conditions they have an estradiol-inducible autostimulatory growth factor activity identified from acid extracts of these cells [Danielpour and Sirbasku, 1983a]. The stock cultures of these cells were grown as described elsewhere [Ikeda et al., 1982]. The in vivo growth properties of the MTW9/PL cells have remained unchanged over 6 years in culture.

The T47D and the MCF-7 cell lines were obtained from the American Type Culture Collection, Rockville, MD. Stock cultures of the T47D cells were grown on 10-cm-diameter plastic petri dishes in Dulbecco's modified Eagle's medium (DME) supplemented with antibiotics, 2 mM glutamine, 15 mM HEPES (pH 7.3), and 10% (vol./vol.) fetal calf serum (FCS). The cells were passaged twice weekly, and these stock cultures were used to initiate growth factor assays under serum-free conditions as described below. The MCF-7 cells were maintained under conditions similar to those of the T47D line. In the cases of the MTW9/PL, the T47D, and the GH3/C14 cells no serum-free hormonally defined culture medium was available for stock culture maintenance. However, defined media are available for the MCF-7 cells [Barnes and Sato, 1979; Allegra and Lippman, 1979], and presumably they could have been used to maintain the stock cultures and assay for new growth factors. We elected to use serum-maintained stock cultures of all cell lines in this study only for the sake of uniformity of the methods.

The GH3/C14 rat pituitary tumor cells were shown previously to form estrogen-responsive [Sorrentino et al., 1976a] and thyroid hormone-responsive [Sorrentino et al., 1976b] tumors in W/Fu rats. Also, these cells have estrogen-specific receptors [Moo et al., 1982]. Stock cultures of GH3/C14 cells were passaged twice weekly in DME supplemented with antibiotics, 2 mM glutamine, 15 mM HEPES (pH 7.3), 12.5% (vol./vol.) horse serum (HS), and 2.5% (vol./vol.) FCS as described before [Ikeda et al., 1982]. After more than 10 years in culture, these cells still form estrogen-responsive tumors in host rats.

Growth Factor Assay Methods

Growth factor activities were assayed by two methods. The first was direct measurement of increase in cell numbers in response to addition of factor to the cells plated under serum-free conditions as described before for the MTW9/PL and GH3/C14 cells [Sirbasku, 1978b], and the MCF-7 line [Sirbasku and Benson, 1980]. While this method of assay provided reliable data clearly establishing logarithmic growth in response to crude [Sirbasku et al., 1981] or purified [Ikeda and Sirbasku, 1984] growth factors, its use in monitoring the purification of growth factors was limited. Among the many problems associated with cell number assays were the difficulties of sterilizing the large number of chromatography fractions without substantial losses of activity owing to binding of the growth factors to the membranes, and the problem that samples from columns often contained high concentrations of salts or acids that inhibited the relatively long, 3- to 6-day cell number assay. Removal of these inhibitors before conducting the assays caused significant losses of total activity, especially in the more purified preparations.

The second method of assay used in our studies was to monitor growth factor-stimulated incorporation of tritium-labeled thymidine into cellular DNA as described in detail elsewhere [Ikeda et al., 1982; Ikeda and Sirbasku, 1984]. This method provided a rapid, reproducible estimation of growth factor-specific activity by determining the concentration of factor protein required to replace one-half of the mitogenic response of cells to an optimum concentration of serum. For example, the MTW9/PL cells responded best to 10% (vol./vol.) FCS; this incorporation was given the designation C_{10}. The specific activity of mammary cell growth factors was then estimated as G_{50}, or one-half the response of the cells to serum $(C_{10} - C_0)$. In all assays the basal level of growth was expressed as C_0, or the amount of label incorporated into DNA in the absence of growth factor or serum. All protein determinations were done by the method of Bradford [1976], bovine serum albumin being used as standard.

The MTW9/PL and GH3/C14 labeled precursor assays were done as described before [Ikeda and Sirbasku, 1984]. The assays with the T47D cells were conducted by a modification of the MTW9/PL method. The T47D cells (10,000) were added to the wells of Costar 24-well cluster plates in a volume of 1.0 ml of DME containing 2% (vol./vol.) FCS and 0.1% bovine serum albumin. After 24 h at 37°C in a CO_2 incubator, the serum-containing medium was removed, and 0.9 ml of DME containing 0.1% bovine serum albumin was added to each well. After an additional 24-h incubation, increasing concentrations of growth factor were added in 0.1-ml volumes, and 22 h later 1.0 μCi of tritium-labeled thymidine was added (70 Ci/mmole) in 0.050 ml of DME. Pulse labeling was continued for 2 h at 37°C, and was terminated as described before [Ikeda and Sirbasku, 1984]. The soluble pools of unincorporated label were washed out with several volumes of 80% methanol, and the label incorporated into DNA was determined as previously described [Ikeda and Sirbasku, 1984]. The assay with MCF-7 cells also was a modification of that used with the MTW9/PL line. MCF-7 cells (10,000) were added to each Costar plate well in 1.0 ml of DME containing 5% FCS (vol./vol.). After 24 h in a CO_2 incubator at 37°C, the serum-containing medium was removed and replaced with serum-free DME. After an additional 24 h, growth factor was added in 0.1 ml of DME, and 22 h later the tritium-labeled thymidine pulse label was done as described above for the T47D cells. The specific activities of growth factors with T47D and MCF-7 cells were estimated as the concentrations of protein required to replace one-half the cells' mitogenic responses to 2% (vol./vol.) FCS and 5% (vol./vol.) FCS, respectively.

Tissue Sources for Growth Factor Isolations

Lyophilized powders of early pregnant sheep uteri, mature ewe kidneys, and whole sheep pituitaries (mixed male and female) were obtained from Waitaki Refrigerating Limited, Christchurch, New Zealand. The growth factor activities of these powders were stable indefinitely at −20°C. The MTW9/B (autonomous) rat mammary tumors used to isolate the mammary tumor autostimulatory activity were grown in male W/Fu rats. We purified the mammary autostimulatory activity from the MTW9/B since these autonomous cells had a twofold higher starting specific activity than the estrogen-responsive MTW9/PL tumors. The GH3/C14 tumors were grown in estradiol-treated ovariectomized W/Fu rats as described before [Sorrentino et al., 1976a]. These were used to isolate the pituitary cell autostimulatory activity and the mammary tumor cell growth-promoting factor. In both cases 1-10-g tumors were harvested and washed extensively with EGTA-saline to remove residual blood. The fresh pig uteri used to isolate the GH3/C14 pituitary cell growth-promoting activity were obtained from a local abattoir. The tissue was washed in running water at the time of collection, and stored at $-20°C$ until used. The activity was stable indefinitely in frozen tissue. Just prior to the beginning of a purification, the uteri were thawed, cut into 2-cm^3 fragments, and washed extensively with EGTA-saline.

RESULTS

Isolation of a Mammary/Uterine/Pituitary Tumor Cell Growth Factor From Lyophilized Powders of Pregnant Sheep Uteri

The methods of preparation of the uterine-derived growth factor (UDGF) have been described in detail by Ikeda and Sirbasku [1984]. Those results will only be summarized here. A total of 500 g of lyophilized powder was added to 5,000 ml of 0.1 M acetic acid; after this mixture was stirred for 24 h at 4°C, the insoluble debris was removed by centrifugation, and the active supernatant was heated (in 200-ml portions) at 93°C for 5 min. This step resulted in a large inactive precipitate. It must be emphasized that the amount of precipitate formed during the high-temperature incubation was pH-dependent. The acetic acid extract of the lyophilized powders was pH 4.5. The available data from all of our studies suggested that as the solution was made more acidic less precipitate formed during heating. Therefore, if the pH of extraction was too low the precipitate that usually formed with heating instead appeared as a protein precipitate in the ammonium acetate-eluted fractions from the SP-Sephadex column. After heating and centrifugation, SP-Sephadex (260 ml of ion exchanger) was added to the supernatant and the mixture was stirred gently overnight at 4°C. The SP-Sephadex was swollen and equilibrated in 0.1 M acetic acid before addition to the heated supernatant. The SP-Sephadex was transfered to a glass column, and the ion exchanger was washed with several column volumes of 0.1 M acetic acid followed by 0.001 M acetic acid. These washes contained little or no UDGF activity. The growth factor activity was eluted from the SP-Sephadex with 0.3 M ammonium acetate, pH 7.2. The most active fractions were pooled and lyophilized to remove the ammonium acetate; the resulting preparation was dissolved in 0.1 M acetic acid and chromatographed on Sephadex G-50 equilibrated and eluted with the same acid.

Pooled active fractions from the Sephadex G-50 were lyophilized, redissolved in 10 mM sodium phosphate (pH 6.0), and chromatographed on CM-Sephadex C-25 equilibrated in the same buffer. The majority (70%) of the UDGF activity became associated with the cation exchanger and was eluted with a linear 0–0.3 M sodium chloride gradient in running buffer. The active fractions were desalted by Sephadex G-25 chromatography in 0.1 M acetic acid.

The final pooled active UDGF fractions were stored at $-20°C$ and were stable indefinitely. A summary of the purification is presented in Table I. From 500 g of powder, 40–50 mg of UDGF was isolated. A concentration of 8 ng/ml UDGF yielded G_{50} for the MTW9/PL cells (1.90×10^{-9} M growth factor). The degree of homogeneity of the preparation was estimated by electrophoresis under nonreducing non-denaturing conditions on 15% acrylamide gels followed by Coomassie blue staining, and by 8M urea, 0.1% SDS polyacrylamide gel electrophoresis, and the same staining. These studies confirmed >95% homogeneity. The results of the urea-SDS gel analysis are shown in Figure 1. Estimation of the molecular weight of UDGF from calibrated urea-SDS gels gave an apparent mass of 4,200 daltons (Fig. 2). Further analysis by reversed-phase high-performance liquid chromatography (HPLC), hydrophobic chromatography, and molecular sieve HPLC all confirmed >90% homogeneity. The estimation of the isoelectric point gave a value of pI = 7.3.

Studies were conducted [Ikeda and Sirbasku, 1984] to determine the cell types that responded to purified UDGF. As shown in Figure 3, UDGF promoted growth of MTW9/PL mammary cells, UCS endometrial tumor cells, and ULMS myometrial tumor cells with estimated values of G_{50} = 10, 36, and 75 ng/ml, respectively. These data, along with the observation that UDGF promoted growth of normal rat uterine cells in short-term monolayer

TABLE I. Purification of Sheep Uterine Mammary Tumor Cell Growth Factor (UDGF)

Steps	Specific activity (G_{50}, ng/ml)	Total protein (mg)
Lyophilized uterine powder	450,000[a]	500,000[b]
0.1 M Acetic acid extraction	1,300	20,600
93°C Treatment	370	4,800
SP-Sephadex chromatography	82	970
Sephadex G-50	21	212
CM-Sephadex C-25	8	40–50

[a]Specific activity of pH 7.2 PBS extract.
[b]Total dry weight of powder used to initiate isolation.

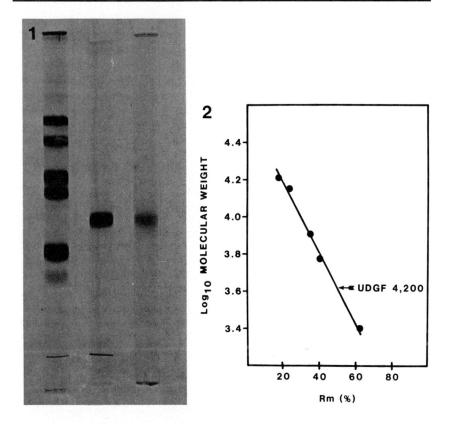

Fig. 1. The 8 M urea-0.1% SDS polyacrylamide gel electrophoresis and Coomassie blue staining analysis of the CM-Sephadex-purified sheep UDGF. The molecular weight standards (left lane) were horse heart myoglobin and sequenced cyanogen bromide-generated fragments of this protein (MW= 16,947, 14,404, 8,159, 6,214, and 2,512 daltons). The middle lane shows the migration position of a single band found after application of 75 μg of UDGF, and the right lane shows analysis of 10 μg of UDGF.

Fig. 2. Estimation of UDGF molecular weight by 8 M urea-0.1% SDS polyacrylamide gel electrophoresis. The data presented in Figure 1 were used to construct a calibration curve from which the molecular weight of sheep UDGF was calculated.

culture (T. Ikeda and D.A. Sirbasku, manuscript in preparation), suggested a role of this activity in neoplastic and normal uterine growth. In addition, we have shown that UDGF was inactive with normal diploid fibroblasts at concentrations of up to 20 μg/ml, and active with mouse 3T3 cells only at high concentrations (i.e., 1 μg/ml). Our initial results suggested that UDGF was a relatively weak mitogen ($G_{50} = 1,400$ ng/ml) for GH3/C14 rat pituitary

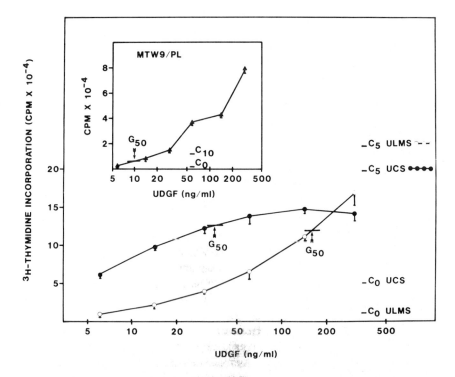

Fig. 3. Growth of tumor cells, derived from MTW9/PL mammary tissue, ULMS uterine smooth muscle (myometrium), and UCS uterine endometrium, in serum-free culture in response to purified sheep UDGF. Growth was monitored by measuring tritium-labeled thymidine incorporation into DNA as described in Materials and Methods. The growth response to serum-free DME without added serum or growth factor is shown as C_0; that promoted by 5% serum is designated C_5. The G_{50} for the UDGF on these cells was calculated from these values.

tumor cells. However, these data were obtained by measuring the incorporation of tritium-labeled thymidine into DNA at 48 h after UDGF addition in serum-free culture. Present data suggest that pulse labeling within 16–24 h after UDGF addition will lead to greater than a tenfold reduction of the estimated G_{50} concentration. Thus, UDGF may be a considerably more potent pituitary cell mitogen than originally estimated. Other studies of cells that respond to purified UDGF are now in progress.

In another study pertinent to the topic of these volumes, we have attempted to supplement the mitogenic action of UDGF on MTW9/PL cells by addition of suboptimal concentrations of serum. The data presented in Figure 4 show the results of these experiments. Addition of even a low concentration

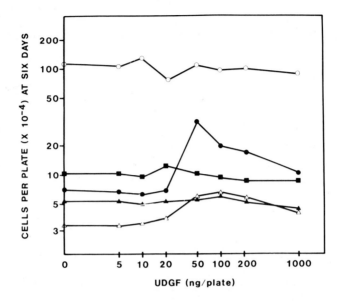

Fig. 4. MTW9/PL cell growth in media supplemented with various components. Growth was measured by the cell number increase assay described in Materials and Methods. Cells (3.0 × 10⁴) were added to 35-mm-diameter dishes containing 3.0 ml DME supplemented with 10% (vol./vol.) FCS. After 24 h the serum-containing medium was removed and replaced with 3.0 ml final volume of serum-free DME only (open triangles), DME plus 0.1% bovine serum albumin (filled triangles), DME containing 1% (vol./vol.) FCS (filled squares), 10% FCS (open circles), or 50 μg/plate (16.7 μg/ml DME) of a phosphate-buffered (pH 7.2) extract of lyophilized pregnant sheep uteri (filled circles). The neutral buffer extract of sheep uteri was prepared as described in Ikeda and Sirbasku [1984]. The designated amounts of UDGF were added to each incubation as the concentration per 3.0 ml of DME. Cell numbers were determined on day 6 and medium was changed on days 2 and 4.

of serum (i.e., 1% FCS) completely suppressed UDGF activity. These data contrasted sharply with those of Figure 3, where the assays showed strong activity under serum-free conditions; clearly, had we sought to purify UDGF by an assay method employing basal serum concentration, we would not have accomplished the task.

Using the purified preparations of UDGF, we have attempted to prepare a serum-free hormonally defined medium for the MTW9/PL rat mammary cells. Despite additions and combinations of many hormones and growth factors we have not yet obtained a completely satisfactory defined medium. Our closest approach to the replacement of the serum requirement for these cells in long-term culture was to use purified UDGF in combination with a non-growth-promoting concentration of neutral buffer extract of sheep uterine

powder (Fig. 5). Under these conditions, logarithmic growth of the MTW9/
PL cells proceeded for 6 days, although fresh UDGF additions were required
every 2 days to sustain the proliferation. These data suggested that UDGF
was rapidly consumed by the cells in culture, and that preparation of a
hormonally defined medium will require frequent additions of purified factors.

Isolation of a Mammary/Pituitary Tumor Cell Growth Factor From Lyophilized Powder of Mature Ewe Kidney

The results described here summarize those to be presented in a more
complete form elsewhere (T. Ikeda and D.A. Sirbasku, manuscript submitted

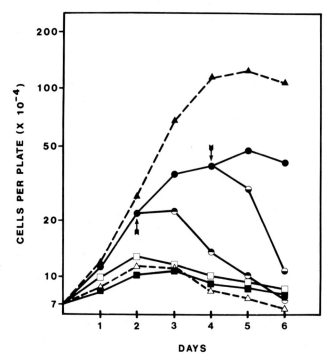

Fig. 5. Demonstration of UDGF as a promoter of cell growth when measured by logarithmic
increase in cell number. The assay was conducted as described in Figure 4, with the exception
that cell numbers were determined daily. MTW9/PL cell growth is shown in response to serum-
free DME only (open triangles), DME containing 33.3 ng/ml UDGF (filled squares), DME with
16.7 μg/ml of neutral buffer extract of lyophilized sheep uteri (open squares), DME supplemented with 10% (vol./vol.) FCS (filled triangles), and finally DME containing the combination
of 3.33 ng/ml UDGF and 16.7 μg/ml neutral buffer uterine extract (filled circles). On days 2
and 4 (shown by the arrows) additional UDGF (33.3 ng/ml) was added to those cultures that
had already received the combination of UDGF and neutral uterine extract. These cultures
continued to grow (filled circles). When additional UDGF was not provided on days 2 or 4, the
effect on the cell numbers is shown by the half-filled circles.

for publication). A total of 500 g of lyophilized powder was added to 5,000 ml of 0.1 M acetic acid; the extraction and 95°C heat-treatment were carried out as described above for the preparation of UDGF. The kidney-derived growth factor (KDGF) was assayed throughout the purification by following the stimulation of tritium-labeled thymidine uptake into DNA of the MTW9/ PL cells in serum-free medium [Ikeda and Sirbasku, 1984]. To the active heated supernatant, 1.0 g of Bio-Rad AG50W-X8 ion exchange resin was added per 100 mg of protein in the heated supernatant. The resin was preswollen and equilibrated in 0.1 M acetic acid before mixing with the KDGF preparation. After stirring at 4°C overnight, the inactive supernatant was discarded, the ion exchanger was transferred to a glass column, and the resin was washed with several column volumes each of 0.1 M and 0.001 M acetic acid. The washes were inactive. The KDGF was eluted with a single step of 0.010 M ammonium hydroxide. While the recovery from this step was not as high as might be desired, the degree of homogeneity of the preparation was improved significantly. The pooled active fractions were lyophilized and redissolved in 10 mM sodium acetate pH 5.8. This solution was applied to a DEAE-Sepharose CL-6B column equilibrated in the same buffer, and eluted with a 0–500 mM sodium chloride linear gradient in running buffer. The active fractions were desalted by Sephadex G-25 chromatography in 10 mM sodium acetate pH 6.2, and applied to a second DEAE-Sepharose CL-6B column equilibrated in the pH 6.2 buffer. KDGF was eluted with a linear gradient of 0–300 mM sodium chloride in running buffer. The pooled active fractions were desalted again, lyophilized, redissolved in 0.1 M acetic acid, and applied to a final Sephadex G-50 column equilibrated and eluted with 0.1 M acetic acid. All of the KDGF activity eluted in a single peak that corresponded to the only fractions containing significant protein. Table II summarizes the results of the KDGF purification.

TABLE II. Purification of Sheep Kidney Mammary Tumor Cell Growth Factor (KDGF)

Steps	Specific activity $(G_{50}, ng/ml)$	Total protein (mg)
Lyophilized kidney powder	345,000[a]	500,000[b]
0.1 M Acetic acid extraction	2,700	31,600
95°C Treatment	310	3,145
Bio-Rad AG50W-X8	58	285
DEAE-Sepharose CL-6B, pH 5.8	41	79
DEAE-Sepharose CL-6B, pH 6.2	29	24
Sephadex G-50	19	11

[a]Specific activity of pH 7.2 PBS extract.
[b]Total dry weight of powder used to initiate isolation.

From 500 g of powder, a total of 8-14 mg of KDGF was isolated, which represented approximately a 5% yield and an overall 18,000-fold purification. The purified KDGF showed G_{50} = 19 ng/ml with MTW9/PL cells in serum-free medium. Characterization of the degree of homogeneity was done by polyacrylamide gel (15%) electrophoresis under nonreducing and nondenaturing conditions, and by 8 M urea, 0.1% SDS gel (12.5%) electrophoresis as decribed for analysis of UDGF [Ikeda and Sirbasku, 1984]. Under these conditions, only one Coomassie blue-stained band was identified even when amounts up to 200 μg were analyzed per gel. Figure 6 shows the results of the urea-SDS gel analysis. The estimated molecular weight of KDGF was 4,200 daltons (Fig. 7), which was the same as estimated for UDGF (Fig. 2.)

Since the apparent molecular weights of KDGF and UDGF were indistinguishable by urea-SDS gel electrophoresis, we attempted to differentiate these two by isoelectric point measurements. As shown in Figure 8, chromatofocusing separated the apparently homogeneous KDGF into two distinct species designated KDGF-I and KDGF-II, which showed pI of 5.2 and 4.8, respectively. The properties of these two forms of KDGF are under study by immunologic and protein chemistry methods to determine whether these have common amino acid sequences. Nevertheless, the pI values of UDGF and both forms of KDGF were clearly different.

Isolation of a Human and Rat Mammary Tumor Cell Growth Factor From Lyophilized Powder of Whole Sheep Pituitaries

Previous data from our laboratory [Sirbasku et al., 1982] demonstrated that the MTW9/PL mammary tumors grew 1.8 to 7.6 times larger in W/Fu female and estradiol-treated male rats bearing developed GH3/C14 pituitary tumors than in control groups of these same animals without the pituitary tumors. Since these tumors secrete both prolactin (PRL) and growth hormone (GH), the experiments implied that the MTW9/PL cells were pituitary hormone-responsive. Leung and Shiu [1981] likewise reported that human T47D mammary tumor formation was stimulated by GH3 tumors in athymic nude mice, and Welsch et al. [1981] described similar but somewhat less pronounced effects of GH3 tumors on human MCF-7 mammary tumor cell growth in athymic nude mice. Despite these clear examples of pituitary hormone responses in vivo we have not been able to demonstrate PRL or GH mitogenic effects on any one of these cell lines in culture [Sirbasku et al., 1982]. While negative data did not prove that these hormones were inactive, our approach became one of examining pituitary extracts for mitogenic activities that might not have been identified before. Early attempts utilized neutral phosphate buffer (pH 7.2) extractions of normal rat pituitaries and GH3/C14

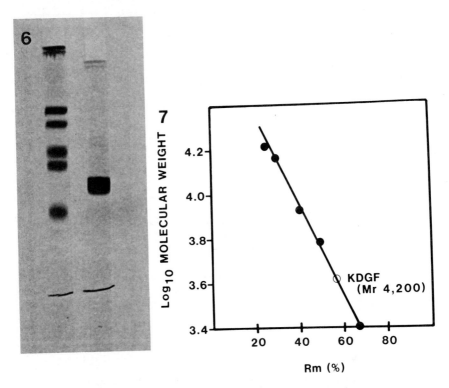

Fig. 6. The 8 M urea-0.1% SDS polyacrylamide gel electrophoresis and Coomassie blue staining analysis of the purified KDGF preparation from the final Sephadex G-50 column step. The migration positions of the known molecular weight markers of myoglobin and sequenced fragments (see legend of Fig. 1) are shown, as is the migration position of a single stained band on another gel that received 50 μg of purified KDGF.

Fig. 7. Molecular weight estimation of purified KDGF. By the same urea-SDS electrophoresis analysis as used for UDGF (see Fig. 2) the molecular weight of KDGF was estimated from calibration curves constructed from the migration positions of myoglobin standards.

tumors [Sirbasku et al., 1982]. A high-molecular-weight growth factor activity (i.e., 50,000–80,000 daltons) was found for MTW9/PL cells; these data were in general agreement with studies by Leung et al. [1983] showing that a similar-size T47D cell growth factor was extracted from the GH3 tumor under nearly neutral pH conditions. However, both of these studies were done under nondissociating conditions, which left open the possibility that the growth factor activity might be associated with various components of the extract. For this reason we undertook a purification of the pituitary mammary cell growth factor under acidic (dissociating) conditions.

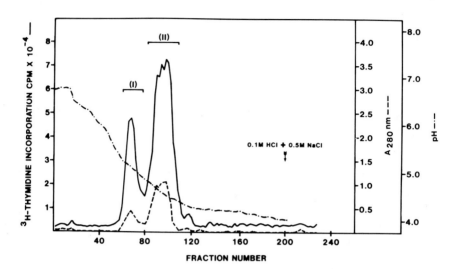

Fig. 8. Determination of the isoelectric point of KDGF by chromatofocusing. The procedure for focusing was based on the manuals of Pharmacia Fine Chemicals, Inc. A column (1.5 × 30 cm) of PBE94 chromatofocusing resin was equilibrated with 25 mM histidine-HCl (pH 6.3) prior to application of the sample (equilibrated in the same buffer). The column was then washed with 50 ml of the histidine buffer, followed by 600 ml of a 1:7 dilution of Polybuffer 74 adjusted to pH 4.0 with 2.0 M HCl. Finally, the column was washed with 0.1 M HCl containing 0.5 M sodium chloride. The flow rate was 15 ml/h, and 3.0-ml fractions were collected.

TABLE III. Purification of Sheep Pituitary Mammary Tumor Cell Growth Factor (PitDGF)

Steps	Specific activity (G_{50}, ng/ml)	Total protein (mg)
Lyophilized pituitary powder	22,000[a]	10,000[b]
0.1 M Acetic acid extraction	702	439
93°C Treatment	176	136
SP-Sephadex chromatography	61	40
Sephadex G-50	29	8–10

[a]Specific activity of pH 7.2 PBS extract.
[b]Total dry weight of powder used to initiate isolation.

Lyophilized powder of sheep pituitaries was used in a one-fiftieth scale purification method based on the first four steps of the UDGF isolation as described above and in Ikeda and Sirbasku [1984]. Table III presents the pertinent data. From only 10 g of powder, 8–10 mg of a potent (G_{50} = 29 ng/ml) MTW9/PL cell growth factor was purified. Under standard assay conditions (Fig. 9) the activity of the acid- and heat-stable pituitary-derived

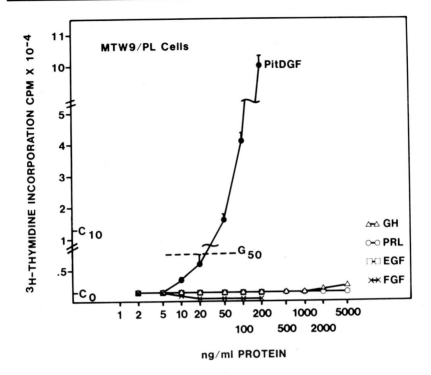

Fig. 9. Effect of PitDGF, bovine GH (growth hormone), bovine PRL (prolactin), mouse EGF (epidermal growth factor), and bovine FGF (fibroblast growth factor) on MTW9/PL cell growth in serum-free DME. Assays were conducted as described in Materials and Methods. Purified EGF and FGF were obtained from Collaborative Research Corp., Lexington, MA.

growth factor (PitDGF) toward MTW9/PL cells was not replaced by high concentrations of either PRL or GH. Experiments with the T47D cells gave similar results, with PitDGF proving to be a much more potent mitogen than either PRL or GH (Fig. 10). An estimation of the homogeneity of the preparation by 8 M urea–0.1% SDS gel electrophoresis, and an estimation of the molecular weight by the same experiments, is shown in Figure 11. The calculated apparent molecular weight was 3,900 daltons, and the preparations appear >90% homogeneous by this method. Other characterizations of the degree of homogeneity are in progress.

In addition to PitDGF's effects on mammary cells, we have assayed its activity with normal diploid fibroblasts and find no response. These data suggest that PitDGF was not any one of the forms of fibroblast growth factor (FGF) also identified in pituitaries [Gospodarowicz, 1975]. Also, FGF activity

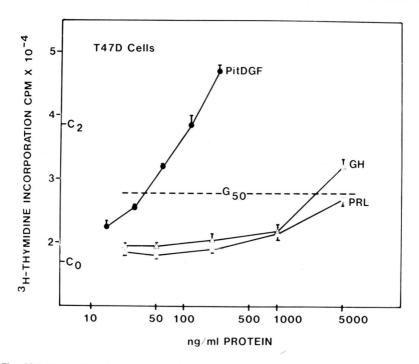

Fig. 10. Effect of PitDGF, bovine GH, and bovine PRL on T47D human mammary tumor cell growth in serum-free DME. Assays were done as described in Materials and Methods. The C_2 value represents growth in response to 2% (vol./vol.) FCS: C_0 shows incorporation in response to DME only.

was destroyed by high temperature, but PitDGF was unaffected by 95°C incubation (see Table III). Surprisingly, when PitDGF was assayed with the GH3/C14 pituitary cells (Fig. 12) the growth factor was a potent mitogen. The significance of this is not clear, but the possibility arises that pituitary-origin factors might exert autocrine or paracrine growth control within that gland.

Partial Purification of a Mammary Tumor Cell Growth Factor and a GH3/C14 Autostimulatory Growth Factor Activity From GH3/C14 Tumors

From the data described above, it is possible to conclude that the GH3/C14 tumor cells were the source of a new growth factor activity and that the methods used to isolate the sheep origin PitDGF might be applicable to the GH3/C14 cell activity. In experiments to be reported elsewhere (D. Daniel-pour et al., manuscript in preparation), we have identified an acetic acid- and

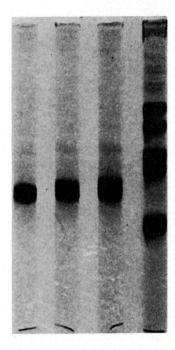 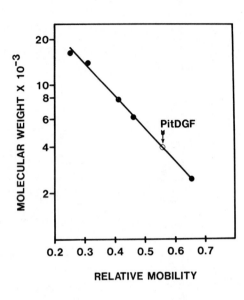

Fig. 11. Estimation of the degree of homogeneity and the molecular weight of sheep PitDGF. The stained gels (left panel) show the results of analysis by urea-SDS polyacrylamide gel electrophoresis of 75, 100, and 150 µg of purified PitDGF (left to right); the far right gel shows migration of the myoglobin and fragments as described in Figure 1. The panel at the right shows the estimation of the molecular weight of sheep PitDGF.

heat-stable polypeptide growth factor from GH3/C14 tumors and from these cells growing in serum-free culture. Also, an acid- and heat-stable activity was identified in the serum-free conditioned medium of the cells in culture. The activity extracted from the cell cultures promoted the growth of the MTW9/ PL rat mammary cells as well as the growth of the T47D and MCF-7 human mammary tumor cells. Since all three of these lines were GH3 tumor-responsive in vivo, our findings suggested that purification of this activity was important. We have partially purified the GH3/C14 mammary tumor growth factor (GH3/C14-MTGF) from tumors grown and washed as described in Materials and Methods.

The isolation of the GH3/C14-MTGF was done by the same methods as those applied to sheep UDGF [Ikeda and Sirbasku, 1984] and sheep PitDGF. Purification was monitored by tritium-labeled thymidine incorporation into MTW9/PL cell DNA as described before [Ikeda and Sirbasku, 1984]. Begin-

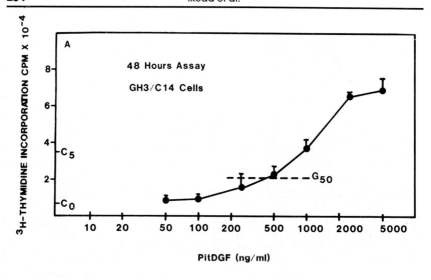

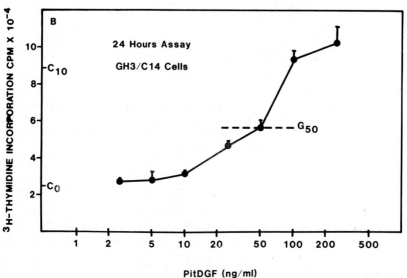

Fig. 12. Effect of PitDGF on GH3/C14 rat pituitary tumor cell growth in serum-free DME. The growth-promoting potency of PitDGF on GH3/C14 cells was estimated at 48 h (A) and 24 h (B) after addition of the designated concentrations of factors. The assay procedures are described in Materials and Methods. In the experiment presented in panel A, the G_{50} of PitDGF was estimated as the concentration of growth factor that replaced one-half of the GH3/C14 cell response to 5% serum, whereas the data in panel B expressed G_{50} as one-half replacement of the response to 10% serum. The reason for the use of two different controls was that these concentrations of serum optimized the cell growth responses at these pulse labeling periods.

ning with 130 g of tumor (wet weight), four steps of 0.1 M acetic acid extraction for 24 h, heating of the active supernatant at 95°C for 5 min, SP-Sephadex chromatography with elution of the activity of 0.3 M ammonium acetate, and finally Sephadex G-50 molecular sieve chromatography in 0.1 M acetic acid were applied to yield a total of 7.2 mg of protein. At this time, no estimations of the degree of homogeneity are available. Table IV presents the partial purification of GH3/C14-MTGF through step four. The yield of activity was high, as was the specific activity of the preparation (G_{50} = 60 ng/ml) Further purification of GH3/C14-MTGF will be done by HPLC reverse-phase methods. When antibody either to sheep PitDGF- or to the GH3/C14 cell-derived activity becomes available, these will be compared for cross-reactivity.

In parallel studies, the same fractions of the GH3/C14-MTGF purification that were assayed for MTW9/PL cell growth activity (Table IV), were also assayed for growth activity with the GH3/C14 cells (Table V). These experiments were suggested by the data showing that the purified sheep PitDGF was mitogenic for GH3/C14 cells in serum-free medium (Fig. 12). As was evident from the data in Table V, the four-step preparation from GH3/C14 tumors was mitogenic (G_{50} = 430 ng/ml) for GH3/C14 cells. Further purification will be necessary to establish whether the MTW9/PL cell growth activity and the GH3/C14 autostimulatory factor are the same molecular species.

TABLE IV. Partial Purification of a Mammary Tumor Cell Growth Factor From GH3/C14 Pituitary Tumors

Steps	Specific activity (G_{50}, ng/ml)	Total protein (mg)
0.1 M Acetic acid extraction	900	316.8
95°C Treatment	725	311.9
SP-Sephadex C-25	225	42.6
Sephadex G-50 in 0.1 M acetic acid	60	7.2

TABLE V. Partial Purification of a GH3/C14 Rat Pituitary Tumor Cell Autostimulatory Growth Factor

Steps	Specific activity (G_{50}, ng/ml)	Total protein (mg)
0.1 M Acetic acid extraction	4,300	316.8
95°C Treatment	2,400	311.9
SP-Sephadex C-25	1,250	42.6
Sephadex G-50 in 0.1 M acetic acid	430	7.2

Partial Purification of a Mammary Tumor-Associated Autostimulatory Growth Factor

Our previous studies [Leland et al., 1981, 1982; Sirbasku and Leland, 1982] showed that neutral buffer (pH 7.2) extracts of MTW9/PL tumors growing in intact females possessed a high-specific-activity autostimulatory factor(s), and that the concentration of the activity in these tumors was related to the estrogen status of the host. These data suggested that, in addition to our original proposal of endocrine estromedins [Sirbasku, 1978b], it was possible that autocrine types of estromedins might also be involved in estrogen-responsive mammary tumor growth in vivo [Sirbasku, 1981]. To further confirm this possibility, we cultured the MTW9/PL cells under serum-free conditions in the presence and absence of physiologic concentrations of estradiol, and prepared acetic acid and 95°C heated extracts of the cells after 3-5 days in the defined medium [Danielpour and Sirbasku, 1983a]. The acetic acid/heated extracts of the cell showed a twofold induction of autostimulatory activity in response to 1.0×10^{-9} to 1.0×10^{-8} M estradiol. Other control studies confirmed the biosynthesis of a mammary tumor-derived growth factor (MTDGF) by the MTW9/PL cells in culture and established the presence of an acid- and heat-stable autostimulatory activity in the serum-free conditioned medium from these cells (D. Danielpour and D.A. Sirbasku, manuscript in preparation). Extending these studies to human MCF-7 cells, we have recently reported the identification of an estrogen-inducible acetic acid-stable and heat-stable (95°C) autostimulatory growth factor in extracts of these cells maintained under serum-free conditions [Danielpour and Sirbasku, 1983b]. Also, an autostimulatory activity has been assayed in the serum-free conditioned medium of the MCF-7 cells. One notable problem has been that while estrogen-elevated autostimulatory activities were readily measured in extracts of both the human and rat mammary cells, we have not been able to find estrogen effects on the levels of the factors in conditioned medium. Several problems were apparent with the bioassay of very low concentrations of growth factors in conditioned medium; our present plan is first to purify the cell-associated activities to homogeneity, raise specific antibodies, and use these in the more sensitive ELISA or radioimmunoassay methods of measurement of the concentration of mitogen in medium versus estrogen treatment.

When considering the possible sources of MTDGF that might yield milligram quantities of homogeneous factor, several facts were taken into consideration. To judge from the data of several investigators [Delarco and Todaro, 1978; Todaro et al., 1980; Roberts et al., 1980] and from our own experience, serum-free conditioned medium was a possible but impractical source. Amounts of hundreds of liters would be required to prepare even microgram quantities of growth factors. Likewise cells from culture presented problems of quantity. Since at best 1.0 g of cells was obtained per large-sized roller bottle, preparation of several hundred bottles might be necessary for even microgram amounts of fully purified activities. The most practical and direct approach appeared to be isolation from solid tumors grown subcutaneously in rats. Applying the same four-step partial purification procedure as used for the sheep PitDGF, MTDGF was isolated in milligram quantities from as little as 46 g (wet weight) of MTW9/B autonomous tumors. Table VI gives the results of this partial purification; from the data it was clear that additional purification was required. However, even at the low overall multiples of purification attained with the first four steps, a high specific-activity growth factor (G_{50} = 84 ng/ml) has been prepared. Estimation of homogeneity of the MTDGF by 8 M urea–0.1% SDS polyacrylamide gel electrophoresis showed this preparation to have many components. At this time we estimate that at most another 100-fold purification may be necessary. If this estimation bears out, several milligrams of MTDGF might be obtained from a kilogram of fresh tumor.

Isolation of a GH3/C14 Rat Pituitary Cell Growth Factor From Pig Uterus

When a survey of the mitogenic activities of neutral buffer extracts of uteri from different species was done (F.E. Leland and D.A. Sirbasku, unpublished data), one interesting observation was made. Both sheep and rat uterine extracts contained more mitogenic activity toward the MTW9/PL cells than toward the GH3/C14 line. Conversely, rabbit and pig uterine extracts contained approximately equal activities toward these two cell lines. Although there were many possible reasons for these results with crude extract activities, one possibility that could be approached by the methods we have developed was that the UDGF molecule was not the same from all species. A study of this possibility was initiated by purification of the GH3/C14 cell UDGF from pig uterus. The assay method used was to follow UDGF stimulation of tritium-

TABLE VI. Partial Purification of MTW9/PL Mammary Tumor-Derived Autostimulatory Growth Factor

Steps	Specific activity (G_{50}, ng/ml)	Total protein (mg)
0.1 M Acetic acid extraction	370 (22,000)[a]	242
95°C Treatment	265	242
SP-Sephadex C-25	240	78
Sephadex G-50 in 0.1 M acetic acid	84	29

[a]The specific activity in parentheses is that of PBS extracts of MTW9/PL tumors.

labeled thymidine into GH3/C14 cell DNA under serum-free culture conditions as described in Materials and Methods. The partial purification procedure was the same as the first three steps used in the sheep uterine factor preparation [Ikeda and Sirbasku, 1984]. As presented in Table VII, the GH3/C14 mitogenic activity was subjected to sixfold purification, to a specific activity of 1,400 ng/ml (G_{50}). The degree of homogeneity of this preparation has not been established, but we anticipate that extensive further purification will be required. We plan to use Sephadex G-50 chromatography in 0.1 M acetic acid, and possibly ion exchange HPLC methods to further purify the pig UDGF. In addition, reverse-phase and molecular sieve HPLC methods are available, and these should be directly applicable since pig UDGF is stable in the conditions required by these procedures. It must be noted, however, that the specific activity of the partially purified pig UDGF preparation shown in Table VII was equal to the G_{50} of the most highly purified sheep UDGF with GH3/C14 cells in serum-free culture [Ikeda and Sirbasku, 1984]. These data support the possibility that UDGFs from different species might not be identical.

When pig UDGF has been purified to homogeneity, it will be compared with sheep UDGF for biologic activity with various cell lines, immunologic cross-reactivity to antibodies raised against sheep UDGF, amino acid sequence (partial) and trypsin digestion maps.

DISCUSSION

By the methods outlined in this report, a new family of mammary and pituitary tumor cell growth factors has been either purified to >90% homogeneity (sheep UDGF, sheep KDGF, and sheep PitDGF) or purified to an extent sufficient for final isolation by HPLC methods. Our estimates are that at least some of these 3,900- to 4,200-dalton polypeptides are distinct (i.e., sheep UDGF and sheep KDGF), although it is recognized that the final proof must come by amino acid sequence determination. The other factors still in the process of final purifications (i.e., GH3/C14-AGF, GH3/C14-MTGF, MTDGF, and pig UDGF) are all high-specific-activity preparations suitable for

**TABLE VII. Partial Purification of a Mammary Tumor
Cell Growth Factor From Pig Uterus**

Steps	Specific activity (G_{50}, ng/ml)	Total protein (mg)
0.1 M Acetic acid extraction	7,550	5,556
95°C Treatment	7,500	5,432
SP-Sephadex C-25	1,300	237

many formulations of hormonally defined media. From the data presented it is readily apparent that this new family of growth factors is available in milligram amounts from either 1,000 g of fresh normal tissue (or fresh tumors) or from 500-g amounts of lyophilized powder of normal tissues. The reasons for this considerable abundance are not understood but from the data presented in Ikeda and Sirbasku [1984], growth factor consumption in culture was rapid, implying that a considerable reservoir might be necessary. Similar data have been obtained with the MTDGF isolated from MTW9/PL tumors (D. Danielpour and D.A. Sirbasku, manuscript in preparation), showing that a large amount of exogenously added factor was consumed by the MTW9/PL cells in culture within 24 h at 37°C.

One other property of the purified factors that merits special emphasis is that their identification and purification are directly the result of using a serum-free assay method. Since serum inactivates these activities (by a mechanism not yet understood), use of serum-free defined conditions represents the ideal environment for characterizing their mechanisms of action. We are now attempting to prepare defined media for the MTW9/PL, T47D, MCF-7, and GH3/C14 cells by using these factors in combination with other hormones and growth factors.

In this report, we have described an approach to the study of cellular physiology based on using tissue culture cells to identify potentially important new polypeptides with effective biologic potencies of 10^{-9} M in completely serum-free medium without the addition of other previously characterized mitogens. This approach, coupled with the animal studies essential to verifying in vivo effects of newly isolated activities, promises to open an entirely new avenue of study of endocrine regulation of growth and differentiation.

ACKNOWLEDGMENTS

The authors thank Ms. Judy M. Roscoe for expert technical assistance, and Mr. Mark W. Kunkel for assistance in the GH3/C14-AGF and GH3/C14-MTGF partial purifications. D.D. is a recipient of a Predoctoral Fellowship in Cancer Research from the Rosalie B. Hite Foundation, Houston, Texas. P.R.G. is supported by a fellowship from the German Program of the Fulbright Commission, the Federal Republic of Germany. D.A.S. is a recipient of an American Cancer Society Faculty Research Award, FRA-212. This work was supported by an American Cancer Society grant, BC-255, and a National Cancer Institute grant, RO1-CA-26617.

REFERENCES

Allegra JC, Lippman ME (1979): Growth of a human breast cancer cell line in serum free hormone supplemented medium. Cancer Res 38:3823–3829.

Ambesi-Impiombato FS, Picone R, Tramontano D (1982): Influence of hormones and serum on growth and differentiation of the thyroid cell strain FRTL. In Sato GH, Pardee AB, Sirbasku DA (eds): "Growth of Cells in Hormonally Defined Media." Cold Spring Harbor, New York: Cold Spring Harbor Laboratory, Book B, pp 483-492.

Barnes D, Sato G (1979): Growth of a human mammary tumor cell line in serum free medium. Nature 281:388-389.

Bradford MM (1976): A rapid and sensitive method for quantification of microgram quantities of protein utilizing the principle of protein-dye binding. Anal Biochem 72:248-254.

Danielpour D, Sirbasku DA (1983a): Autocrine control of estrogen-responsive mammary tumor cell growth. In Vitro 19:252.

Danielpour D, Sirbasku DA (1983b): Estrogen-inducible autostimulatory growth factors found in human breast cancer cells. J Cell Biol 95 (Part 2):394a.

Delarco JE, Todaro GJ (1978): Growth factors from murine sarcoma virus transformed cells. Proc Natl Acad Sci USA 75:4001-4005.

Gospodarowicz D (1975): Purification of a fibroblast growth factor from bovine pituitary. J Biol Chem 250:2515-2520.

Ikeda T, Sirbasku DA (1984): Purification and properties of a mammary/uterine/pituitary tumor cell growth factor from pregnant sheep uterus. J Biol Chem 259:4049-4064.

Ikeda T, Liu QF, Danielpour D, Officer JB, Iio M, Leland FE, Sirbasku DA (1982): Identification of estrogen-inducible growth factors (estromedins) for rat and human mammary tumor cells in culture. In Vitro 18:961-979.

Kirkland WL, Sorrentino JM, Sirbasku DA (1976): Control of cell growth. III. Demonstration of the direct mitogenic effect of thyroid hormones on an estrogen-dependent rat pituitary tumor cell line. J Natl Cancer Inst 56:1159-1164.

Leland FE, Iio M, Sirbasku DA (1981): Hormone-dependent cell lines. In Sato GH (ed): "Functionally Differentiated Cell Lines." New York: Alan R. Liss, pp 1-46.

Leland FE, Danielpour D, Sirbasku DA (1982): Studies of the endocrine, paracrine, and autocrine control of mammary tumor cell growth. In Sato GH, Pardee AB, Sirbasku DA (eds): "Growth of Cells in Hormonally Defined Media." Cold Spring Harbor, New York: Cold Spring Harbor Laboratory, Book B, pp 741-750.

Leung CKH, Shiu RP (1981): Required presence of both estrogen and pituitary factors for the growth of human breast cancer cells in athymic nude mice. Cancer Res 41:546-551.

Leung CKH, Rowe JM, Shiu RPC (1983): Characterization of a pituitary derived growth factor for human breast cancer cells. J Cell Biol 97 (Part 2):393A.

Moo JB, Stancel GM, Heindel JJ, Sirbasku DA (1982): Effects of estradiol on the cell cycle of a rat pituitary tumor cell line containing estrogen receptors. In Sato GH, Pardee AB, Sirbasku DA (eds): "Growth of Cells in Hormonally Defined Media." Cold Spring Harbor, New York: Cold Spring Harbor Laboratory, Book A, pp 429-444.

Roberts AB, Lamb LC, Newton DL, Sporn MB, Delarco JE, Todaro GJ (1980): Transforming growth factors: Isolation of polypeptides from virally and chemically transformed cells by acid/ethanol extraction. Proc Natl Acad Sci USA 77:3493-3498.

Sirbasku DA (1978a): Hormone-responsive growth in vivo of a tissue culture cell line established from the MT-W9A rat mammary tumor. Cancer Res 38:1154-1165.

Sirbasku DA (1978b): Estrogen-induction of growth factors specific for hormone-responsive mammary, pituitary, and kidney tumor cells. Proc Natl Acad Sci USA 75:3786-3790.

Sirbasku DA (1981): New concepts in control of estrogen-responsive tumor growth. Banbury Rep 8:425-443.

Sirbasku DA, Benson RH (1980): Proposal of an indirect (estromedin) mechanism of estrogen-induced mammary tumor cell growth. In McGrath CM, Brennan MJ, Rich MA (eds): "Cell Biology of Breast Cancer." New York: Academic, pp 289-314.

Sirbasku DA, Leland FE (1982): Estrogen-inducible growth factors: Proposal of new mechanisms of estrogen-promoted tumor growth. In Litwack G (ed): "Biochemical Actions of Hormones." New York: Academic, pp 115-140.

Sirbasku DA, Leland FE, Benson RH (1981): Properties of a growth factor activity present in crude extracts of rat uterus. J Cell Physiol 107:345-358.

Sirbasku DA, Officer JB, Leland FE, Iio M (1982): Evidence of a new role for pituitary-derived hormones and growth factors in mammary tumor cell growth in vivo and in vitro. In Sato GH, Pardee AB, Sirbasku DA (eds): "Growth of Cells in Hormonally Defined Media." Cold Spring Harbor, New York: Cold Spring Harbor Laboratory, Book B, pp 763-778.

Sorrentino JM, Kirkland WL, Sirbasku DA (1976a): Control of cell growth. I. Estrogen-dependent growth in vivo of a rat pituitary tumor cell line. J Natl Cancer Inst 56:1149-1153.

Sorrentino JM, Kirkland WL, Sirbasku DA (1976b): Control of cell growth. II. The requirement of thyroid hormones for the in vivo estrogen-dependent growth of rat pituitary tumor cells. J Natl Cancer Inst 56:1155-1158.

Soule HD, Vazquez J, Long A, Albert J, Brennan M (1973): A human cell line from a pleural effusion derived from a breast carcinoma. J Natl Cancer Inst 51:1409-1413.

Todaro GJ, Fryling C, Delarco JE (1980): Transforming growth factors produced by certain human tumor cells: Polypeptides that interact with epidermal growth factor receptors. Proc Natl Acad Sci USA 77:5258-5262.

Welsch CW, Swim EL, McManus MJ, White AC, McGrath CM (1981): Estrogen-induced growth of human breast cancer cells (MCF-7) in athymic nude mice is enhanced by secretions from a transplantable pituitary tumor. Cancer Lett 14:309-316.

Index

Acetic acid, 217, 229, 230, 232–233, 235, 238

Acid phosphatase, prostatic epithelial cultures, 57

Acini. *See* Prostatic epithelium in serum-free defined medium

ACTH, adrenocortical cell cultures, 15, 23–25

Adhesion, prostatic epithelial cultures, 53

Adrenal cell cultures, 30

Adrenocortical cell cultures, bovine, 15–25
  ACTH, 15, 23–25
  antibiotics, 18
  ascorbic acid, α-tocopherol, selenium, 15, 18, 21–23
  culture methods, 19–20
  fatty acid-free BSA, 15, 16, 18–21
  FGF, 15, 16, 19–21, 23
  fibronectin-coated substrate, 15–16, 18, 21
  growth in defined medium, 20–23
    antioxidants, 22, 30
    concentration effects, 21
  Ham's F12 and DMEM (1:1) medium, 15, 16, 18
  HDL, 17, 23
  insulin, 15, 17, 21
  LDL, 15–21, 23, 24
  medium components, use of 18–19
  oxygen, 19
  quantitation, 20
  support of adrenal-specific steroid production, 23–25
  HPLC, 24–25
  thrombin, 15, 17, 19, 21
  transferrin, 15, 17, 19, 21
  from zona fasciculata-reticularis, 15, 19

Albumin, fatty acid-free, mammary epithelium culture on collagen, 139; *see also* Bovine serum albumin

Aldosterone and mammary organ culture, 146, 154, 155, 156, 159

Alveolar lesions, mammary hyperplastic nodules (HAN), 153, 155, 159, 163
  nodule-like, 158–160, 163–165

α-Amanitin, ovary cell cultures, rat, 68

β-Aminoproprionitrile, 110

Androgen(s)
  -binding protein, 33, 39–41
  breast cancer cell culture, 188–189

Animal models, cf. in vitro, 48
  breast cancer cell culture, 184–185

Antibiotics
  adrenocortical cell cultures, 18
  GH_3 rat pituitary line in defined medium, 7

Antioxidants and growth of
adrenocortical cultures, 22, 30
Ascorbic acid
adrenocortical cell cultures, 15, 18,
21-23
mammary epithelium culture on
collagen, 132
solution, 117-118

Basal lamina and mammary
epithelium culture on collagen,
105-106
modulation of collagen production
in vitro, 113-118
BHK cells, 69, 71, 72
Biotin, mammary epithelium culture
on collagen, 131, 135
Blood meal, GH_3 rat pituitary line in
defined medium, 4, 7
Bovine pituitary extract, 175
Bovine serum albumin (BSA)
fatty acid-free, adrenocortical cell
cultures, 15, 16, 18-21
fraction V, mammary epithelium
culture on collagen,
131-133, 135-139
and mammary tumor cell line (rat
64-24), 97-98
Breast. See Mammary
BSA. See Bovine serum albumin

CAMA-1 cell line, 187
Carcinogens
and mammary organ culture, 144,
145
testing, 47-48
see also Mammary cancer, human,
optimal supplementation;
Transformation, cell, in
culture; specific carcinogens
β-Carotene, chemoprevention of
transformation, 165
Caseins and gene expression, 148,
149, 151-152

Cell counting (Coulter), ovarian cell
cultures, 67, 75
Cell growth. See Growth, cell
Cell proliferation, granulosa cell
culture, 74-75
Cell transformation. See
Transformation, cell, in culture
Charcoal-extract FCS, GH_3 rat
pituitary line in defined medium,
2-3, 5, 6
Cholera toxin
mammary epithelium culture on
collagen, 131, 133
mammary tumor cell line (rat 64-
24), 99, 100
Chromatography, HPL, steroid
production, adrenocortical cell
cultures, 24-25
Chromosome stability, testicular
somatic cells, primary culture, 31
Collagen. See Mammary epithelium,
culture on collagen in SFM
Collagenase
/dispase digestion, testicular
somatic cells, primary culture,
34-37
dispersal method, prostatic
epithelial cultures, 50-52
mammary epithelium culture on
collagen, and cell isolation,
128-129
prostatic epithelial cultures, 49-50
Concentration and growth of
adrenocortical cultures, 21
Cortisol
and mammary organ culture, 155,
156
production, adrenocortical cell
cultures, 24-25
Coulter cell counting, ovary cell
cultures, rat, 67, 75
Culture models, cf. in vivo animal, 48
breast cancer cell culture, 184-185
Cyclic AMP

granulosa cell culture, 67, 79-83
mammary epithelial cell culture
        (human), 179
solution, 118
α-Cyclodextrin, 98
Cycloheximide, ovary cell cultures, rat,
        68
Cysteine, GH_3 rat pituitary line in
        defined medium, 12
Cytokinesis, ovary cell cultures, rat,
        69, 70, 72

Defined medium
    and growth of adrenocortical
        cultures, 20-23
    prostatic epithelial cultures
        preparation, 53-55
        sources of materials, 55-56
    see also GH_3 rat pituitary cell line in
        defined medium; Prostatic
        epithelium in serum-free
        defined medium
3-β-ol-Dehydroxysteroid
    dehydrogenase staining, 32
Densitometry, prostatic epithelium in
    culture, 56-57
Dexamethasone
    and mammary epithelium culture
        on collagen, 112, 113, 121
    prostatic epithelium in culture,
        53-55, 59
DMBA, 185, 190
    and transformation in culture,
        154-159, 162-164
DMEM
    GH_3 rat pituitary line in defined
        medium, 9-10
    ovary cell cultures, with F12 and
        HEPES, rat, 64, 68, 73,
        83-84
    -Ham's F12, mammary tumor cell
        culture
    MCF-7, 202, 204, 206
    rat 64-24, 90-93, 99

mammary epithelium culture on
        collagen, 127, 131, 135, 137
testicular somatic cells, primary
        culture, 39, 42
DNase I, and mammary epithelium
        culture on collagen, 107
DNA synthesis
    breast cancer cell culture, 187
    and transformation in culture,
        155-156, 160
Dose-response studies, mammary
        epithelium culture on collagen,
        132

EGF
    mammary epithelium culture on
        collagen, 112, 113, 121,
        131-133, 135-137, 140
    mammary tumor culture, 190
        MCF-7, 203, 205, 206, 210
        rat 64-24, 91, 99, 100
    cf. PitDGF, 231, 232
    prostatic epithelial cultures, 49,
        53-55, 59
    testicular somatic cells, primary
        culture, 41, 42
EHS sarcoma, 111
Electron microscopy, prostatic
        epithelial cultures, 57
Electrophoresis. See SDS-PAGE
Embryonin, 113
Engelbreth-Holm-Swarm (EHS)
        sarcoma, 111
Epithelial cell culture, cf. whole
        isolated mammary organ, 144;
        see also Mammary epithelial
        cells, monolayer culture (human)
Epithelial tree, mammary, 106
Estradiol
    MCF-7 cell culture, 208, 211, 214
    and ZR-75-1 cells, 193, 194, 196,
        197
Estrogens
    breast cancer cell culture, 186-188

and mammary organ culture,
145-147, 149, 150, 154, 155
receptors, ZR-75-1 cells, 197
Estromedins, 236
Ewe. *See* Sheep, GFs from lyophilized powder

F10, F12. *See* Ham's F12 medium
Fatty acid-free albumin
BSA, adrenocortical cell cultures,
15, 16, 18-21
mammary epithelium culture on collagen, 139
see also Bovine serum albumin
Fetal calf serum
charcoal-extract, GH_3 rat pituitary line in defined medium, 2-3, 5, 6
MCF-7 cell culture, 205, 206
FGF
adrenocortical cell cultures, 15, 16, 19, 20, 21, 23
GH_3 rat pituitary line in defined medium, 5, 12
cf. PitDGF, 231, 232
Fibroblast
contamination, prostatic epithelial cultures, 49, 51-52
outgrowth, 29
Fibronectin
-coated substrate, adrenocortical cell cultures, 15, 16, 18, 21
and granulosa cell culture, 73, 78
MCF-7 cell culture, 203, 205, 210
ovarian cell cultures, 68-72
purification, 64-65
solution, 120
4F medium and granulosa cell culture, 77, 80, 81
FSH
and granulosa cell cultures,
response to, 73-77, 83
estrogen formation, 81

serum suppression of FSH-induced function, 78-83
ovarian cell cultures, 63, 68
testicular somatic cells, primary culture, 41, 42

Gene expression, milk proteins,
148-151
GH
and mammary organ culture,
145-147, 149, 150, 154
cf. PitDGF, 231, 232
GH_3/C14 GF
autostimulatory, 232-235, 238
partial, purification, 235
isolated from pig uterus, 237-238
partial, purification, 238
GH_3 rat pituitary cell line in defined medium, 1-13
antibiotics, 7
blood meal, 4, 7
culture methods, 6-11
cysteine, 12
FCS, 2-3, 5, 6
FGF, 5, 12
hormone supplements, 8, 9
insulin, 4-10, 12
long G1 period, 12
medium, 9-10
parathyroid hormone, 4-5, 7, 10
PDGF, 12
prolactin, 1, 12
serum depletion, 11-12
serum-free medium derivation, 1-6
somatomedin C, 4, 5, 10, 12
thyroid-hormone depleted medium, 1-7, 10
transferrin, 4-7, 10
Glucocorticoids
breast cancer cell culture, 188
and milk protein gene expression, 149-151
and transformation in culture, 155
see also specific glucocorticoids

Glycine/collagenase, testicular somatic
    cells, primary culture, 37–38
Glycosaminoglycans, 122
G1 period, GH_3 cells, 12
Granulosa cell culture, growth and
    function, 66, 72–83
  cAMP, 67, 79–83
  cell proliferation, 74–75
  fibronectin, 73, 78
  4F medium, 77, 80, 81
  FSH, response to, 73–77, 83
    induced estrogen formation, 81
  hydrocortisone, 73–74
  IBMX, 68, 79–80, 82
    phosphodiesterase inhibition,
        79, 83
  insulin, 73
  LH, 77, 78, 80, 81, 83, 84
  20-α-OH-P, 67, 74, 75, 78
  serum suppression of FSH-induced
      function, 78–83
  simplicity of isolation, 73
  ^{3}H-thymidine incorporation, 75–76
  see also Ovary cell cultures, rat
      functional, in SFM
Growth, cell
  mammary epithelial cell culture
      (human), 175–176
    on collagen, nutritional
        requirements, 132–135
    MCF-7 cell culture, 205–213
    quantitation, prostatic epithelium
        in culture, 56–57
    solution, 112–113
    and ZR-75-1 cells, 191–195
Growth factors. See specific growth
    factors
Growth factors for mammary and
    pituitary tumor cells, isolation,
    217–239
  acetic acid- and heat-stable, 217,
      229, 230, 232–233, 235,
      238
  GH_3/C14 autostimulatory GF,
      232–235, 238

partial purification, 235
GH_3/C14 GF isolation from pig
    uterus, 237–238
  partial purification, 238
growth factor assay methods,
    219–220
  ^{3}H-thymidine uptake, 219
from lyophilized powder of mature
    ewe kidney (KDGF),
    226–228, 238
  purification, 227
  SDS-PAGE, 228–229
from lyophilized powder of
    pregnant sheep uterus
    (UDGF), 221–227, 230, 233,
    237, 238
  purification, 222
  SDS-PAGE, 222–223
from lyophilized powder of whole
    sheep pituitaries (PitDGF),
    228–235, 237
  purification, 230
  SDS-PAGE, 231–233
MCF-7 mammary tumor cell line
    (human), 218–220, 228,
    233, 236, 239
MTW9/PL autostimulatory GF
    (MTDGF), 236–239
  partial purification and SDS-
      PAGE, 237
MTW9/PL rat mammary tumor
    cells, 218–221, 223,
    228–229, 232, 234, 239
T47D mammary tumor cell line
    (human), 218, 220, 228,
    229, 231, 233, 239
tissue sources, 220–221
TSH, 217–218

Ham's F12 medium
  and DMEM
    adrenocortical cell cultures, 15,
        16, 18
    MCF-7 cell culture, 208

and F10, GH₃ cell line, 9-10
mammary epithelium culture on
    collagen, 127, 131, 135, 137
ovarian cell cultures, rat functional,
    with DMEM and HEPES, 64,
    68, 73, 83-84
testicular somatic cells, primary
    culture, 39, 42
Hamster, BHK cells, 69, 71, 72
Heat stability, GFs, 217, 229, 230,
    232-233, 235, 238
Heparan sulfate proteoglycan, 105,
    106, 120
HEPES buffer
    mammary epithelium culture on
        collagen, 129, 131
    MCF-7 cell culture, 203
    ovarian cell cultures, with DME and
        F12, 64, 68, 73, 83-84
    testicular somatic cells, primary
        culture, 39
HMEC. *See* Mammary epithelium,
    monolayer culture
Hydrocortisone
    granulosa cell culture, 73-74
    mammary organ, 146, 148, 149
Hyperplastic alveolar nodules, 153,
    155, 159, 163
Hyperplastic mammary cell
    outgrowths, 162, 163

IBMX, ovary cell cultures, rat, 68,
    79-80, 82
    phosphodiesterase inhibitor, 79, 83
IMEM-HS, ZR-75-1 cells, 192-197
Inoculum density, testicular somatic
    cells, primary culture, 37
Insulin
    adrenocortical cell cultures, 15, 17,
        21
    GH₃ rat pituitary line in defined
        medium, 4-10, 12
    granulosa cell culture, 73, 78

mammary epithelium culture on
    collagen, 131-133, 135-137,
    140
mammary organ culture, 145, 146,
    148-150, 154-156, 159
mammary tumor cells, 189
    MCF-7 cell culture, 203,
        205-206, 209
    rat 64-24, 99, 100
prostatic epithelial cultures, 49, 59
    zinc-free, 52-55
testicular somatic cells, primary
    culture, 41, 42
and ZR-75-1 cells, 193-194
In vitro models, cf. animal models, 48
    breast cancer cell culture, 184-185
3-Isobutyl-1-methylxanthine. *See*
    IBMX, ovary cell cultures, rat
Isolation, cell (dispersion, dissociation)
    collagenase method. *See*
        Collagenase
    granulosa cell culture, simplicity of
        isolation, 73
    mammary epithelium, 106-110,
        127-129
        Nitex membrane filtration, 108
        separation from stromal cells,
            129
        solutions, 108-110
    prostatic epithelium, 49-52
        fibroblast contamination, 49,
            51-52

Keratin, mammary epithelial cell
    culture (human), 181
Kidneys
    BHK cells, 69, 71, 72
    ewe, GF from lyophilized powder,
        226-228, 238

α-Lactalbumin, 101
Lactogenesis, 151
Laminin, 105, 106, 120
LDH, breast cancer cell culture, 186

Leydig cells, 30–32, 42, 43
  3-β-ol-dehydroxysteroid
        dehydrogenase staining, 32
LH
  and granulosa cell culture, 77, 78,
        80, 81, 83, 84
  ovarian cell cultures, 63
Linoleic acid, 135, 139; see also
        Bovine serum albumin
Lipoproteins and adrenocortical cell
        cultures
  HDLs, 17, 23
  LDLs, 15–21, 23, 24
Liposomes, 98, 102
Lobuloalveolar structure and
        transformation in culture, 154,
        156, 157
Lyophilization. See under Growth
        factors for mammary and
        pituitary tumor cells, isolation

α_2-Macroglobulin, 113, 117
Mammary cancer, human, optimal
        supplementation, 183–198
  androgens, 188–189
  CAMA-1 cell line, 187
  culture conditions select cells, 184
  EGF, 190
  estrogens, 186–188
        DNA synthesis and enzymes,
              187
  glucocorticoids, 188
  insulin, 189
  in vitro vs. in vivo, 184–185
  MDA-MB-231 cell line, 190
  PRL, 191
  progestins, 191
  retinoids, 190
  source of cell lines from malignant
        effusions, 184
  species differences, 185
  T_3, 189
  T47D cell line, 187
  vitamin D, 190–191

ZR-75-1 cell line, 183, 187, 189,
        191
  growth regulation and PR,
        195–197
  growth requirements, 191–195
  IMEM-HS, 192–197
  source, 192
Mammary carcinoma MCF-7 cell line,
        184–185, 187–195, 201–214,
        218–220, 228, 233, 236, 239
  cell characteristics, 201
  EGF, 203, 205, 206, 210
  estradiol effect, 208, 211, 214
  fibronectin, 203, 205, 210
  growth characteristics in vitro,
        205–213
        FCS, 205, 206
        F12:DME, cf. separately, 208
  insulin, 203, 205–206, 209
  $PGF_{2\alpha}$, 203–206, 211
  preparation of medium and
        supplements, 202–204, 206
  PRL, 208, 212
  serum spreading factor, 204, 213
  somatomedin, 212
  source, 201
  transferrin, 203, 205, 206, 212
  trypsinization and plating, 204–205
  urokinase, 208–209
Mammary epithelium, culture on
        collagen in SFM, 105–123,
        127–140
  ascorbic acid, 117–118, 132
  basal lamina, 105, 106
        modulation of collagen
              production in vitro,
              113–118
  biotin, 131, 135
  BSA, fraction V, 131–133,
        135–139
  cAMP, 118
  cholera toxin, 131, 133
  collagen
        gel culture, 129–131

purification, 110-111, 112
substrates modify mammary cell
    GF responsiveness,
    118-122
type I, 120, 121, 123
type II, 120
type III, 120
type IV, 105-106, 120-123
dexamethasone, 112, 113, 121
dose-response studies, 132
EGF, 112, 113, 121, 131-133,
    135-137, 140
fatty acid-free albumin, 139
fibronectin, 120
GAGs, 122
growth of cells in SFM, 112-113
heparan sulfate proteoglycan, 105,
    106, 120
insulin, 131-133, 135-137, 140
isolation (dissociation), 106-110,
    127-129
    ducts, 106-107
    epithelial tree, 106
    Nitex membrane filtration, 108
    separation from stromal cells,
      129
    solutions, 108-110
laminin, 105, 106, 120
linoleic acid, 135, 139
medium
    DMEM, 127, 131, 135, 137
    Ham's F12, 127, 131, 135, 137
    HEPES buffer, 129, 131
    199, 129, 131
    supplements, 112-114
MTF, 115-117
nutritional requirements, 132-135
organoids, 108-109, 119
Pedersen fetuin, 112-113
proline analogs, 105-106, 115,
    118, 122, 123
putrescine, 135, 139
selenous acid, 131, 132, 137
T_3, 132, 138

α-tocopherol succinate, 131, 135
transferrin, 131, 133, 135-137
Waymouth's medium, 127, 130,
    131
Mammary epithelium, monolayer
    culture (human), 171-182
cAMP, 179
characterization of cell populations,
    181
cobblestone morphology, 180
initiation of cell growth, 175-176
medium, 174-176
    serum-free MCDB170, 175-181
    objectives of system
      development, 171-172
    organoids, 173-175, 177
    processing of tissue, 172-174
    propagation of HMEC, 178-181
STV, 176
subculture of HMEC, 176-178
tissue collection, 171, 172
Mammary organ, isolated whole
    (mouse), serum-free culture,
    143-165
aldosterone, 146, 154-156, 159
carcinogens and neoplastic
    transformation, 144-145
cortisol, 155, 156
cf. epithelial cell culture, 144
estrogen and progesterone,
    145-147, 149-152, 154, 155
cf. explant system, 144
GH, 145-147, 149, 150, 154
hydrocortisone, 146, 148, 149
insulin and PRL, 145, 146,
    148-150, 154-156, 159
milk
    -like secretion, 146
    protein gene expression,
      148-151, 152
two-step culture method, 145-148
Waymouth medium, 145, 154
see also Transformation, cell, in
    culture

Mammary tumor cell line (rat 64-24),
    growth in SFM, 89-102
  BSA, growth-promotion, 97-98
    cf. other fatty-acid carriers, 98
  cells, source, 90
  cholera toxin, 99-100
  clonal growth conditions, 102
  EGF, 91, 99, 100
  ethanolamine and
      phosphoethanolamine,
      89-90, 100-101
    growth promotion, 95-97
    cf. other cell types, 96-97, 101
  insulin, 99-100
  medium composition, 91-92
    DME-Ham's F12, 90-93, 99
    without HEPES, 90
  PRL, 90-91
    growth-promotion, 92-95
    -responsive, 89
  T_3, 91
  transferrin, 91, 100
Mammary tumor factor, solution,
    115-117
Mammary tumor virus. See MTV
MCA and transformation in culture,
    153-154, 160
MCDB170, serum-free, mammary
    epithelial cell culture (human),
    175-181
MCF-7 cells. See Mammary carcinoma
    MCF-7 cell line
MDA-MB-231 cell line, 190
Medium 199, mammary epithelium
    culture on collagen, 129, 131
3-Methyl-cholanthrene, and
    transformation in culture, 153,
    154, 160
Milk
  fat globule antigen, mammary
      epithelial cell culture
      (human), 181
  -like secretions, cultured mammary
      organ, 146

protein gene expression, 148-151,
    152
MM, medium for mammary epithelial
    cell culture (human), 174-181
MtT/W5 pituitary tumor, 1
MTV
  and progesterone, cultured
      mammary organ, 151
  and transformation in culture,
      153-155
MTW9 cell line, 96, 97
MTW9/PL autostimulatory GF,
    236-239
  SDS-PAGE and partial purification,
    237
MTW9/PL rat mammary tumor cells,
    218-221, 223, 228-229, 232,
    234, 239
Myoid cells, peritubular, 33, 34, 38,
    39, 41-43

NEM, 110, 111
Neoplastic transformation. See
    Transformation, cell, in culture
Nitex membrane filtration
  and mammary epithelium
      culture on collagen, 108
  solution, 108-110

20α-OH-P, granulosa cell culture, 67,
    74, 75, 78
Organoids, mammary epithelial cell
    culture, 108-109, 119,
    173-175, 177
Ovary cell cultures, rat functional, in
    SFM, 63-87
  α-amanitin, 68
  cell counting, 67, 75
  culture media (DME, F12, HEPES),
    64, 68, 73, 83-84
  cycloheximide, 68
  fibronectin, 68-72, 83
    purification, 64-65
  FSH, 63, 68

insulin, transferrin, hydrocortisone,
64, 68, 69, 71-72, 83-84
IBMX, 68, 79-80, 82
phosphodiesterase inhibitor, 79,
83
LH and PRL, 63
PGs, 63
primary cells, 64
rats, 66
RF-1 ovarian cell line (rat follicular),
64-66
cytokinesis, 69-70, 72
growth, 68-72
see also Granulosa cell culture,
growth and function
Oxygen and adrenocortical cell
cultures, 19

Parathyroid hormone, GH$_3$ rat
pituitary line in defined medium,
4-5, 7, 10
PDGF, GH$_3$ rat pituitary line in defined
medium, 12
Pedersen fetuin and mammary
epithelium culture on collagen,
112-113
Peritubular myoid cells, 33, 34, 38,
39, 41-43
Perphenazine stimulation and
mammary epithelium culture on
collagen, 107
Phosphodiesterase inhibition by IBMX,
79, 83
pI, KDGF, 230
Pituitary extract, bovine, 175
Plasminogen activator
breast cancer cell culture, 187
prostatic epithelial cultures, 57, 58
Platelet-derived growth factor, GH$_3$ rat
pituitary line in defined medium,
12
Plating
density, testicular somatic cells,
primary culture, 39-40

MCF-7 cell culture, 204-205
medium, serum-free, prostatic
epithelial cultures, 52
PMSF, 110
Progesterone
and mammary organ culture,
145-147, 149, 150, 154, 155
production, adrenocortical cell
cultures, 24-25
receptor, breast cancer cell culture,
186
Progestins, breast cancer cell culture,
191
Prolactin
GH$_3$ rat pituitary line in defined
medium, 1, 12
and mammary organ culture, 145,
146, 148-150, 154-156, 159
mammary tumor cell culture, 191
MCF-7 cells, 208, 212
rat 64-24, 89, 90-91
rat 64-24, growth promotion,
92-95
ovarian cell cultures, 63
cf. PitDGF, 231, 232
Proline analogs, 105-106, 115, 118,
122, 123
Prostaglandins
F$_{2\alpha}$, MCF-7 cell culture, 203-206,
211
ovarian cell cultures, 63
Prostate cancer, carcinogen testing,
47-48
in vitro vs. animal models, 48
Prostatic epithelium in serum-free
defined medium, 47-59
acid phosphatase, 57
adhesion, 53
characterization and differentiated
cell function, 57-58
chemically defined medium, 53
dexamethasone, 53-55, 59
EGF, 49, 53-55, 59
growth quantitation, 56-57

insulin, 49, 59
  zinc-free, 52-55
isolation of epithelium, 49-52
  estimation of viable acini, 52
  fibroblast contamination, 49,
    51-52
  source, 50
medium preparation, 53-55
  sources of materials, 55-56
need for model system, 47-48
plasminogen activator, 57, 58
RPMI-1640, 49, 51, 53-54
seeding the acini, 52-53
spermine tetrahydrochloride, 55
transferrin, 53-55, 59
vitamin A, 49, 54, 55
$ZnCl_2$, 54, 55
Proteoglycan, heparan sulfate, and
  mammary epithelium culture,
  105, 106, 120
Putrescine, 135, 139
Pyridoxal 5'-phosphate, 152

Quantitation
  adrenocortical cell cultures, 20
  rat ovary cell culture, Coulter
    counter, 67, 75

Retinoids, breast cancer cell culture,
  190; see also Vitamin A
RF-1 rat follicular ovarian cell line,
  64-66
RPMI-1640, 49, 51, 53-54

Saline, trypsin, versene, 176
Sarcoma, EHS, 111
SDS-PAGE
  KDGF, 228, 229
  MTW9/PL autostimulatory GF,
    237
  PitDGF, 231, 233
  UDGF, 222-223
Selenium

adrenocortical cell cultures, 15, 18,
  21-23
chemoprevention of transformation,
  165
Selenous acid, 131, 132, 137
Sertoli cells, 31-33, 38, 41-43
  androgen-binding protein, 33,
    39-41
Serum
  depletion, GH_3 rat pituitary line in
    defined medium, 11-12
  -free defined medium, derivation,
    GH_3 rat pituitary line, 1-6
  spreading factor, MCF-7 cell
    culture, 204, 213
  supplementation, testicular somatic
    cell culture, 40
Sheep, GFs from lyophilized powder
  ewe kidneys, 226-228, 238
  pituitary, 228-235, 237
  uterus, 221-227, 230, 233, 237,
    238
Somatomedins
  C, GH_3 rat pituitary line in defined
    medium, 4, 5, 10, 12
  MCF-7 cell culture, 212
Species differences, breast cancer cell
  culture, 185
Spermine oxidase, 51-52, 57
Spermine tetrahydrochloride, 55
Steroidogenesis, 15; see also specific
  steroids
Storage, medium components, 16-18
Stromal cells, separation of mammary
  epithelium from, 129

Tamoxifen and ZR-75-1 cells, 195-197
Testicular somatic cells, primary
  culture, 29-43
  chromosome stability, 31
  culture conditions, 39-43
    Ham's F12, 39, 42
    HEPES, 39

insulin, transferrin, EGF, FSH,
41, 42
MEM, 39, 42
serum supplementation, 40
substrate and plating density,
39–40
Leydig cells, 30–32, 42, 43
3-β-ol-dehydroxysteroid
dehydrogenase staining,
32
peritubular myoid cells, 33–34, 38,
39, 41–43
preparation of cells for culture,
32–38
amount of digestion, 36–37
glycine/collagenase, 37–38
inoculum density, 37
purity, 32–33
successive collagenase/dispase
digestion, 34–37
washing, 37
selection of model system,
31–32
Sertoli cells, 31–33, 38, 41–43
androgen-binding protein,
33, 39–41
T47D mammary tumor cell line
(human), 96, 97, 187, 218, 220,
228–229, 231, 233, 239
Thrombin, adrenocortical cell cultures,
15, 17, 19, 21
[3]H-Thymidine incorporation
GF assay, 219
and granulosa cell culture, 75–76
Thymidine kinase, breast cancer cell
culture, 186
Thyroid hormones, depletion from
GH$_3$ rat pituitary line defined
medium, 1–7, 10; *see also*
specific hormones
α-Tocopherol
adrenocortical cell cultures, 15, 18,
21–23
succinate, mammary epithelium
culture on collagen, 131, 135

Transferrin
adrenocortical cell cultures, 15, 17,
19, 21
GH$_3$ rat pituitary line in defined
medium, 4–7, 10
mammary epithelium culture on
collagen, 131, 133, 135–137
and mammary tumor cell lines
MCF-7 cells, 203, 205, 206,
212
rat 64-24, 91, 100
prostatic epithelial cultures, 53–55,
59
testicular somatic cells, primary
culture, 41, 42
Transformation, cell, in culture,
152–165
alveolar lesions, nodule-like,
158–160, 163–165
chemoprevention of transformation,
164–165
DMBA, 154–159, 162–164
DNA synthesis, 155–156, 160
expression of preneoplastic and
neoplastic characteristics,
161–164
glucocorticoids, 155
HAN, 153, 155, 159, 163
hyperplastic mammary cell
outgrowth, 162, 163
influence of different hormone
mixtures, 159
cf. in vitro development, 154
lobuloalveolar structures, 154, 156,
157
mammary fat pad transplantation of
transformed cell in vivo, 161
mammary organ culture, 144–145;
see also Mammary organ,
isolated whole, serum-free
culture
MCA, 153, 154, 160
MTV, 153–155
need for epithelial cell models,
152–153

TRH, GH$_3$ rat pituitary line in defined
    medium, depleted medium, 1-7,
    10
Triiodothyronine (T$_3$)
    breast cancer cell culture, 189
    GH$_3$ rat pituitary line in defined
        medium, depleted medium,
        1-7, 10
    mammary epithelium culture on
        collagen, 138
    and mammary tumor cell line (rat
        64-24), 91
    and ZR-75-1 cells, 193-194
Trypsin, 176
Trypsinization, MCF-7 cell culture,
    204-205
TSH, 217-218
TURP, prostatic epithelial cultures, 50
22-1 cells, 96, 97

Urokinase, MCF-7 cell culture, 208-
    209
Uterus, sheep, GF from lyophilized
    powder, 221-227, 230, 233,
    237, 238

Versene, 176
Vitamin A
    chemoprevention of transformation,
        165

prostatic epithelial cultures, 49, 54,
    55
    see also Retinoids
Vitamin C. See Ascorbic acid
Vitamin D, breast cancer cell culture,
    190-191
Vitamin E. See α-Tocopherol

Washing, testicular somatic cells,
    primary culture, 37
Waymouth's medium
    mammary epithelium culture on
        collagen, 127, 130, 131
    and mammary organ culture, 145,
        154
Whey acid protein, 148, 150
WRK-1 cells, 96, 97

Zinc
    chloride, prostatic epithelium in
        culture, 54, 55
    -free insulin, prostatic epithelial
        cultures, 52-55
Zona fasciculata-reticularis, 15, 19
ZR-75-1 cell line, 183, 187, 189, 191